Design and Analysis of Clinical Trials for Predictive Medicine

Chapman & Hall/CRC Biostatistics Series

Published Titles

Adaptive Design Methods in Clinical Trials, Second Edition
Shein-Chung Chow and Mark Chang

Adaptive Design Theory and Implementation Using SAS and R, Second Edition
Mark Chang

Advanced Bayesian Methods for Medical Test Accuracy
Lyle D. Broemeling

Advances in Clinical Trial Biostatistics
Nancy L. Geller

Applied Meta-Analysis with R
Ding-Geng (Din) Chen and Karl E. Peace

Basic Statistics and Pharmaceutical Statistical Applications, Second Edition
James E. De Muth

Bayesian Adaptive Methods for Clinical Trials
Scott M. Berry, Bradley P. Carlin, J. Jack Lee, and Peter Muller

Bayesian Analysis Made Simple: An Excel GUI for WinBUGS
Phil Woodward

Bayesian Methods for Measures of Agreement
Lyle D. Broemeling

Bayesian Methods in Epidemiology
Lyle D. Broemeling

Bayesian Methods in Health Economics
Gianluca Baio

Bayesian Missing Data Problems: EM, Data Augmentation and Noniterative Computation
Ming T. Tan, Guo-Liang Tian, and Kai Wang Ng

Bayesian Modeling in Bioinformatics
Dipak K. Dey, Samiran Ghosh, and Bani K. Mallick

Benefit-Risk Assessment in Pharmaceutical Research and Development
Andreas Sashegyi, James Felli, and Rebecca Noel

Biosimilars: Design and Analysis of Follow-on Biologics
Shein-Chung Chow

Biostatistics: A Computing Approach
Stewart J. Anderson

Causal Analysis in Biomedicine and Epidemiology: Based on Minimal Sufficient Causation
Mikel Aickin

Clinical and Statistical Considerations in Personalized Medicine
Claudio Carini, Sandeep Menon, and Mark Chang

Clinical Trial Data Analysis using R
Ding-Geng (Din) Chen and Karl E. Peace

Clinical Trial Methodology
Karl E. Peace and Ding-Geng (Din) Chen

Computational Methods in Biomedical Research
Ravindra Khattree and Dayanand N. Naik

Computational Pharmacokinetics
Anders Källén

Confidence Intervals for Proportions and Related Measures of Effect Size
Robert G. Newcombe

Controversial Statistical Issues in Clinical Trials
Shein-Chung Chow

Data and Safety Monitoring Committees in Clinical Trials
Jay Herson

Design and Analysis of Animal Studies in Pharmaceutical Development
Shein-Chung Chow and Jen-pei Liu

Design and Analysis of Bioavailability and Bioequivalence Studies, Third Edition
Shein-Chung Chow and Jen-pei Liu

Design and Analysis of Bridging Studies
Jen-pei Liu, Shein-Chung Chow,
and Chin-Fu Hsiao

Design and Analysis of Clinical Trials for Predictive Medicine
Shigeyuki Matsui, Marc Buyse,
and Richard Simon

Design and Analysis of Clinical Trials with Time-to-Event Endpoints
Karl E. Peace

Design and Analysis of Non-Inferiority Trials
Mark D. Rothmann, Brian L. Wiens,
and Ivan S. F. Chan

Difference Equations with Public Health Applications
Lemuel A. Moyé and Asha Seth Kapadia

DNA Methylation Microarrays: Experimental Design and Statistical Analysis
Sun-Chong Wang and Arturas Petronis

DNA Microarrays and Related Genomics Techniques: Design, Analysis, and Interpretation of Experiments
David B. Allison, Grier P. Page,
T. Mark Beasley, and Jode W. Edwards

Dose Finding by the Continual Reassessment Method
Ying Kuen Cheung

Elementary Bayesian Biostatistics
Lemuel A. Moyé

Frailty Models in Survival Analysis
Andreas Wienke

Generalized Linear Models: A Bayesian Perspective
Dipak K. Dey, Sujit K. Ghosh,
and Bani K. Mallick

Handbook of Regression and Modeling: Applications for the Clinical and Pharmaceutical Industries
Daryl S. Paulson

Inference Principles for Biostatisticians
Ian C. Marschner

Interval-Censored Time-to-Event Data: Methods and Applications
Ding-Geng (Din) Chen, Jianguo Sun,
and Karl E. Peace

Joint Models for Longitudinal and Time-to-Event Data: With Applications in R
Dimitris Rizopoulos

Measures of Interobserver Agreement and Reliability, Second Edition
Mohamed M. Shoukri

Medical Biostatistics, Third Edition
A. Indrayan

Meta-Analysis in Medicine and Health Policy
Dalene Stangl and Donald A. Berry

Mixed Effects Models for the Population Approach: Models, Tasks, Methods and Tools
Marc Lavielle

Monte Carlo Simulation for the Pharmaceutical Industry: Concepts, Algorithms, and Case Studies
Mark Chang

Multiple Testing Problems in Pharmaceutical Statistics
Alex Dmitrienko, Ajit C. Tamhane, and Frank Bretz

Noninferiority Testing in Clinical Trials: Issues and Challenges
Tie-Hua Ng

Optimal Design for Nonlinear Response Models
Valerii V. Fedorov and Sergei L. Leonov

Patient-Reported Outcomes: Measurement, Implementation and Interpretation
Joseph C. Cappelleri, Kelly H. Zou, Andrew G. Bushmakin, Jose Ma. J. Alvir, Demissie Alemayehu, and Tara Symonds

Quantitative Evaluation of Safety in Drug Development: Design, Analysis and Reporting
Qi Jiang and H. Amy Xia

Randomized Clinical Trials of Nonpharmacological Treatments
Isabelle Boutron, Philippe Ravaud, and David Moher

Randomized Phase II Cancer Clinical Trials
Sin-Ho Jung

Sample Size Calculations for Clustered and Longitudinal Outcomes in Clinical Research
Chul Ahn, Moonseong Heo, and Song Zhang

Sample Size Calculations in Clinical Research, Second Edition
Shein-Chung Chow, Jun Shao and Hansheng Wang

Statistical Analysis of Human Growth and Development
Yin Bun Cheung

Statistical Design and Analysis of Stability Studies
Shein-Chung Chow

Statistical Evaluation of Diagnostic Performance: Topics in ROC Analysis
Kelly H. Zou, Aiyi Liu, Andriy Bandos, Lucila Ohno-Machado, and Howard Rockette

Statistical Methods for Clinical Trials
Mark X. Norleans

Statistical Methods in Drug Combination Studies
Wei Zhao and Harry Yang

Statistics in Drug Research: Methodologies and Recent Developments
Shein-Chung Chow and Jun Shao

Statistics in the Pharmaceutical Industry, Third Edition
Ralph Buncher and Jia-Yeong Tsay

Survival Analysis in Medicine and Genetics
Jialiang Li and Shuangge Ma

Theory of Drug Development
Eric B. Holmgren

Translational Medicine: Strategies and Statistical Methods
Dennis Cosmatos and Shein-Chung Chow

Chapman & Hall/CRC Biostatistics Series

Design and Analysis of Clinical Trials for Predictive Medicine

Edited by
Shigeyuki Matsui
Marc Buyse
Richard Simon

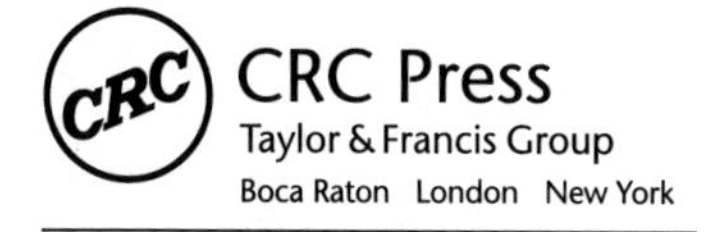

CRC Press is an imprint of the
Taylor & Francis Group, an **informa** business
A CHAPMAN & HALL BOOK

CRC Press
Taylor & Francis Group
6000 Broken Sound Parkway NW, Suite 300
Boca Raton, FL 33487-2742

Printed on acid-free paper
Version Date: 20150204

International Standard Book Number-13: 978-1-4665-5815-1 (Hardback)

Visit the Taylor & Francis Web site at
http://www.taylorandfrancis.com

and the CRC Press Web site at
http://www.crcpress.com

Contents

Section III Phase III Randomized Clinical Trials Using Biomarkers

Section IV Analysis of High-Dimensional Data and Genomic Signature Developments

Section V Randomized Trials with Biomarker Development and Validation

Section VI Evaluation of Surrogate Biomarkers

Preface

The foundation of modern clinical trials was laid many years before modern developments in biotechnology and genomics. Drug development in many diseases is now shifting to molecularly targeted treatment. At the same time, pretreatment prediction of patients' clinical outcomes and responsiveness to treatment based on reliable molecular biomarkers or diagnostic tests is becoming an essential component of modern medicine. Confronted with such a major break in the evolution toward personalized or predictive medicine, the methodologies for design and analysis of clinical trials also have to evolve.

This book is one of the first attempts to provide a systematic coverage of all stages of clinical trials for the codevelopment of therapeutics and diagnostics for predictive medicine. Chapter 1 provides a detailed listing of the contents of this book. The target audience includes researchers, practitioners, and students of clinical biostatistics. Many chapters may also be beneficial for clinical investigators, translational scientists, and others who are involved in clinical trials.

As the new paradigm toward predictive medicine continues to evolve, we hope that this book will contribute to its development through the use of appropriate statistical designs and methods in future clinical trials. We also hope the book will stimulate active statistical research in this area.

We sincerely express our thanks to all of the contributors to this book, who are leading experts in academia, the pharmaceutical industry, or government organizations for providing an overview of the current state of the art in this area.

Shigeyuki Matsui

Marc Buyse

Richard Simon

Editors

Shigeyuki Matsui, PhD, is professor in the Department of Biostatistics, Nagoya University Graduate School of Medicine, Nagoya, Japan. He is also a visiting professor at the Institute of Statistical Mathematics. He has served as council and nominating committee member of the International Biometric Society. He is currently council of the Biometric Society of Japan (BSJ) and editor-in-chief of the *Japanese Journal of Biometrics*. He is the recipient of the 2014 BSJ Award. Dr. Matsui is also a frequent reviewer commissioned by the government and advisor to pharmaceutical companies in Japan. He holds degrees in engineering from the Tokyo University of Science, Japan.

Marc Buyse, ScD, is the founder of the International Drug Development Institute (IDDI), Louvain-la-Neuve, Belgium, and of CluePoints Inc., Cambridge, Massachusetts. He is associate professor of biostatistics at Hasselt University in Belgium. He was president of the International Society for Clinical Biostatistics, president of the Quetelet Society, and fellow of the Society for Clinical Trials. He worked at the EORTC (European Organization for Research and Treatment of Cancer) in Brussels and at the Dana Farber Cancer Institute in Boston. He holds degrees in engineering and statistics from Brussels University (ULB), management from the Cranfield School of Management (Cranfield, United Kingdom), and a doctorate in biostatistics from Harvard University (Boston, Massachusetts).

Richard Simon, DSc, is chief of the Biometric Research Branch of the National Cancer Institute, where he is head statistician for the Division of Cancer Treatment and Diagnosis and leads the Section on Systems and Computational Biology. He is the author or coauthor of more than 450 publications. He has been influential in promoting excellence in clinical trial design and analysis. He has served on the Oncologic Advisory Committee of the U.S. Food and Drug Administration and is recipient of the 2013 Karl E. Peace Award for Outstanding Statistical Contributions for the Betterment of Society. He leads a multidisciplinary group of scientists developing and applying methods for the application of genomics to cancer therapeutics. He is the architect of BRB-ArrayTools software used for the analysis of microarray and digital expression, copy number, and methylation data.

Contributors

Ariel Alonso
Interuniversity Institute for Biostatistics and Statistical Bioinformatics (I-BioStat)
Leuven University
Leuven, Belgium

Robert Becker, Jr.
Office of In Vitro Diagnostic Devices and Radiological Health
United States Food and Drug Administration
Silver Spring, Maryland

Thomas Bengtsson
Biostatistics, Genentech
South San Francisco, California

Harald Binder
Division Biostatistics
University Medical Center Mainz
Mainz, Germany

Tomasz Burzykowski
International Drug Development Institute
Louvain-la-Neuve, Belgium
and
Interuniversity Institute for Biostatistics and Statistical Bioinformatics (I-BioStat)
Hasselt University
Hasselt, Belgium

Marc Buyse
International Drug Development Institute
Louvain-la-Neuve, Belgium
and
Interuniversity Institute for Biostatistics and Statistical Bioinformatics (I-BioStat)
Hasselt University
Hasselt, Belgium

Yuki Choai
Department of Statistical Science
The Graduate University for Advanced Studies
Tokyo, Japan

John Crowley
Cancer Research And Biostatistics
Seattle, Washington

Takashi Daimon
Department of Biostatistics
Hyogo College of Medicine
Hyogo, Japan

Paul Delmar
Biostatistics, Roche
Basel, Switzerland

Shinto Eguchi
Department of Mathematical Analysis and Statistical Inference
The Institute of Statistical Mathematics
Tokyo, Japan

Boris Freidlin
Biometric Research Branch
National Cancer Institute
Bethesda, Maryland

Jane Fridlyand
Biostatistics, Genentech
South San Francisco, California

Thomas Gerds
Department of Public Health
University of Copenhagen
Copenhagen, Denmark

Akihiro Hirakawa
Center for Advanced Medicine and Clinical Research
Graduate School of Medicine
Nagoya University
Nagoya, Japan

Antje Hoering
Cancer Research And Biostatistics
Seattle, Washington

Sally Hunsberger
National Institute of Allergy and Infectious Diseases
National Institutes of Health
Bethesda, Maryland

Osamu Komori
Department of Mathematical Analysis and Statistical Inference
The Institute of Statistical Mathematics
Tokyo, Japan

Edward Korn
Biometric Research Branch
National Cancer Institute
Bethesda, Maryland

Mike LeBlanc
Fred Hutchinson Cancer Research Center
Seattle, Washington

Grazyna Lieberman
Regulatory Policy, Genentech
South San Francisco, California

Howard Mackey
Biostatistics, Genentech
South San Francisco, California

Sumithra Mandrekar
Department of Health Sciences Research
Mayo Clinic
Rochester, Minnesota

Shigeyuki Matsui
Department of Biostatistics
Graduate School of Medicine
Nagoya University
Nagoya, Japan

Lisa McShane
Biometric Research Branch
National Cancer Institute
Bethesda, Maryland

Stefan Michiels
Service de Biostatistique et d'Epidémiologie
Gustave Roussy
Université Paris-Sud
Villejuif, France

Geert Molenberghs
Interuniversity Institute for Biostatistics and statistical Bioinformatics (I-BioStat)
Hasselt University
Hasselt, Belgium

and

Leuven University
Leuven, Belgium

Hisashi Noma
Department of Data Science
The Institute of Statistical Mathematics
Tokyo, Japan

Takahiro Nonaka
Department of Statistical Science
The Graduate University for Advanced Studies
and
Pharmaceuticals and Medical Devices Agency
Tokyo, Japan

Federico Rotolo
Service de Biostatistique et d'Epidémiologie
Gustave Roussy
Université Paris-Sud
Villejuif, France

Daniel Sargent
Department of Health Sciences Research
Mayo Clinic
Rochester, Minnesota

Martin Schumacher
Center for Medical Biometry and Medical Informatics
University Medical Center Freiburg
Freiburg, Germany

Richard Simon
Biometric Research Branch
National Cancer Institute
Bethesda, Maryland

Greg Spaniolo
GPS, Genentech
South San Francisco, California

Peter Thall
Department of Biostatistics
MD Anderson Cancer Center
The University of Texas
Houston, Texas

Ru-Fang Yeh
Biostatistics, Genentech
South San Francisco, California

Section I

Introductory Overview

1

Clinical Trials for Predictive Medicine: New Paradigms and Challenges

Richard Simon, Shigeyuki Matsui, and Marc Buyse

CONTENT

Randomized clinical trials have played a fundamental role in modern medicine. For many treatments, the variation in prognosis among patients exceeds the size of the treatment effect and evaluation of the treatment is very error-prone without large randomized clinical trials. In oncology, developments in biotechnology and advances in understanding tumor biology have provided a better understanding of this variability. In many cases, tumors of a given primary site appear to be heterogeneous with regard to the mutations that cause them, their natural course, and their response to therapy. The heterogeneity in response to therapy is likely to be an important component of the observed small average treatment effects seen in many phase III randomized clinical trials. Small average treatment effects in common diseases for inexpensive and well-tolerated drugs like aspirin can be worthwhile and of public health importance. Small average treatment effects for very expensive drugs with serious adverse effects are much less acceptable for patients and for health care economics. Small average effects imply large NNT values, where NNT denotes the number of patients needed to treat in order to save one life or benefit one patient, on average. When the average treatment effect is small, it is likely that most patients do not benefit but are at risk for the adverse effects of the drug and may have missed the opportunity to receive a drug that might have helped them. Detecting small treatment effects requires large randomized clinical trials as the sample size is approximately inversely proportional to the square of the treatment effect to be detected.

The ideal approach to dealing with heterogeneity in response is to understand it, not just to average outcome for large number of patients so that a small treatment effect can be reliably distinguished from a null effect. Some drugs that are in common use today have long been known, because of their mechanism of action, to exert their effects in a subset of patients. For instance, tamoxifen and aromatase inhibitors are only indicated for the treatment of hormone-responsive breast cancer. But most anticancer drugs are not targeted at well-characterized patient subsets and are therefore administered to all patients with a given tumor type, which may be justified if all patients have a chance of deriving a benefit from these drugs, but not if the benefit is confined to a small subset of *responding* patients. Developments in biotechnology have provided genome-wide assays for characterizing disease tissue, and these tools have been utilized to obtain better understanding of disease pathology. In cancer, high-throughput DNA sequencing has identified somatically mutated genes whose protein products serve as new molecular targets for therapy. In fact, the majority of current drug development in oncology involves the development of inhibitors of protein products of deregulated genes. These drugs are not expected to be as broadly active as early chemotherapy DNA toxins. Their antitumor effect is likely to be restricted to patients in whom deregulation of the drug target is driving the invasion of the tumor.

Success with this approach depends on having a drug target that is important to the disease, having a drug that can be delivered in high enough concentration that it can strongly inhibit the target, adequately understanding the biology of the tumor and the target to be able to identify a predictive biomarker that identifies the patients who are likely to benefit from the drug, and developing a technically accurate test to measure the predictive biomarker.

Some people think of personalized medicine as consisting of post hoc analyses of registries to determine how outcome depends on demographic, staging, and other factors. This approach has serious deficiencies, however. First, treatment selection is not primarily about understanding *prognostic* factors, it is about understanding factors that result in a patient benefiting from one treatment more than another (factors *predictive* of treatment effects). Because the bias in treatment selection for observational registry data can rarely be adequately disentangled based on measured baseline factors, such registry data are rarely, if ever, adequate for identifying predictive biomarkers, particularly for new drugs. In order to effectively develop new treatments, one ideally needs to identify the predictive biomarker prior to the phase III pivotal trials performed to evaluate the drugs. In reality, however, many predictive factors for the treatment of cancer patients have so far been identified post hoc using data from large randomized clinical trials in unselected patients. Population-based registries can sometimes be used to identify patients with such good prognosis on standard therapy that substantial benefit from a new drug is not likely. That type of prognostic biomarker could be used to deselect or exclude such good prognostic patients from clinical trials of the new drug.

In most cases, the codevelopment of a drug and a predictive biomarker must be based on appropriately designed prospective clinical trials.

This represents a quantum increase in the complexity of drug development and of clinical trials. Given the fact that cancers of many or most primary sites are heterogeneous in their underlying biology and responsiveness to therapy, the approach of codevelopment of new drug and companion diagnostic is scientifically compelling but practically difficult. Industry perspectives on the codevelopment of drug and companion diagnostic are described in Chapter 2.

In cases where the drug is relatively specific and the importance of the molecular target in disease pathogenesis is well established, the process can be relatively straightforward. Examples include trastuzumab for breast cancer, vemurafenib for melanoma, and crizotinib for lung cancer (Slamon et al., 2001; Chapman et al., 2011; Shaw et al., 2013). In the case of vemurafenib, drug development was driven by the discovery of the V600E *BRAF* point mutation in approximately half of melanoma cases; hence, the existence of the mutation served as the predictive biomarker. For crizotinib, a translocation in the *ALK* gene served the same role. For trastuzumab, overexpression of the *HER2* protein was found to be prognostic in breast cancer and led to the development of inhibitors of the protein. There was uncertainty over whether overactivation of *HER2* should be measured based on an immunohistochemistry (ICH) test for protein overexpression or a fluorescence in situ hybridization (FISH) test for amplification of the *HER2* gene and on what threshold of positivity should be used for these tests. In cases such as these, however, the drug was screened to work for biomarker positive tumors and clinical development was focused from the start on test-positive patients. If there is some uncertainty as to what assay to use for assessing *biomarker positivity* as there was in the case of trastuzumab, this should be resolved during phase I and phase II trials if possible. By the time of initiation of phase III trials of the new drug, one should have a single *analytically validated* assay that will be used. Analytically validated means technically accurate for measuring the analyte that the assay is purported to measure. If there is no gold standard for measuring the analyte, then the assay should be robust and reproducible. Chapter 3 of this volume provides more information about analytical validation. In clinical trials, the question often arises as to whether patient selection can be based on an assay performed by a local laboratory, or whether a central laboratory should review all local assay results as part as the patient eligibility. The decision to use a local or a central laboratory depends on the availability, reproducibility, and validity of the assay. Even when assays are well established and widely used, their results may come into question and trigger the need for an interlaboratory reproducibility study. Such a study was recently conducted on the ICH and FISH tests for amplification of the *HER2* gene, after patients with nonamplified tumors appeared to derive benefit from trastuzumab in two large adjuvant trials conducted by major U.S. cooperative groups (Perez et al., 2013).

The phase III designs for trastuzumab, vemurafenib, and crizotinib were *enrichment designs* for which only test-positive patients were eligible.

The test-positive patients were randomized to a regimen containing the new drug versus a control regimen. For initiating such a clinical trial, one needs a threshold of positivity for the analytically validated assay used to define the test. This is generally not a problem for mutation-based tests but it can be an issue for tests based on gene amplification, protein expression, or RNA abundance. One can try to evaluate the relationship of assay value to tumor response in the phase II development period. This requires, however, (1) that one is not stringent in restricting eligibility for the phase II trials based on assay value, (2) that the phase II trials are large enough for this analysis, and (3) that the assay used for phase II is the assay that will be used for phase III. The assay versus response analysis will be based on a phase II endpoint. The particular endpoint used will depend on the disease and on whether the phase II trials are randomized or single arm. The phase II trials should be designed with this objective in mind. An alternative to using phase II data to define the assay threshold of positivity is to conduct the phase III trial initially without such a restriction and to adaptively define the optimal threshold in the phase III study (Jiang et al., 2009; Simon and Simon, 2013).

In some cases, there will be less preclinical evidence that the effectiveness of the drug will be through a mechanism measured by the selected biomarker. These include cases where the biomarker is not so tightly linked to the drug target or where the drug has several targets whose role in disease pathogenesis is not fully understood. The early development period, including phase I and II trials, is the time to evaluate candidate biomarkers as described in Chapters 4 through 7 of this volume. Markers that identify the patients who respond to the drug need to be identified in phase II trials. This requires that these trials be conducted in such a way that all patients have tissue available for all of the candidate biomarkers to be measured and that the sample sizes be increased to provide for adequately powered analyses. These analyses are likely to result in one of three conclusions: (1) No good predictive biomarker is identified and the drug does not have sufficient activity for phase III development. (2) No good predictive biomarker is identified, but the drug has sufficient activity for phase III development. (3) A promising predictive biomarker is identified. In the latter case, the evidence for the biomarker may not be strong enough to use an enrichment design in phase III and one of the *all-comers* designs may be more appropriate. These designs enroll both test-positive and test-negative patients and evaluate the treatment effect overall, in test-positive and in test-negative patients (Karuri and Simon, 2012; Simon, 2013) while controlling for the multiple tests. Designs of this type are described in Chapters 8 through 10 of this volume. The evidence for the predictive biomarker at the end of phase II should be relatively strong to warrant the substantial complexity of proceeding on this path. It requires that one have an analytically validated test for the phase III trial and that the phase III trial be sized for an adequately powered separate analysis of the test-positive patients. If the evidence for the biomarker is too weak after phase II, it may not be deemed worthwhile to proceed in this way. If the evidence is too strong, then there may be ethical difficulties to a phase III trial that includes test-negative patients.

If no single promising predictive biomarker has been identified by the time of initiation of the phase III trial, three approaches are available for continuing the search. The first is the usual approach of designing the phase III trial in the usual way with broad eligibility, using all of the 5% type I error for the test of treatment effect for the intention to treat (ITT) population, and then conducting post hoc hypothesis generation subset analyses on the final results. Any subset finding would have to be confirmed in a subsequent phase III clinical trial. The second approach is to reserve part of the 5% type I error to identify and validate a predictive biomarker or predictive biomarker signature within the phase III trial. These methods, including the adaptive signature design and cross-validated adaptive signature design (Simon, 2013) and the continuous adaptive signature method (Matsui et al., 2012), involve partitioning the patients in the clinical trial into a training set and a test set, developing a candidate predictive biomarker or biomarker signature on the training set using any prospectively defined algorithm, and then testing the treatment effect in the subset of patients in the test set that are positive for the biomarker or biomarker signature developed on the training set. The cross-validated versions of these approaches improve statistical power by using cross-validation of the development-validation process rather than simple sample splitting. These methods are described in Chapters 16 and 17 of this volume. The third approach is to utilize the prospective–retrospective analysis approach of Simon et al. (2009). With this approach, one would reserve some of the 5% type I error for a single test of treatment effect in a subset to be determined in the future. The subset must be identified based on data external to the phase III clinical trial. The biomarker defining the subset can be identified by the time of final analysis of the clinical trial or later. For example, accumulating external evidence on an association between *K-ras* mutation status and responsiveness of a colorectal tumor to anti-EGFR (epidermal growth factor receptor) antibody, cetuximab helped in identifying a subset of patients without *K-ras* mutations after the primary analysis in a phase III clinical trial to evaluate the efficacy of cetuximab for advanced colorectal cancer (Karapetis et al., 2008). The approach requires archiving tissue for all randomized patients and measuring the biomarker using an assay analytically validated for use with archived tissue, although the assay need not be available until the biomarker is subsequently defined. If tissue is not available on all patients, tissue should be collected before randomization to ensure that *missingness* is independent of treatment assignment. The size of the phase III trial should be somewhat increased to adjust for the treatment effect in the ITT population being conducted at a somewhat reduced significance level.

We have used the term *analytical validation* in the previous paragraphs to indicate that the test accurately measures the analyte it is supposed to measure or is robust and reproducible. Analytical validation is distinguished from *clinical validation* and *medical utility* (Simon et al., 2009). Clinical validation means that the assay correlates with a clinical outcome. For example, demonstrating that a marker correlates with outcome for a population of patients heterogeneous with regard to stage and treatment represents clinical validation. One can clinically validate a prognostic signature by showing that it is prognostic on a dataset not used for developing the signature or by proper use of cross-validation (Subramanian and Simon, 2010). Medical utility means that the biomarker is actionable for informing treatment selection in a manner that benefits the patients by either improving outcome or by reducing adverse effects for equivalent outcome. Most prognostic factors are not actionable, particularly when they are developed using data for a population mixed with regard to stage and treatment. For example, to show that a prognostic signature identifies a subset of patient with stage I estrogen receptor–positive (ER+) breast cancer who have such good prognosis that they do not require cytotoxic chemotherapy, one needs to study patients with stage I ER+ breast cancer who did not receive cytotoxic chemotherapy. The phrase *medical utility* as used here does not imply analysis of costs versus benefits or benefits versus adverse effects. We use the term to indicate establishing that the biomarker can inform the aforementioned treatment selection using only standard prognostic factor–based clinical guidelines in a manner that results in patient benefit in terms of survival or some other well-defined endpoint. Further details for assessing the medical utility of prognostic signatures are described in Chapter 11 of this volume.

There is a misconception that the gold standard for evaluating medical utility of a predictive biomarker requires a clinical trial in which patients are randomized to either have or not have the biomarker measured. With this *marker strategy design*, physicians make their treatment selections either informed by the marker value or using standard of care selections. There are several serious problems with this design, the greatest of which is that many, if not most, patients in both arms of the randomization will receive the same treatment. This induces a dramatic reduction in the statistical power of the clinical trial, and the trial will need to have an enormous sample size in order to detect a treatment effect. A second problem is that since the biomarker is not measured for one arm of the trial, one cannot focus the analysis on patients who receive different treatments on the two strategies and cannot dissect the patient population into biomarker-based subsets for separate analysis.

In many settings, there are much better clinical trial designs for evaluating medical utility of a predictive biomarker. A predictive biomarker must be defined with regard to a specific therapy and a specific control. For example, the V600E *BRAF* mutation is predictive for benefit from vemurafenib in melanoma patients but not for benefit from cytotoxic chemotherapy. The simple all-comers designs in which we measure the marker on all patients, and then randomize all patients to the new drug or control can establish medical utility in a much more efficient way than the marker strategy design. For example, Let $S_+(T)$ and $S_+(C)$ denote the 5-year survival probability of biomarker-positive patients receiving the new treatment or the control, respectively. For biomarker-negative patients, let these survival probabilities be $S_-(T)$ and $S_-(C)$. Let x denote the proportion of patients who are biomarker positive. If all patients receive the standard of care control without measuring the marker, then the 5-year survival probability would be $xS_+(C) + (1 - x)S_-(C)$. A biomarker-based treatment strategy in which marker-positive patients receive the new treatment and marker-negative patients receive the control has expected survival probability $xS_+(T) + (1 - x)S_-(C)$. The treatment effect for comparing the marker-based strategy to the standard of care not using the marker is thus $x[S_+(T) - S_+(C)]$. This treatment effect can be efficiently estimated by the all-comers design, because the treatment effect in the marker-positive subset is $[S_+(T) - S_+(C)]$ and the proportion of marker positive is easily estimated. Hence, the all-comers design in which the marker is measured in all patients and all patients are randomized to the treatment or control provides a more efficient estimate of the treatment effect with use or non-use of the biomarker than does the marker strategy design. Since $x[S_+(T) - S_+(C)]$ depends only on the treatment effect in the marker-positive subset, using the enrichment design and excluding test-negative patients provides an even more efficient way of estimating the treatment effect than with the marker strategy design.

As we have seen so far, prognostic and predictive biomarkers or signatures are an essential element in the new paradigm of clinical trials for personalized or predictive medicine. Recent advances in biotechnology and genomics have opened a new field to develop genomic signatures based on data-driven analytical approaches to high-dimensional genomic data from high-throughput technologies. These topics are covered in Chapters 12 through 15 of this volume.

So far, we have discussed prognostic and predictive biomarkers. There are also early detection biomarkers and endpoint biomarkers. Endpoint biomarkers themselves are of several types. Pharmacodynamic biomarkers are used to determine whether a drug inhibits its target. Intermediate endpoints are used in phase I and II studies to optimize the treatment regimen and the target population without any claim that the intermediate endpoint is a valid surrogate for the phase III endpoint. Surrogate endpoints are sometimes used in phase III trials as alternatives for survival. For a surrogate to be valid, one must have previously demonstrated that for the class of drugs being evaluated, a treatment effect on the surrogate provides a good prediction of the treatment effect on survival (Burzykowski et al., 2005). This is discussed in detail in Chapter 18 of this volume.

References

Burzykowski T, Molenberghs G, Buyse M (eds.). *The Evaluation of Surrogate Endpoints*. Springer, New York, 2005, 408pp.

Chapman PB, Hauschild A, Robert C et al. Improved survival with vemurafenib in melanoma with *BRAF* V600E mutation. *New England Journal of Medicine* 364: 2507–2516, 2011.

Jiang W, Freidlin B, Simon R. Biomarker adaptive threshold design: A procedure for evaluating treatment with possible biomarker-defined subset effect. *Journal of the National Cancer Institute* 99: 1036–1043, 2007.

Karapetis CS, Khambata-Ford S, Jonker DJ et al. *K-ras* mutations and benefit from cetuximab in advanced colorectal cancer. *New England Journal of Medicine* 359: 1757–1765, 2008.

Karuri S, Simon R. A two-stage Bayesian design for co-development of new drugs and companion diagnostics. *Statistics in Medicine* 31: 901–914, 2012.

Matsui S, Simon R, Qu P, Shaughnessy JD, Barlogie B, Crowley J. Developing and validating continuous genomic signatures in randomized clinical trials for predictive medicine. *Clinical Cancer Research* 18: 6065–6073, 2012.

Perez EA, Press MF, Dueck AC et al. Round-robin clinico-pathological review of *HER2* testing in the context of adjuvant therapy for breast cancer (N9831, BCIRG 006, and BCIRG 005). *Breast Cancer Research Treatment* 138: 99–108, 2013.

Shaw AT, Kim DW, Nakagawa K et al. Crizotinib versus chemotherapy in advanced *ALK*-positive lung cancer. *New England Journal of Medicine* 368: 2385–2394, 2013.

Simon N, Simon R. Adaptive enrichment designs for clinical trials. *Biostatistics* 14: 613–625, 2013.

Simon RM. *Genomic Clinical Trials and Predictive Medicine*. Cambridge University Press, Cambridge, U.K., 2013.

Simon RM, Paik S, Hayes DF. Use of archived specimens in evaluation of prognostic and predictive biomarkers. *Journal of the National Cancer Institute* 101: 1446–1452, 2009.

Slamon DJ, Leyland-Jones B, Shak S et al. Use of chemotherapy plus a monoclonal antibody against *HER2* for metastatic breast cancer that overexpresses *HER2*. *New England Journal of Medicine* 344: 783–792, 2001.

Subramanian J, Simon R. Gene expression-based prognostic signatures in lung cancer: Ready for clinical use? *Journal of the National Cancer Institute* 102: 464–474, 2010.

2

An Industry Statistician's Perspective on Personalized Health Care Drug Development

Jane Fridlyand, Ru-Fang Yeh, Howard Mackey, Thomas Bengtsson, Paul Delmar, Greg Spaniolo, and Grazyna Lieberman

CONTENTS

2.1 Introduction

Much of historical drug development has been based on a one-size-fits-all paradigm. However, as the slowdown in the number of the new drug approvals demonstrates, this strategy is becoming less viable [1]. The FDA Critical Path Initiative [2] calls for a focus on personalized medicine approaches. Such an approach is enabled by recent developments in molecular profiling techniques. To meet the challenge of personalized medicine, clinical development plans must include strategies incorporating patient selection, and as statisticians, we must embrace these expanded clinical strategies. Drug companies have set ambitious goals around the delivery of personalized medicines to the patients. These goals have created an environment in which an increased focus is being given to the incorporation of predictive biomarkers into clinical development plans. Here we present some issues arising when evaluating diagnostics (Dx) in clinical development programs. One approach to such development is to incorporate the known biomarker (single or complex) into the clinical development program from the beginning, and design appropriate proof of concept (POC) experiments evaluating drug activity in diagnostically defined patient subsets. Alternative scenarios include performing retrospective analyses on clinical and biomarker/genomic data of the approved drug and, if appropriate, updating the drug label to include information on a biomarker/drug–response relationship. A significantly less desirable but in theory possible situation includes late emergence of the biomarker hypotheses and needing to use pivotal trial for both discovery and confirmation. Thus, one could expect a significant impact on many aspects of drug development. Examples include defining clinical and regulatory strategies, clinical trial design, development decision criteria, and utilizing classification approaches and exploratory analyses.

The overview begins with introducing key personalized health care (PHC)-related concepts and terms, summarizing regulatory codevelopment paradigm and outlining underlying philosophy. We then describe general principles for considering drug/Dx codevelopment. These high-level principles are followed by summary of specific challenges that come up in the design of POC trials with the diagnostic component, with a focus on oncology. These challenges are broadly divided into strategic, operational, and statistical issues. Due to less experience with drug/Dx codevelopment in non-oncology, many of the specific points raised are more directly relevant to oncology but broader concepts apply across all therapeutic areas. A brief section stating some recent regulatory considerations for phase III trials with diagnostic question follows. Finally, the analytics issues section focuses on good statistical practices related to exploratory analyses; the topics discussed in this document range from data generation, analysis planning and execution, to interpretation, and validation strategy.

This overview chapter is targeted toward industry biostatisticians involved in projects that incorporate predictive biomarkers. The intent is to enable the biostatistician to be a valuable strategic partner on such projects. This chapter is intended to provide biostatistician with an understanding of key questions that need to be asked throughout the PHC drug development program.

2.1.1 Introductory Concepts and Philosophy

An excellent discussion with extensive references of the basic concepts utilized in this chapter can be found in [3–5], and also described in detail in Chapters 1 and 18 of this book. To remind the reader, a *prognostic biomarker* provides information about the patient overall outcome, regardless of therapy. A *predictive biomarker* provides information on the effect of a therapeutic intervention in a patient, and is often a target for therapy. One can distinguish baseline and early predictive (pharmacodynamics or PD) biomarkers, with the first being used for patient selection and the second for providing information on the therapeutic activity. This manuscript is restricted to the discussion of the baseline biomarker.

Following basic principles of the clinical trial design, it is necessary to have a reliable estimate of the behavior of the efficacy endpoint of interest under standard of care in order to judge a relative activity of the investigational agent. This estimate may come from the historic data or from a control arm in a randomized trial. When evaluating a predictive biomarker along with the drug activity, the role of randomized trials becomes even more important. Single-arm trials may not be able to distinguish between prognostic and predictive contributions of the biomarkers in the absence of reliable historical data.

With the advent of the novel therapies, the prognostic and predictive biomarker categories are heavily intermingled [6,7]. For example, a target may be viewed as attractive for a drug development because it was shown to be important in prognosis, for example, Her2 overexpression. Thus, a negative prognostic factor can be neutralized with a new therapy, targeted to the same marker (e.g., Herceptin for Her2-positive breast cancer patients). Conversely, ER/PR status has been shown to be a positive prognostic factor and thus treatments that target hormonally dependent tumors further improve outcome for ER-/PR-positive patients in comparison to patients with triple negative tumors. In the future, the advent of therapies for triple negative breast tumors may eliminate the differential prognosis with the evolving standard of care.

In parallel with conducting clinical trials with the drug and the biomarker, it is imperative to initiate studies/conduct research evaluating real-world population-level data to put forward/verify clinical team assumptions with regard to the prevalence or distribution of the biomarker in the target population, the expected direction, magnitude and form of the prognostic association, and generalizability of the patient population. Some of these questions fall under the expertise of an epidemiologist rather than a biostatistician, and we encourage team statisticians to bring together relevant quantitative functions for the discussion.

2.1.2 Basics of Drug/Diagnostics Codevelopment

Companion diagnostic is a molecular test, which is essential for determination of patient's eligibility for treatment. In the following texts, we discuss initial questions when considering companion diagnostic plan.

2.1.2.1 PHC Assessment versus Development Strategy

As shown in Figure 2.1, there are three main possibilities for PHC/development strategy: *selected (or enriched)*, *stratified*, and *AllComers (traditional approach without using the biomarker)* [8]. *Stratified* and *AllComers* approaches are sometimes grouped together as *AllComers*, since in contrast to the *enriched* approach, patient enrollment is not restricted by the diagnostic in either scenario but having a Dx hypothesis (*stratified* approach) affects the trial endpoints and analysis plan. Note that PHC assessment may be reevaluated as program progresses and new information emerges. There should be a duality between the PHC assessment and the development strategy.

Having a strong Dx hypothesis is highly advantageous in drug/Dx codevelopment. In the absence of such a hypothesis, a clinical team may often plan to include biomarkers as exploratory endpoints for hypothesis generation but generally not for planning primary or secondary analyses. From a development perspective, a *stratified strategy* is the most challenging and comprehensive one. Additional considerations (e.g., development speed and cost) may lead the team to choose a *selected* over a *stratified* approach in the early stages even when some activity in Dx-negative patients is not unlikely, in which case a staged development plan may be considered. With such a plan, the drug will be first tested in the Dx-positive patients believed most likely to benefit, followed by the evaluation in Dx-negative patients.

PHC ASSESSMENT		
• **Strong Dx hypothesis** • **No activity in Dx neg**	• **Strong Dx hypothesis** • **Possibly some activity in Dx neg**	• **No strong Dx hypothesis** • **Exploratory Stage**
DEVELOPMENT STRATEGY		
Selected	**Stratified**	**AllComers**
• **Patient selection through all phases of development**	• **Complex, larger phase IIs with stratification** • **Complex phase IIIs**	• **No selection or stratification** • **Data exploration**
Dx test prior to randomization Dx+ Placebo Active	Dx test prior to randomization Dx- Dx+ Placebo Placebo Active Active	Randomize all subjects Placebo Active

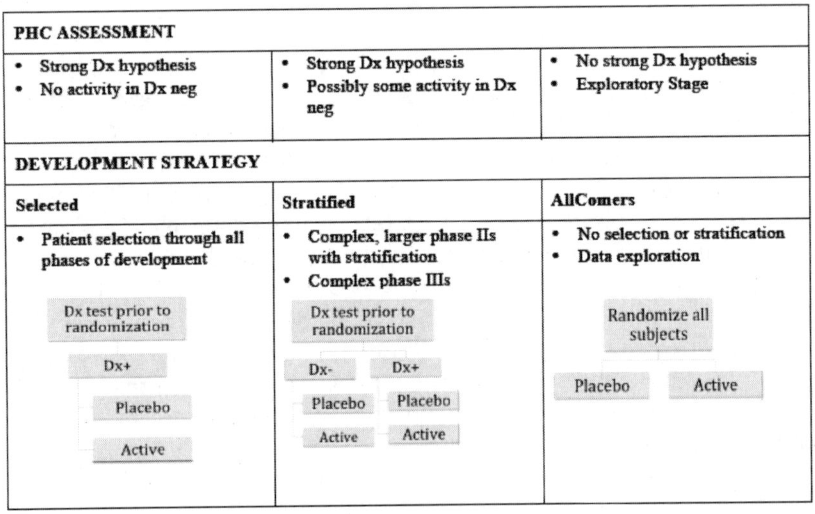

FIGURE 2.1
PHC assessment versus development strategy, and associated trial designs. *Notes*: (1) The Stratified strategy may be limited to pre-planned stratified analysis only. (2) In the Stratified scenario, stratification on the biomarker can be done either prospectively (as shown here) or retrospectively, as long as biomarker analysis is pre-planned.

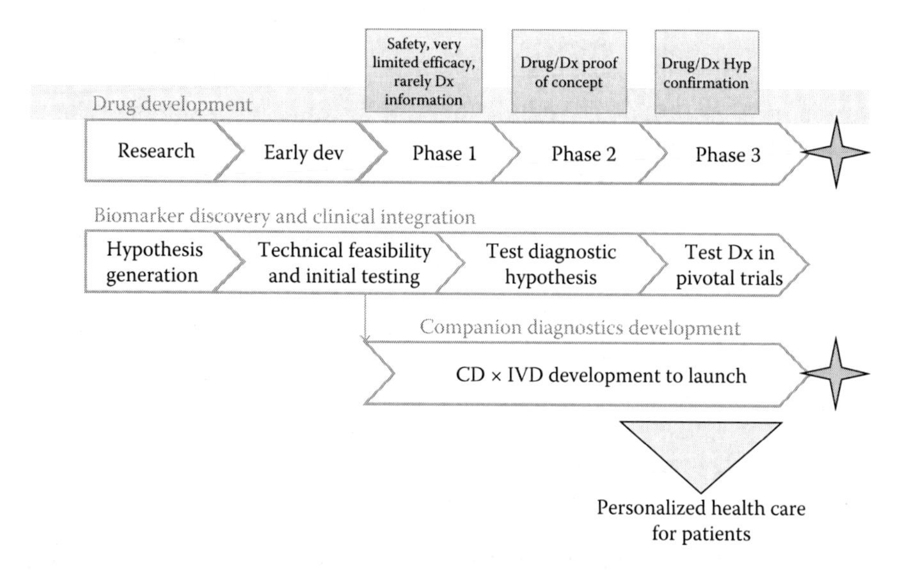

FIGURE 2.2
Typical development milestones for the drug/Dx codevelopment process. (Adapted from FDA draft concept paper on drug diagnostic codevelopment, April, 2005. Demonstrates need for synchronization between drug and diagnostic development timelines.)

Potential regulatory considerations of *selected* development are discussed in the FDA draft enrichment guidance [9].

Typical development milestones for the general drug/Dx codevelopment process are shown in Figure 2.2. These milestones are closely aligned with current regulatory requirements outlined in [10]. It is evident from Figure 2.2 that the currently accepted development paradigm needs a Dx hypothesis to be formulated well in advance of a pivotal trial, and generally prior to the POC trial. FDA draft guidance on in vitro diagnostic [11] further addresses this point. *Biomarker-related* interaction with health authorities should be planned and fully incorporated in the development plan, just as is the case with the other regulatory interactions. Interestingly, recent draft guidance [9] suggests that this paradigm may be changing going forward (see Section 2.3).

In the early development, especially for a drug belonging to the class of molecules not previously evaluated in clinic (*First in Class* or FIC), the clinical experience prior to the pivotal study is likely to be very limited, and a PHC assessment may be based nearly exclusively on literature and preclinical data. Key considerations include understanding of the biological rationale of the PHC hypothesis (e.g., based on the mechanism of drug action) and summary of supporting data and experiments.

To pursue Dx in clinical development for *stratified* or *selected* scenario, there needs to be a relatively well-defined diagnostic hypothesis using tissue, tumor, or blood-borne markers, for example, patients harboring a certain mutation are more likely to respond to the treatment. The single-analyte Dx is common (e.g., a single gene mutation, amplification, expression); however, composite measures also represent possible Dx, for example, serving as a pathway activation indicator or expression signature.

Designing a composite measure could involve performing exploratory analyses using high-dimensional microarray data generated using the cell lines and xenograft models. Approaches to performing these types of analyses are briefly outlined by the analytic portion of this chapter, and are also discussed in more detail in Chapters 12 through 15 of this book. Here, we assume the existence of a well-defined summary measure across multiple assays. Assay measurement issues are an important area for an industry statistician to understand, and challenges connected with analytical validation of biomarker assays are discussed in Chapter 3.

Additionally, as discussed in the introduction, understanding the biomarker prevalence/distribution in the targeted indication is of paramount importance for development decision making and for planning the phase II trial. The expected prevalence can be estimated based on multiple sources of information including in-house experience (cell lines and purchased archival samples [tumors or fluids] or potentially archival samples collected on previous clinical trials), public databases (e.g., Sanger Mutational database), and literature reports. The confidence in these estimates should be assessed by the development team. It is possible that a dedicated marker distribution study may be needed prior to the start of the first POC or a pivotal trial. This may be done by collaborating with the academic centers with well-established tumor banks in the tumor type of interest or by purchasing samples for in-house tumor bank enriched for the specific tumor type. Issues like drift over time in marker status (e.g., changing status between primary and metastatic samples) and its prognostic significance need to be taken into account when planning sample collections.

In summary, it is essential for a statistician to understand the nature of both biological rationale and preclinical experiments, as well as, where available, epidemiological and clinical data, in order to aid the team with reliable evaluation of the strength of evidence contained in the data and, hence, robustness of the proposed development plan.

2.2 POC Designs

In this section, we focus on the *stratified* development strategy scenario (see Figure 2.2), in which a POC phase II trial needs to allow for simultaneous drug/Dx evaluation leading to an informative decision with regard to a label-enabling phase III trial design, that is, it should address a question about a relative activity of a drug at a recommended phase II dose in the diagnostically defined patient subsets versus unselected population. As can be seen in Figure 2.1, the other two development scenarios clearly defined target population in which a primary activity question is being asked.

2.2.1 Overall Considerations

The team needs to balance the probability of success, speed, and cost considerations when designing a POC trial. Since all three parameters cannot be optimized simultaneously, the strength of scientific evidence for the biomarker hypothesis, timeline goals, the competitive landscape, and overall portfolio considerations will dictate a balance.

It is important to be explicit regarding the decisions that will need to be made based on the outcome of a phase II POC trial. In the context of *stratified* PHC, POC does not only need to enable a pivotal (phase III) trial, but also determine its design with regard to the Dx (see Figure 2.2). If the biomarker threshold for positivity is not well understood (e.g., the biomarker is not naturally bimodal such as mutation), it may also be necessary to use phase II data to define a biomarker threshold for defining Dx-positive patients subset in phase III, as described later in Section 2.2. Most often, a randomized trial against a control will be needed to distinguish predictive and prognostic effects of the putative biomarker. Unless stated otherwise, the discussion in the following text pertains to randomized trial designs.

2.2.2 Operational Considerations

Here we focus on operational issues specific to oncology. However, much of what is presented in the following text is applicable to other therapeutic areas in which diagnosis is determined by assaying a particular marker(s) on a patient sample.

Key operational issues potentially impacted by the decision to mandate tissue testing for patients entering the trial include projected enrollment rate and number of eligible sites. Additional questions with regard to operational conduct of the trial may include the following:

1. What is the assay-failure proportion (marginal and joint if more than one assay)? The trial size needs to account for the patients without the interpretable assay.
2. Is tissue testing going to be retrospective or prospective? If prospective:
    a. Is the assay robust enough that single batch analysis is not required for comparability of the measurements?
    b. Will the results be used for randomization? If yes, is the expected turnaround time for test results compatible with how long patients may be willing to wait to receive treatment?

The total trial size may in part be driven by the prevalence of the Dx-positive patients. A statistician needs to work closely with the team to determine whether it may be necessary to decrease the trial size by switching to enrolling Dx-positive patients only, once sufficient number of diagnostically unselected patients is enrolled. This may be necessitated, for example, by a lower than expected Dx prevalence. A possibility of restricting enrollment to marker-positive patients later in the trial needs to be reflected in the protocol and randomization algorithm, and assay regulatory requirements need to be carefully considered.

The sensitivity of timing of trial efficacy analyses to the assumptions such as sites start-up, effective enrollment rate, time to event, Dx marker prevalence, and potential prognostic significance of the Dx marker needs to be evaluated to obtain realistic timelines.

2.2.3 Statistical Considerations

PHC evaluation using *stratified* clinical development plan should be focused on answering the question of how to best design the phase III without unduly delaying the program. Typically, the phase III design choices (see Figure 2.2) considered are the following:

1. AllComers (AC)
2. *Stratified* for Dx with the coprimary endpoints (Dx, AC)
3. *Selected* for Dx
4. *Stop* the development in that indication

Some key parameters necessary for the design of the trial include

1. Description of the target population(s), including relevant Dx subsets
2. Clinically relevant effect size in individual subsets to be evaluated
3. Dx prevalence and prognostic attributes
4. Expected behavior of a control arm
5. Understanding attributes of the proposed Dx assay such as sensitivity and specificity

With a randomized controlled study, an underlying statistical model to estimate the main effects of treatment and the biomarker as well as the interaction between the treatment and the biomarker is the following:

$$\text{Outcome} \propto f(\boldsymbol{\alpha}\text{Treatment} + \boldsymbol{\beta}\text{Marker} + \boldsymbol{\gamma}\text{Treatment} \times \text{Marker})$$

Testing the null hypotheses for an interaction term of $\boldsymbol{\gamma} = 0$ gets at the question of the predictiveness of the biomarker, that is, dependence of the treatment effect of the biomarker level. The specific model used depends on the type of outcome and the assumptions (e.g., Cox proportional hazards model for time-to-event data in oncology; logistic model with logit link for the response rate, or a linear model for a continuous readout in inflammation and other nononcology indications).

Most phase II and even phase III studies are generally not powered to formally test for an interaction—such tests often require significantly higher number of subjects than in a typical clinical trial. A variety of approaches, ad hoc and other, are used to arrive at a point estimate for parameters of interest. For example, targeting estimation to parameter contrasts of clinical significance will often yield smaller sample sizes *versus* inference on the interaction term alone [14]. All of the tests to be performed and decision rules need to be prespecified in the statistical analysis plan prior to data unblinding. When the biomarker is bimodal, semiquantitative approaches include modeling effect individually in the prespecified subgroups and qualitatively comparing the two effects to assess predictiveness of the biomarker. With the continuous biomarker, it is often helpful to visualize and quantify effect size in the patient subgroups defined by prespecified biomarker percentiles to ensure that effect size changes as expected with the biomarker value. Development decision will always depend on the observed data as well as effect size deemed to be *clinically meaningful* defined in what is often called *diagnostic target profile* for a drug describing desired effect size in biomarker subgroups and clarifying the strength of the predictive relationship between the treatment effect and the biomarker required for the clinical development program.

2.2.3.1 Defining Decision Rules

A simplistic way to think about the outcome of the POC trial is in terms of the phase III decision criterion for unselected patients (AllComers) and each of prespecified subsets (Dx positive). Each of the subsets needs to pass a set criterion in order to be considered as a coprimary endpoint in phase III trial. An example of a decision strategy for a single Dx marker is presented in Table 2.1.

The operational characteristics of any decision rule and the robustness of outputs should be assessed analytically and/or via simulations under a variety of the scenarios. Given the total number of events and fixed trial design, examples of parameters to vary in the simulations include marker prevalence, their prognostic and predictive effect, treatment effect in Dx-negative patients, and patient enrollment pattern. Simulations should help quantify the balance between the risk of taking an inactive drug forward and not advancing an active compound. The exact decision rules would depend on many considerations including the commercial ones.

2.2.3.2 Sample Size Considerations

In the following text, we discuss two main scenarios for the biomarker that affect sample size projections: biomarkers with clear prespecified cutoff (e.g., bimodal biomarkers, such as mutation) versus biomarkers where the

TABLE 2.1

Decision Criteria Based on Phase II Result

Phase II Results	Effect Is Unfavorable in AllComers	Effect Is Favorable in AllComers
Effect is favorable in Dx-positive patients	Selected	AllComers if effect in Dx positive and Dx negative is similar
		Stratified with coprimary endpoint (e.g., Dx positive and all patients) if effect in Dx positive meaningfully exceeds effect in Dx negative
		Selected if effect is not favorable in Dx negative
Effect is not favorable in Dx-positive patients	Stop	Investigate if not false positive; possibly Go to AllComers

Note: Concept of *favorable* versus *unfavorable* may be different in AllComers versus Dx-positive patients.

cutoff needs to be determined (e.g., continuous, such as gene expression as described later in this section).

2.2.3.2.1 Categorical or Ordinal Markers (with Prespecified Cutoffs)

For each Dx subset that is of primary interest, it is necessary to have a sufficient number of events in the relevant subset(s) to provide an informative assessment for further evaluation. The standard approach to sizing a study with a time-to-event endpoint involves Schoenfeld's approximation [12], with inference taking the form of a test of H_0: $\beta=0$ versus H_a: $\beta<0$, where β equals the log of the hazard ratio, HR_{true}, between the two treatment groups. It can be shown that $\log(HR_{observed})$ is approximately distributed as Gaussian with the mean of $\log(HR_{true})$ and variance of $4/N$ (N is the number of events), and the sample size calculations are done accordingly. In a typical POC trial, Dx subsets of interest may contain 30–50 events or less if a very strong treatment effect is targeted. Under a range of commonly targeted hazard ratios, each additional 10 events typically corresponds to small (less than 5%) absolute improvement in type I and II error rates for a prespecified decision boundary. The decision boundary depends on what is considered to be a target effect for the drug and often set so type I and type II errors are about 20%–35% given a reasonable sample size. Here type I error refers to advancing inactive or marginally active drug into phase III, whereas type II error refers to stopping development of a drug whose activity would be clinically meaningful. See Table 2.2 for an example showing probability of phase III G_o when the decision rule is observed for HR of less than 0.75. One can see that with 30 events and above, probability of G_o is mainly driven by the true underlying HR and changes very little as number of events increases. In the example shown, 40–50 events in the subset of interest would be appropriate for the drug with the true HR of close to 0.60. Note that unlike phase III trials, phase II trials are

TABLE 2.2

Example: Probability of G_o to Phase III (Observed HR < 0.75) Given True HR and Number of Events

True HR (Rows) and Number of Events (Columns)	10	20	30	40	50	60	70
0.3	0.93	0.98	0.99	1.00	1.00	1.00	1.00
0.4	0.84	0.92	0.96	0.98	0.99	0.99	1.00
0.5	0.74	0.82	0.87	0.90	0.92	0.94	0.96
0.6	0.64	0.69	0.73	0.76	0.78	0.81	0.82
0.7	0.54	0.56	0.57	0.59	0.60	0.61	0.61
0.8	0.46	0.44	0.43	0.42	0.41	0.40	0.39
0.9	0.39	0.34	0.31	0.28	0.26	0.24	0.22
1.0	0.32	0.26	0.22	0.18	0.15	0.13	0.11

focused on estimation rather than testing, and the sample size is driven not by exact type I and type II error rates but rather by feasibility, timelines, and ability to obtain clinically meaningful estimates. So, one may say that sizing and decision making in phase II trials is more of an art than an exact science.

An additional consideration for sample size planning is rooted in regulatory discussions and overall development plan. In the event that POC trial leads the team to believe that the benefit is concentrated in Dx-positive patients only, suggesting selecting only such patients for the phase III trial, regulatory agencies may be interested in seeing some evidence that the drug is not active in Dx-negative patients. One way to provide such evidence is to plan for a sufficient number of Dx-negative patients in the phase II trial. *Sufficient* may be defined semirigorously with regulatory consultation, in addition to statistical, operational, and ethical considerations. Current FDA enrichment draft guidance [9] provides some guidelines on the number of Dx-negative patients evaluated prior to phase III in order to restrict phase III to selected population. Totality of prior clinical experience, including patients from the phase I trials, may be used toward the selection argument. In particular, it is generally not expected that the number of Dx-negative patients would be large enough to make a statistical argument with regard to lack of activity in these patients.

Even in the situation described earlier, which assumes that a marker cutoff is prespecified prior to the trial start (e.g., a patient is Dx positive if at least 50% of the tumor cells stain with the 2+ or 3+ immunohistochemistry (IHC) score), the team may consider remaining flexible with regard to updating the cutoff prior to the start of the phase III trial.

2.2.3.2.2 *Continuous Markers (No Predefined Cutoff)*

Many potential diagnostic biomarkers are inherently continuous (e.g., gene expression) or ordered categorical (e.g., protein expression by immunohistochemistry) rather than bimodal (e.g., mutation) and without an evident cutoff defining the *Dx-positive group*. In such cases, a cutoff must be defined through the use of the explicit criteria, which should be discussed with the development team. The challenge will be how to efficiently power a study to determine whether the treatment is efficacious as well as whether the biomarker is necessary to select patients. In addition, it would also be valuable to reliably estimate the biomarker threshold value, which separates patients deriving meaningful clinical benefit from those who do not.

To date, widely accepted statistical approaches to design and power a clinical study to estimate a continuous biomarker with an unknown threshold are not available. It should be noted that the FDA prefers prospectively designed studies as a regulatory requirement, although prospective retrospective options may not be completely ruled out (unpublished materials and presentations, e.g., by O'Neil [13], new FDA draft enrichment guidance [9]). In particular, it is advised in [9] that phase III data can be used to define the diagnostic for the final label as long as statistical validity of the phase III trial is preserved.

Mackey and Bengtsson [14] recently presented a strategy for sample size determination that hierarchically evaluates drug efficacy, a diagnostic's necessary for patient selection, and the diagnostic threshold. Their approach targets inference on clinically meaningful contrasts versus raw interaction terms, and highlight potential efficiency gains through randomization in cases where the biomarker has no effect in the control arm (i.e., is not prognostic). The setup assumes the effect of treatment effect is adequately described by the model $\boldsymbol{\beta}+f(C)\boldsymbol{\theta}$, where f is a specified monotonic function and C a patient's biomarker value within the interval [0, 1]. As a result, $\boldsymbol{\beta}+f(0)\boldsymbol{\theta}$ represents the effect of treatment in patients with the lowest biomarker values (i.e., *minimal treatment effect*) and $\boldsymbol{\beta}+f(1)\boldsymbol{\theta}$ represents the effect of treatment in patients with the highest biomarker values (*maximal treatment effect*). If the interaction effect of the biomarker on the log-hazard function is assumed to be linear, f can be taken to be the identity function, and $\boldsymbol{\beta}$ and $\boldsymbol{\beta}+\boldsymbol{\theta}$ represent the *minimal* and *maximal treatment effects*, respectively. In addition, if the biomarker is mapped uniformly to [0, 1] (e.g., using the empirical CDF), $\boldsymbol{\beta}+c\boldsymbol{\theta}$ can represent treatment effects at particular percentiles of the biomarker population. For example, a reduction in the risk for disease progression among patients with biomarker values at the 75th percentile can be expressed as $\boldsymbol{\beta}+3/4\boldsymbol{\theta}$. The average effect among patients in the upper quartile of biomarker values can also be calculated as $\boldsymbol{\beta}+(3/4+1)/2\boldsymbol{\theta}$ or $\boldsymbol{\beta}+7/8\boldsymbol{\theta}$ (see Section 6.1, [14], and Chapter 17 of this book for related discussions).

The required number of events in a one-sided test for various contrasts under H_a: $\boldsymbol{\beta}+l\boldsymbol{\theta}<a_l$ at the α level with power $1-\delta$ can be estimated by $v^2(Z_{1-\alpha}+Z_{1-\delta})^2/(\boldsymbol{\beta}+l\boldsymbol{\theta}-a_l)^2$, where v^2 is the approximate unscaled variance of the contrast estimate, l is a scalar value in [0, 1] (e.g., 3/4 or 7/8), a_l is a specified value under the alternative, and $Z_{1-\alpha}$ and $Z_{1-\delta}$ are quantiles of the standard normal distribution. If the biomarker is not prognostic, contrast variances will be smaller than when the biomarker is prognostic and randomization can be exploited to provide more efficiency by randomizing

more than 50% of patients to the treatment arm due to variance asymmetry in the randomization ratio, $\boldsymbol{\pi}$. For example, when the biomarker is continuous, $v2 = [(4-3\boldsymbol{\pi})/(1-\boldsymbol{\pi})+12(l2-l)]/\boldsymbol{\pi}$ (see [14] for more details). If we wish to size a phase II study targeting the upper quartile where $a_l = 0.80$, and desire to achieve 80% power for an average effect of log(0.40) in this group, approximately 95 progression events would be required with a 0.10 type I error rate under 2:1 randomization versus 100 under 1:1 randomization. In addition, the interaction term estimate (which is the typical parameter of interest in discussions regarding predictive biomarkers) will have larger variance than all estimated contrasts of the form $\boldsymbol{\beta}+l\boldsymbol{\theta}$ where $0<l<1$.

Mackey and Bengtsson [14] also advocate the mapping of continuous biomarkers to uniform [0, 1] as a standard across biomarker studies to allow for intuitive interpretability, and allow *apples to apples* comparability of treatment effects across studies. Further, threshold estimation can be approached by anchoring to a clinically relevant treatment effect, as suggested by regulators [15]. However, Mackey and Bengtsson [14] illustrate the significant (sample size) challenges of threshold estimation prior to phase III. Considering the previous example, if log(0.80) is specified as the smallest effect considered clinically meaningful, a 95% confidence interval for the *target effect threshold* (i.e., the biomarker value producing $\log(HR)=0.8$)) illuminates this difficulty with extremely wide confidence bounds (c.f., Section 5.1, [14]). Factors contributing to such wide intervals include: the magnitude of $\boldsymbol{\theta}$, the sample size, and/or linearity of the log risk as a function of the biomarker. Unless biomarker effects are pronounced, or strongly nonlinear, typically sized phase II studies will be inadequate for *target effect threshold* estimation. While, significant linear effects are sometimes seen in phase II as exemplified in [16,17], both cases involve a large positive intercept (i.e., low biomarker patients are harmed by treatment) and a large negative slope (i.e., high biomarker patients benefit). A biomarker producing a linear effect becomes less useful, however, when the intercept is positive due to its inability to discriminate into clinically useful biomarker-positive and biomarker-negative subgroups. This fact highlights the need for biomarkers, or biomarker signatures, that sharply discriminate subgroups (e.g., logistic or step function).

An alternative to threshold estimation via anchoring to a target effect is due to [18] whose approach consists of likelihood ratio maximization under a step function relationship between the biomarker and the log hazard ratio. This method does not require the specification of a functional form for the biomarker effect as described earlier; however, likelihood maximization is performed under a step function relationship between the biomarker and log hazard. While it has been shown that this approach yields a consistent estimate of the threshold when the true f is a step function [19], the operating characteristics of this procedure with respect to a threshold estimand have not been reported when f is not a step function. For example, a *natural* threshold does not exist when f is linear and it is not apparent what the threshold estimand will be under this procedure.

2.3 Brief Phase III Considerations

As discussed in the previous section, POC study needs to enable key decisions with regard to the phase III design (see Figure 2.1). In some instances, the target population as defined by the diagnostic will be clear based on the analyses of the prior clinical data. However, in other cases, enough ambiguity will remain to require the use of pivotal trial to further refine diagnostic hypothesis and thus to define target population. Recently, a draft FDA guidance for industry on enrichment strategies for clinical trials [9] has been released, addressing for the first time the questions with regard to suitability of using a pivotal trial for both exploratory and confirmatory purposes. Potential approaches include reserving type I error for testing the genomic subset (e.g., refining the proposed biomarker cutoff or finding a new biomarker subgroup entirely) to be identified based on the initial proportion of the enrolled patients, or, alternatively, on randomly sampled subset upon enrolment completion [20,21] (see Chapter 16 of this book for the discussion of adaptive signature designs). Such late emergence of the diagnostic subset would make current contemporaneous paradigm of drug/Dx codevelopment (see Figure 2.2) difficult and will likely require further adaptations to the current regulatory recommendations. Additional key points in the new draft guidance [9] with respect to predictive diagnostics include confirmation by the FDA that the decisions to conduct a pivotal trial in diagnostically restricted (enriched) population are a sponsor's decision and that prospective stratification on the biomarker is not always possible and, in general, not essential (see [22] for statistical justification).

2.4 Performing Exploratory Analyses

This section focuses on statistical considerations for exploratory analysis of a potentially large number of candidate biomarkers using clinical trial data. Likely applications include, but are not limited to, evaluation of phase II data to support phase III planning, and hypothesis generation on mechanism of action from phase III data to aid the development of new molecules. We describe the main analytic issues teams should address in such settings and make general recommendations following established good statistical practices as a sensible starting point. *Exploratory* should never be equated with *unplanned*, and the key requirements of exploratory and primary/secondary PHC analyses are similar (see Table 2.3).

TABLE 2.3
PHC Checklist

	Key Requirements Are Similar between Primary/Secondary and Exploratory Analyses			
	Primary/Secondary PHC Analyses		Exploratory PHC Analyses	
	Required?	**Main Risk if Not Available**	**Required?**	**Main Risk if Not Available**
PHC subset clinical efficacy requirements	Yes	Misalignment of PHC and clinical strategy	Can be helpful	Result interpretation, stopping rule
Assay readiness	Yes	Reproducibility, regulatory	Yes	Reproducibility, interpretation of assay outputs
Biomarker analysis plan	Yes	Regulatory, appropriate data collection	Scope and priority	Misalignment within team, uncontrolled scope, results, interpretation, and stopping rule
Type I error control/ multiplicity	Yes, usually requires adequate type I error control	Regulatory	Yes, usually in the form of multiplicity	Inability to judge strength of hypotheses
Cutoff selection	Yes	Regulatory, commercial, labeling	Can be helpful	Planning for future testing/samples/datasets
Validation strategy	Yes	Suboptimal phase III design	Good to have	Planning, data collection, stopping rules
Good statistical practice	Yes	Reproducibility, regulatory, lack of appeal to regulatory and investigators	Yes	Reproducibility, lack of scientific planning

2.4.1 Planning, Documentation, and Communications

Given the complexity and potentially open-ended nature of exploratory predictive biomarker analyses, it is crucial to devise a biomarker analysis plan at the project initiation in order to align key stakeholders on the scope and prioritization of analyses. Doing so will aid resource planning and help prevent low value-added data-mining traps. Key elements of a biomarker analysis plan include the analysis objectives, ranked priorities of analysis, statistical methods, definition of key variables, and description of outputs. Additional topics that may enhance the clarity of the project include: study background, rationales of the biomarker analysis, and data specification.

In addition, documentation and version control of programming code and all data manipulation steps are indispensible to ensuring reproducibility of findings [23]. This issue is further underscored by a recent episode where three clinical trials that implemented genomic signatures to choose patients' cancer therapies were suspended after independent reanalyses failed to reproduce published results and severe errors were identified [24,25]. Tools such as *Sweave* can be used to create and update dynamic analysis reports in LaTeX with embedded *R* code [26], or *CVS* [27] may be used for keeping track of all changes to a set of files.

During and following the analysis, statisticians are encouraged to communicate issues and analysis results with the biomarker/clinical scientists to ensure proper interpretation in the right context, and highlight caveats of analysis, such as potential bias of biomarker datasets from convenience samples.

2.4.2 Data Generation

Each assay technology has different issues that require attention. To be able to assess the impact of assay-specific issues on the interpretation of biomarker analysis in relation to clinical outcomes, statisticians should proactively work with the biomarker scientist, and acquire a basic understanding of the science, sample collection and handling, data processing, performance characteristics, and limitations of the specific biomarker assays relevant to their study.

2.4.3 Fit-for-Purpose Statistical Analysis and Criteria

The statistical analysis plan and biomarker selection criteria should always be guided by project objectives and clinical significance of the development program, and should be prospectively specified as much as possible. It is also important to characterize the prognostic versus predictive effect of a biomarker with respect to the study design and key assumptions, and perform additional analysis that adjusts for known prognostic factors. When devising criteria to select candidates for further evaluation from a large number of biomarkers, effect-size-based criteria should also be considered in addition to statistical significance filters to reflect clinical significance.

2.4.4 Assessing and Interpreting Statistical Evidence

One distinct feature of many exploratory biomarker analyses is the large number of biomarker hypotheses tested simultaneously. As a result, it is imperative and often nontrivial to assess the statistical strength of findings in aggregate over all biomarkers under investigation to either control for, or estimate, the overall error rate. False discovery rates (FDRs) are often useful in these settings in addition to generalization of p-values. For a comprehensive review of this topic, see Chapter 13 of this book, and also [28]. One should clearly specify the type and interpretation of overall error rate under consideration, as well as the method and assumptions used for calculation. Choice of methods should be guided by project objectives and follow-up plans. Permutation tests can be very useful to provide a more realistic estimate of the FDR especially when complex statistical criteria are applied. In addition, approaches to reduce the burden of multiple testing by limiting number of candidate markers (e.g., including only markers on certain disease pathways) could also help.

2.4.5 Cutoff Selection for Continuous Biomarkers

Most biomarkers are measured quantitatively and yield continuous scores. However, it is often necessary to dichotomize, or categorize, a continuous predictive biomarker to facilitate treatment decisions. This area is underdeveloped, with sparse literature and examples. In principle, if a cutoff is required for the development, the distribution of a biomarker and the relationship between outcomes and cutoffs should be described to inform a choice of cutoff that is guided by study objectives, overall risk–benefit assessment as described in project objectives, and underlying biology of a biomarker. The goal of cutoff selection should be clearly defined by the team in order to determine the most appropriate measures to describe in relation to varying cutoffs. In general, the cutoff selection should be viewed as a subjective/strategic decision, instead of an analytical question with a correct answer (see Section 2.2.3.2.2).

If natural cutoffs with biological justification are not available, common practices are to take data-dependent approaches, including the use of data-dependent percentiles as splits (e.g., median split; top quartile versus bottom quartile), or optimization strategy by searching for a cutoff that optimizes an objective function (e.g., treatment effect differences between the two subsets as delimited by given cutoffs). Note that these methods will likely yield different results with dataset updates. The optimization approach for cutoff selection can also be viewed as a special case of complex predictor development, and hence, methods and issues for development of complex predictors may also apply (e.g., CV).

2.4.6 Developing a Complex Predictor

Biology is fundamentally complicated, and it is rare to attribute treatment efficacy to a single factor, leading to hopes that better predictive performance may be achieved by combining information in a complex predictor. To date, there are no examples of complex predictor-based companion diagnostics that have been approved by health authorities. However, there are FDA-cleared tests for breast cancer prognosis of tumor recurrence, such as Oncotype Dx (based on 21-gene RT-PCR panel; [29]) and MammaPrint (a 70-gene array; [30–32]). Both assays have been tested using multiple independent clinical datasets.

The development of a complex predictor usually involves many steps with sometimes hidden decisions and optimization, including feature selection, model building, and performance evaluation. Numerous methods and options are available in the statistical and machine learning literature [33]. Choices of options in the process such as distance metrics for similarity, restriction on model complexity, and metrics of predictor performance should be guided by project objectives and nature of datasets. Some issues are discussed in Chapters 12, 14, and 15 of this book.

When team is interested in pursuing a complex predictor, statisticians should help the team set realistic expectation given the sample size, data quality, and potential impact. High variance and overfitting are often a major concern in this setting, and one should consider simple, highly regularized approaches [34] and the *less fitting is better* principle. Ideally, predictor performance should be assessed by independent datasets, if available, and by CV or bootstrapping as internal validation. One should be conscious about all selection, optimization, and potentially hidden decisions made during the complex predictor development process to ensure subsequent performance evaluation is not unknowingly biased due to untested selections. See references [34,35] for additional discussion.

2.4.7 Validation Strategy

In principle, the validation strategy for candidate biomarkers and complex predictors derived from exploratory analyses should be carefully prespecified in the project clinical development plan and proactively communicated to the stakeholders. The ultimate goal is to validate them in independent clinical studies designed to test the biomarker/predictor hypothesis. However, in most cases, clinical datasets are sparse and important decisions often need to be made in the absence of additional information. One can make the best use of the existing datasets to estimate prediction performance by using methods such as CV [36–39]. A common and serious mistake when applying

CV methods is failing to include all tuning/selection/optimization steps of predictor training inside the CV loop. Such a failure results in biased (and optimistic) estimates of prediction errors [40]. Chapters 12, 14, and 15 of this book contain additional discussion on this topic.

At the molecule program level, the team should also consider different resource allocation strategies to increase overall development success rate (e.g., one bigger biomarker study with more power for discovery versus two small studies, one for discovery and the other for independent validation).

2.5 Summary

The role of an industry clinical biostatistician requires increasing levels of awareness of complexities surrounding drug development in today's world. In this chapter, we have outlined a number of challenges and considerations relevant to concurrent evaluation of drug and diagnostic hypotheses. These challenges go far beyond statistical issues and include strategic, scientific, regulatory, and operational considerations. We hope that this high-level overview will be of use to any biostatistician embarking on drug development projects where diagnostic hypothesis is considered.

References

1. Herper M. The truly staggering cost of inventing new drugs. *Forbes*, 2012; 189(4):38–39.
2. FDA. *Innovation or Stagnation: Challenge and Opportunity on the Critical Path to New Medical Products*. FDA website, Washington, DC, 2004.
3. Oldenhuis CN, Oosting SF, Gietema JA et al. Prognostic vs predictive value of biomarkers in oncology. *European Journal of Cancer*, 2008; 44:946–953.
4. Atkinson AJ, Colburn WA, DeGruttola VG et al. Biomarkers and surrogate endpoints: Preferred definitions and conceptual framework. *Clinical Pharmacology Therapy*, 2001; 69:89–95.
5. Kleinbaum DG, Sullivan KM, and Barker ND. *A Pocket Guide to Epidemiology*. Springer, New York, 2007.
6. NIH consensus conference. Treatment of early-stage breast cancer. *Journal of the American Medical Association*, 1991; 265(3):391–395.
7. Buyse M, Loi S, van't Veer L et al. Validation and clinical utility of a 70-gene prognostic signature for women with node-negative breast cancer. *Journal of the National Cancer Institute*, 2006; 98(17):1183–1192.
8. Kaiser L, Becker C, Kukreti S, and Fine BM. Decision making for a companion diagnostic in an oncology clinical development program. *Drug Information Journal*, 2011; 45(5):645–655.

9. FDA. Draft guidance for industry: Enrichment strategies for clinical trials to support approval of human drugs and biological products. http://www.fda.gov/downloads/Drugs/GuidanceComplianceRegulatoryInformation/Guidances/UCM332181.pdf, 2012.
10. Woodcock J. Assessing the clinical utility of diagnostic used in drug therapy. *Clinical Pharmacology and Therapeutics*, 2010; 88(6):765–773.
11. FDA. Draft guidance for industry and FDA staff: In vitro companion diagnostics devices. http://www.fda.gov/downloads/MedicalDevices/DeviceRegulationandGuidance/GuidanceDocuments/UCM262327.pdf, 2011.
12. Schoenfeld DA. Sample-size formula for the proportional-hazards regression model. *Biometrics*, 1983; 39:499–503.
13. O'Neil, R. Some considerations for statistical design, analysis and interpretation for biomarker classifier based clinical trials in establishing efficacy in support of regulatory, marketing and promotional claims. http://www.fda.gov/ohrms/dockets/ac/08/slides/2008-4409s1-03-FDA-O'Neill.pdf, 2008.
14. Mackey H and Bengtsson T. Sample size and threshold estimation for clinical trials with predictive biomarkers. *Contemporary Clinical Trials*, 2013; 36:664–672.
15. FDA. Guidance for industry and review staff: Target product profile—A strategic development process tool. http://www.fda.gov/downloads/Drugs/GuidanceComplianceRegulatoryInformation/Guidances/ucm080593.pdf, 2007.
16. Spigel DR, Ervin TJ, Ramlau RA et al. Randomized phase II trial of onartuzumab in combination with erlotinib in patients with advanced non–small-cell lung cancer. *Journal of Clinical Oncology*, 2013; 31(32):4105–4114.
17. Makhija S, Amler LC, Glenn D et al. Clinical activity of gemcitabine plus Pertuzumab in platinum-resistant ovarian cancer, fallopian tube cancer, or primary peritoneal cancer. *Journal of Clinical Oncology*, 2010; 28(7):1215–1223.
18. Jiang W, Freidlin B, and Simon R. Biomarker-adaptive threshold design: A procedure for evaluating treatment with possible biomarker-defined subset effect. *Journal of the National Cancer Institute*, 2007; 99(13):1036–1043.
19. Pons O. Estimation in cox-regression model with a change-point according to a threshold in a covariate. *The Annals of Statistics*, 2003; 31(2):442–463.
20. Freidlin B and Simon R. Adaptive signature design: An adaptive clinical trial design for generating and prospectively testing a gene expression signature for sensitive patients. *Clinical Cancer Research*, 2005; 11:7872–7878.
21. Freidlin B, Jiang W, and Simon R. The cross-validated adaptive signature design. *Clinical Cancer Research*, 2010; 16:691–698.
22. Kaiser LD. Stratification of randomization is not required for a pre-specified subgroup analysis. *Pharmaceutical Statistics*, January–February 2013; 12(1):43–47.
23. Dupuy A and Simon RM. Critical review of published microarray studies for cancer outcome and guidelines on statistical analysis and reporting. *Journal of the National Cancer Institute*, January 17, 2007; 99(2):147–157.
24. Baggerly KA and Coombes KR. Deriving chemosensitivity from cell lines: Forensic bioinformatics and reproducible research in high-throughput biology. *Annals of Applied Statistics*, 2009; 3:1309–1334.
25. *The Cancer Letter*, October 2, 9, and 23, 2009, January 29, May 14, July 16, 23, 30, 2010.

26. Leisch F. Sweave: Dynamic generation of statistical reports using literate data analysis. In Härdle W and Rönz B., eds., *Compstat 2002—Proceedings in Computational Statistics*, Physica Verlag, Heidelberg, Germany, 2002, pp. 575–580.
27. CVS: http://www.nongnu.org/cvs/.
28. Dudoit S, Shaffer JP, and Boldrick JC. Multiple hypothesis testing in microarray experiments. *Statistical Science*, 2003; 18(1):71–103.
29. Paik S, Shak S, Tang G et al. A multigene assay to predict recurrence of tamoxifen-treated, node-negative breast cancer. *The New England Journal of Medicine*, 2004; 351:2817–2826.
30. Van de Vijver MJ, He YD, van't Veer LJ et al. A gene-expression signature as a predictor of survival in breast cancer. *The New England Journal of Medicine*, 2002; 347(25):1999–2009.
31. Glas AM, Floore A, Delahaye LJMJ et al. Converting a breast cancer microarray signature into a high-throughput diagnostic test. *BMC Genomics*, 2006; 7:278.
32. FDA CDRH. Class II special controls guidance document: Gene expression profiling test system for breast cancer prognosis. http://www.fda.gov/MedicalDevices/DeviceRegulationandGuidance/GuidanceDocuments/ucm079163.htm, 2007.
33. Hastie T, Tibshirani R, and Friedman J. *The Elements of Statistical Learning*. Springer, Dordrecht, the Netherlands, 2009.
34. Simon R. Roadmap for developing and validating therapeutically relevant genomic classifiers. *Journal of Clinical Oncology*, 2005; 23:7332–7341.
35. Subramanian J and Simon R. Gene expression-based prognostic signatures in lung cancer: Ready for clinical use? *Journal of the National Cancer Institute*, April 7, 2010; 102(7):464–474.
36. Huang Y, Pepe MS, and Feng Z. Evaluating the predictiveness of a continuous marker. *Biometrics*, 2007; 63:1181–1188.
37. Pepe MS. *The Statistical Evaluation of Medical Tests for Classification and Prediction*. Oxford University Press, Oxford, U.K., 2003.
38. Gu W and Pepe M. Measures to summarize and compare the predictive capacity of markers. *The International Journal of Biostatistics*, October 1, 2009; 5(1):Article27.
39. Molinaro A, Simon R, and Pfeiffer R. Prediction error estimation: A comparison of resampling methods. *Bioinformatics*, 2005; 21:3301–3307.
40. Varma S and Simon R. Bias in error estimation when using cross-validation for model selection. *BMC Bioinformatics*, February 23, 2006; 7:91.

3

*Analytical Validation of In Vitro Diagnostic Tests**

Robert Becker, Jr.

CONTENTS

3.1 Introduction

This chapter focuses on analytical validation of in vitro diagnostic devices (IVDs), as the foundation for IVDs' clinical use. In broadest terms, analytical validation is the process through which one gains assurance that the data

* The views expressed in this chapter are those of the author and do not necessarily represent the official views or policy of the United States Food and Drug Administration.

rendered by IVDs are reliably correct. With the expectation that each specimen has a *true value* (truth) for any measured quantity (measurand), analytical validity concerns the ability of the IVD to yield that value as a test result. Notably, though the expectation of a *true value* for any measurand agrees with our intuitive ideal, that value is unknowable in a formal sense (Joint Committee for Guides in Metrology, 2008b).

Since no measurement method is perfect, attention focuses on understanding the manner and degree to which test results deviate from the truth that a perfect test would yield. Bias is one form of deviation, wherein the test results systematically differ from truth. Results also differ from truth because of measurement errors that are reflected in dispersion of results upon repeated testing. Dispersion of test results arises both from variation among measurements that are repeated with all known factors held constant (e.g., *duplicate testing*; repeatability) and from variation that is attributable to known changes in testing conditions (e.g., *interlaboratory variation*; reproducibility).

Control and minimization of these errors is useful across the continuum of basic, translational, and clinically applied science. Correct test results underlie insights for definition and understanding of disease processes and for accurate diagnosis and treatment. Poor tests can prevent beneficial insights. They can also be a distraction, as "Conclusions reached based on studies of a system in analytical flux may yield results reflective of testing artifact and whimsy rather than actual pathophysiological phenomenon of medical interest" (Mansfield et al., 2007a).

Robust analytical validation assumes additional importance in the context of continuing product development—that is, with changes ranging from modest updates in the measurement process, to incorporation of new measurands for the product, and even to validation of an entirely new device. For example, if validation of the original device relied on results from interventional trials that are impractical or unethical to duplicate using the changed or new device, then analytical performance characteristics of the latter assume increased importance in evaluating safety and effectiveness of that device.

Numerous publications treat the analytical validation of IVDs, whether in a general sense (Westgard and Darcy, 2004) or in a more applied manner (Linnet and Boyd, 2006). Analytical validation specifically in the context of pharmacogenetic and pharmacogenomic testing has also received attention (Mansfield et al., 2007a,b). The treatment given in this chapter introduces the kinds of studies that are necessary for analytical validation of any IVD and notes special considerations for multianalyte tests that are of high interest for predictive medicine. At the same time, attention is focused on the critical link (Westgard and Darcy, 2004) between analytical validation and issues arising from the clinical use of IVDs for predictive medicine.

3.2 Prerequisites for Analytical Validation

Before undertaking analytical validation of a test, several important issues should be settled. To begin, there should be unambiguous identification of the measurand and of the units or kind of result that the test reports. Though international units (système international, SI) are defined for many analytes, provisional or arbitrary units are used for many others. Some tests combine intermediate results for multiple measurands to yield the reported result. For many tests, intermediate numerical data are reduced to qualitative (e.g., positive or negative) test results. The design of suitable analytical validation studies greatly depends upon these test features.

Analytical validation also requires a sufficiently detailed specification of the test's components: instruments and nondisposable equipment, reagents/disposable supplies, software and the method by which they are used to generate test results. Together with the identified measurand, these elements define the test that is the object of an analytical validation effort.

Understanding the clinical context for the test's use is the final prerequisite to satisfy before undertaking analytical validation of the test. Analytical validation demonstrates the test's analytical performance characteristics,* but those characteristics have meaning only insofar as they relate to the clinical implications of *right* and *wrong* test results. In other words, an assurance that the test results are *reliably correct* is made with reference to the test's intended use.

Attention to the test's intended use does not mean that a new technology (or platform supporting it) must be initially validated for all possible intended uses. For many new technologies, the range of intended uses increases with time. Analytical validation for one intended use can lead to rapid adoption of the platform for a host of uses that have similar analytical requirements. As with a recently developed DNA sequencing platform, an initial analytical validation might be sufficient to support a wide range of intended uses (U.S. Food and Drug Administration, 2013; Bijwaard et al., 2014). Still, consideration of the platform's analytical validity remains appropriate as more specific intended uses are brought forward. Data from the initial analytical validation can greatly assist such consideration.

* An apt definition of "performance characteristics" is in the Code of Federal Regulations (CFR) for the Clinical Laboratory Improvement Amendments of 1988, at 42CFR493.2: "Performance characteristic means a property of a test that is used to describe its quality, e.g., accuracy, precision, analytical sensitivity, analytical specificity, reportable range, reference range, etc." Though the properties cited in the definition are analytical performance characteristics, the term is often used with regard to clinical performance. The two meanings are distinguished by the appropriate adjective or (less reliably) by the usage context.

3.3 Analytical/Clinical Interface

Given that an analyte has medical relevance, adequate quality in its detection or measurement is essential for achieving the clinical results that are expected from using the test in medical practice. In ascertaining quality, selection of the right performance characteristics to examine (along with their acceptance criteria) is a key to assurance that the test is adequate for its intended use. This selection depends partly on the test's design and partly on the clinical issues that attend the test's use. For example, a qualitative test that drives a medical decision based simply on detection of an analyte requires a different approach to analytical validation than does a quantitative test for which various levels of the measurand carry distinct clinical implications. As another example, a measurand with clinical importance related to a narrow range of analyte levels (e.g., for a drug with a *narrow therapeutic window*) requires special attention to performance characteristics across that measurement range.

Development of an adequate and efficient analytical validation plan often rests greatly on the test developer's prior experience and good judgment. This is especially true for *first-of-a-kind* tests. Agreement on best practices for analytical validation is greatest when there is extensive biological insight and clinical experience relating an analyte to beneficial medical decisions. Such is the case, for example, with analytical validation of tests that measure serum electrolytes or blood glucose. However, with cancer, the linkage between test results and clinical results often is less well understood. Though collections of performance characteristics are routinely identified for study, results from their examination often are more *descriptive* than *prescriptive*. Compare, for example, a general treatment of analytical performance characteristics for tumor-associated antigens (U.S. Food and Drug Administration, 1997) with the prescriptive set of analytical specifications for tests used to monitor blood glucose (U.S. Food and Drug Administration, 2014a). There is much work yet to be done in settling on best practices for analytical validation of many cancer-related tests.

A prevalent approach to analytical validation is simply to focus on performance characteristics and acceptance criteria matching those that have previously served well for validation of analytically similar IVDs. This *state-of-the-art* approach (Westgard, 1999) is often taken for tests based on technologies that are already well established for medical use. Two drawbacks are that it does not account for analytical challenges that are peculiar to the new test and it ignores the clinical implications of those challenges. Consider, for example, testing for prostate-specific antigen (PSA) in serum. New kinds of analytical validation studies (i.e., for equimolarity) became necessary when tests distinguishing free PSA from complexed PSA were brought forward as an aid in distinguishing between prostate cancer and benign prostatic disease. More stringent acceptance criteria (e.g., for the limit of detection and limit of quantitation) were necessary for measurement of PSA as a prognostic marker after prostatectomy. Clearly, the pursuit of new intended uses has implications for analytical validation, whether the measurand is novel or one that is repurposed.

A robust approach to analytical validation is one that explicitly takes account of the anticipated clinical effect of test results, especially when setting the acceptance criteria for performance characteristics (e.g., ahead of a pivotal clinical study for a drug and a companion diagnostic device). Though increasing attention is being paid (Model, 2012), this approach is often challenging—most importantly because some knowledge of the measurand's clinical significance (e.g., for therapeutic effect) is first needed in order to estimate the allowable bias and imprecision for the test. Data that can provide this knowledge, for example, from early-phase therapeutic product trials (including substantial numbers of marker-positive and marker-negative subjects), are often not obtained.* Other approaches to estimating the biomarker's clinical significance, for example, based on preclinical data, have unproven value. Nevertheless, some proposed approaches to codevelopment of therapeutic products and IVDs for cancer hold hope for analytical validation that is clinically informed (Freidlin and Simon, 2005; Beckman et al., 2011).

3.4 Analytical Validation of Tests Based on Novel Biomarkers and Measurement Technologies

For some novel IVDs, the practicality of traditional approaches to analytical validation is stretched to its limit. One reason is the growing trend in the use of cutting edge technologies to search for pathophysiological variations in patients' (or tumors') DNA. A result is that the biomarker consists of an open-ended set of mutations that is empirically defined (e.g., according to the prevalence of particular mutations among the genetic loci that draw investigators' attention). The roles of particular mutations might be less important than is their effect as a (perhaps interacting) group. These features have implications for how analytical validation can be accomplished.

Activating mutation in gene XXX as an analyte of interest is an instructive example. Along with a functional definition of the analyte comes the possibility that multiple mutations qualify as *activating*. Early test development efforts might focus on a small set of well-defined mutations (as happened for single nucleotide sequence variants (SNVs) in the Kirsten rat sarcoma viral oncogene homolog (KRAS) in colorectal cancer), such that in-depth

* The drawbacks of marker-selective trial designs, in terms of understanding the predictive implications of the test results, have been well described (Težak et al. 2010; Janes et al. 2011; Pennello 2013).

analytical validation for detection of each mutation is practical. For other genes (e.g., the epidermal growth factor receptor gene [EGFR]), activation might initially be attributed to a class of mutations (i.e., deletions within certain exons), encompassing a larger set of DNA sequence changes. When multiple specific mutations comprise the analyte of interest, performing the analytical validation studies on relevant subsets of those mutations might be a necessary and satisfactory practice. To draw the strongest conclusions from studies that are performed, one should select the mutation subset members according to their prevalence, biological significance, and known analytical challenges.

Other analytical validation issues arise for composite test results (e.g., quantitative scores or class assignments, derived from results for the members of a clearly specified set of measurands). When the composite result deals with only a few measurands, full-fledged analytical validation for each of them remains feasible (U.S. Food and Drug Administration, 2011b; Kondratovich, 2012). The demonstration of suitable repeatability and reproducibility for the composite result across its range of reportable values (and, especially, near a cutoff value if one applies) is highly recommended. The usual studies of repeatability (see Section 3.6.1) might be extended to include simulations of precision for the composite result, based both on known (experimental) precision results for individual measurands and on various combinations of measurand results that can lead to selected composite results. Comprehensive analytical validation reaching back to individual measurands requires much more effort when the composite test result deals with tens or hundreds of measurands. In such cases, allocation of effort for analytical validation at the measurand level might necessarily be more selective. Ultimately, decisions about analytical validity are framed in terms of performance characteristics for the composite result (McShane et al., 2013b).

Technical advances for analytical methods and platforms often help drive the recognition and clinical application of novel biomarkers. The analytical validation issues for new technology are not new in principle; however, the pace of technical development creates challenges for completing analytical validation (according to traditional approaches) on a scale and in a timeframe matching those intended for biomarker-driven drug development. To manage analytical validation in a fast-paced setting, some developers implement new tests on already validated platforms, applying extant data about the platform for validation of the new test. This approach is commonly practiced for some types of IVD products targeting specific analytes (U.S. Food and Drug Administration, 2009). Prior validation data for analytes that are similar to analyte(s) under development might also be useful. For example, an approach for analytical validation of a next-generation sequencing (NGS) platform for certain classes of analyte (i.e., germ-line SNV and indel DNA variants) has recently been used (U.S. Food and Drug Administration, 2013; Bijwaard et al., 2014).

3.5 Analytical Validation Resources

Principles and recommendations for the validation of measurements in science and industry extend to analytical validation of IVDs primarily through activities of the Clinical Laboratory Standards Institute (CLSI, formerly the National Committee on Clinical Laboratory Standards [NCCLS]) in the United States and the International Organization for Standardization (ISO) overseas. Where feasible, these efforts are based on concepts of metrology (the field of knowledge concerned with measurement [Joint Committee for Guides in Metrology, 2008a]) that are agreed upon internationally. The National Institute of Standards and Technology (NIST), the American National Standards Institute (ANSI), and the American Society for Testing and Materials (ASTM) are major governmental and private proponents of metrological principles in the United States.

Scientific, industrial, and regulatory bodies all participate in developing documents concerning best practices for analytical validation. Published *standards* typically reflect a consensus both on terminology (sometimes varying somewhat from official international definitions) and on designs and methods recommended for use in analytical validation studies. Those designs and methods often are adapted for local use (e.g., by a product's manufacturer). In addition, the published documents continually evolve, with new practices developed from time to time in order to meet changing needs.

For emerging technologies, efforts by interested bodies and stakeholders (often as consortia) can identify analytical issues that need attention, describe or provide useful test materials, and establish analytical validation practices. One example is in work reported by the *Microarray Quality Consortium* (MAQC) concerning performance characteristics of high-dimensional gene expression platforms (MAQC Consortium, 2006) and with subsequent attention to bioinformatics issues (MAQC Consortium, 2010; Slikker, 2010). MAQC work is in progress toward analytical validation of NGS platforms (U.S. Food and Drug Administration, 2011a). Recent and ongoing work from the *Genome in a Bottle Consortium* provides reference materials and datasets (*arbitrated integrated genotypes*) of substantial value for analytical validation of genomic assays (Zook et al., 2014). Associations of end users (Association for Molecular Pathology, 1999; Pont-Kingdon et al., 2012; Rehm et al., 2013) provide recommendations addressing many aspects of analytical validation for clinical DNA sequencing assays. For some specific diagnostic applications, end users and other bodies collaborate directly for standardization of test methods and materials (White et al., 2010). Finally, for specific IVDs and classes of IVDs that are cleared or approved by the *Center for Devices and Radiologic Health* in the U.S. Food and Drug Administration, nonproprietary information concerning analytical validation methods and results is published in review decision summaries (U.S. Food and Drug Administration, 2014b) and guidance documents (U.S. Food and Drug Administration, 2014c).

3.6 Practical Analytical Validation

Analytical validation involves experiments, yielding measurements and illustrations of *performance characteristics* that can be affected by systematic and nonsystematic sources of error. Some widely accepted experimental designs and practices for experiments are cited in the following text, grouped according to higher-order concepts of analytical validity.

3.6.1 Precision

Obtaining consistent results, when the test is applied under constant or controlled conditions, is a fundamental aspect of analytical validity. Multiple measurements of material from the same specimen within the same test *run* typically yield a best-case perspective on the test's imprecision (i.e., the "dispersion of independent results of measurements obtained under specified conditions" [NCCLS, 2004]). Imprecision under conditions that better match the scope of variation in day-to-day use of the test is naturally of high interest. The term *intermediate precision* is put forth in CLSI guidance (NCCLS, 2004) to describe imprecision measurements under conditions that include variation of time, calibration, operator, and equipment among the repeated measurements. Imprecision measurements under conditions that examine higher-order variates (e.g., laboratories and reagent lots) typically give the broadest view of test results' dispersion and are considered to represent the test's *reproducibility* rather than merely its *repeatability*.

Results from repeatability or reproducibility studies that start each measurement at a very early step of the testing process (e.g., cutting sections or extracting material from tissue) can be affected by biological variability of the measurand within the specimen. Studies that begin measurements at a later testing step (e.g., after extracting the analyte[s] from tissue) can give a more focused portrayal of precision, at the cost of leaving unexamined some aspects of the test's precision.

3.6.2 Interference

Biological specimens have many substances, beside the analyte(s) of interest that can affect measurements. The presence of such substances is a source of bias in test results that degrades the analytical specificity of the test. Interference studies, as part of analytical validation, aim to "evaluate interfering substances in the context of medical needs and to inform … customers of known sources of medically significant error" (CLSI, 2005a).

Well-accepted practices are described for evaluating interference in measurements from any of the commonly studied body fluids (e.g., serum, plasma, whole blood, cerebrospinal fluid, and urine). The most commonly employed study design involves adding interfering substances to samples. With this spike-in design, interfering substances selected from a large menu can be studied for their effects across wide ranges of controlled concentrations. Use of this design presumes that a suitable preparation is available for each substance and that the spike-in procedure adequately mimics the natural presence of the substance in clinical specimens.

Genomic tests often are highly multiplexed systems, containing combinations of probes; amplification reagents; and detection reagents for tens, hundreds, or more analytes in the same reaction vessel. Depending on test design, interactions among test components and analytes that limit the rate or extent of reactions can alter the results for some or all measurands. Studies should be performed to ensure that results for measurands at relatively low levels are not impaired when other measurands are at high levels (CLSI, 2008a).

Tissue, as a specimen type, presents interference testing issues beyond those encountered with body fluids. Interfering substances (e.g., melanin) that are specific to the tissue or tumor type might need consideration. Interference can depend on the distribution of the interfering substance in the specimen. For some tests, considering a gross pathophysiological change (e.g., hemorrhage or necrosis) as analogous to an *interfering substance* is sensible. Studies with that perspective can inform conclusions about preprocessing (e.g., dissecting) tissue specimens or rejecting them for analysis.

3.6.3 Recovery of Expected Values

Bias in test results can also be evaluated in terms of the response to known changes in the measurand. A common type of study involves evaluating the effect of adding known amounts of the analyte to test samples (CLSI, 2005b). The *percent recovery* is calculated by comparing the observed change to the expected change in test results, with 100% recovery indicating the absence of detectable bias. Studying recovery across a wide range of the measurand is especially useful for detecting proportional bias. In planning recovery experiments, important considerations include the selection of an appropriate sample matrix (i.e., the *components of a material system, except the analyte* [ISO, 2009a]), the availability of reference materials for the analyte(s), and the suitability of the technique for adding the reference materials to the test samples.

3.6.4 Cross-Reactions/Nonspecific Binding

Cross-reactivity is interference due to a degree of structural similarity between the analyte and the interfering substance (CLSI, 2005a). It deserves separate consideration, because it can be hard to evaluate through a spike-in approach that is applied to the complete test as described in Section 3.6.2. Techniques (e.g., Western blots) providing sharper insight about physico-chemical differences can help. Often the issue to be addressed is obvious, as with ensuring the ability of the test to distinguish clinically important SNVs. Accounting for potential cross-reaction with nucleotide sequences at different genetic loci also draws attention. Subtler cross-reactions might involve derivative forms of the analyte of interest (e.g., differing through phosphorylation or methylation) or associations between the analyte of interest and other substances (e.g., for free versus bound forms of the analyte). Knowledge of the presence and clinical significance of these analytical distinctions must be applied during the early phases of test development.

3.6.5 Linearity

It is common practice to design tests so that "there exists a mathematically verified straight-line relationship between the observed values and the true concentrations or activities of the analyte" (CLSI, 2003). One reason is that linearity aids in result interpolation (between calibrated reference levels). Another is that departure from linearity can be a sign of practical limitations in achieving the conditions that underlie the theory of the test. An example is the high dose hook effect that emerges in immunochemical assays at high analyte concentrations (ISO, 2009b). Linearity studies help in establishing the range of reportable values for the measurand. Reportable range is an important performance characteristic for any IVD.

It is perhaps worth noting that linearity is generally relevant for individual measurands, and not for composite results (i.e., results derived from multiple measurands). Algorithms that combine measurands' values typically have nonlinear features. Occasionally, test developers endeavor to establish analytical linearity for a composite result as a performance characteristic supporting clinical interpretation of the test result. Such efforts appear to be misguided.

3.6.6 Performance When Measurands' Values Are near Medical Decision Point(s)

It is a common practice to evaluate tests' performance characteristics using some samples for which the measurands' true values are near clinically important decision points. For tests that report quantitative results, these studies are naturally conducted along with (or as part of) studies that are described earlier. When medical management relies on quantitative determination of a measurand with a stated accuracy, establishing the *limit of quantitation* (CLSI, 2012) provides assurance as to the lowest level of the measurand for which that accuracy can be obtained.

For tests that render a qualitative result (e.g., *positive* or *negative*, derived by interpreting a quantitative signal in terms of a cutoff value for the measurand), it is appropriate to evaluate performance characteristics when the measurand is near the cutoff value. When a medical decision point or cutoff value concerns the presence of any detectable level of the measurand, determinations of *limit of blank* and *limit of detection* should be made according to well-established experimental designs (CLSI, 2012; Pennello, 2013).

Additional studies (CLSI, 2008b) are appropriate for tests reporting qualitative results based on a cutoff other than the limit of detection. These include a finding of measurand values (e.g., the C_{50} and the C_5–C_{95} interval) that are associated with specific distributions of qualitative results. C_{50} is "the analyte concentration near the cutoff that yields 50% positive results and 50% negative results when many replicates of a single sample at that concentration are tested." C_5–C_{95} interval is "the range of analyte concentrations around the cutoff such that observed results at concentrations *outside* this interval are consistently negative (concentrations <C5) or consistently positive (concentrations >C95)" (CLSI, 2008b). A narrow C_5–C_{95} interval is associated with superior analytical performance.

As mentioned already, analytical validation at the level of individual measurands might be abbreviated when a composite test result deals with many measurands. Even so, when a cut-point is used to interpret a composite result, robust assessment of the test's performance characteristics near the cut-point is essential for analytical validation of the test.

3.6.7 Method Comparison

While studies of the kinds already described do much to identify and quantify test systems' analytical strengths and weaknesses, a comparison of results between one test system and another at various levels of their measurand(s) is often employed as well. Ideally, one of the two tests is a reference method, in which case "the difference between the two methods measures the trueness of the new method, measured as bias" (CLSI, 2010).

Though a suitable design for conducting a method comparison study is relatively straightforward, variations on such design are commonplace, and attention must be paid to details about the specimens that are tested. Clinical specimens should be from patients who adequately represent the intended use population. Data acquisition requires duplicate determinations by both methods for a collection of at least 40 clinical samples. Commonsense and simple measures are recommended to avoid spurious correlation between the methods due to artifacts arising from the timing and order by which samples are tested. It is also important to ensure that measurands in the clinical samples used for the study span the range of clinically significant and reportable results for the two methods.

The data analysis first involves visual and computed checks to ensure that the dataset is suitable for calculations that can support conclusions about bias between the methods. The calculations that often draw greatest interest are the coefficients from linear regression (by appropriate technique) of paired results from the two methods. However, these statistics alone do not provide a complete evaluation of bias between the methods across levels of the measurand (CLSI, 2010).

Several practical issues often limit the value of method comparison studies for analytical validation of novel genomic tests. First among these typically is the absence of a reference method. For tests involving multiple measurands, there might be no test available for use as a single *comparator* method. Finally, there might be little or no understanding of the implications, from observed analytical bias, for performance of the test as a clinical predictor.

Despite these limitations, the experimental approach used for method comparison studies can be valuable for *bridging studies*. From these studies, and with outcome data from a clinical trial that includes both marker-positive and marker-negative subjects, the degree of concordance between two versions of the test (one, a version used in the clinical trial, and the other, a new version proposed for marketing) can be used to estimate the clinical effect of the therapeutic product for patients tested using the new version of the IVD (U.S. Food and Drug Administration, 2012).

3.6.8 Additional Analytical Validation Studies

Depending on the design of the test and its platform, additional studies might be needed for analytical validation. For example, if the test uses specimens from various sources (e.g., blood and plasma, or fresh and frozen tissue), then matrix comparison studies are appropriate (CLSI, 2005c). Results are needed from studies that establish instrument stability and (especially for highly automated test platforms) the extent and effect of carryover or contamination between samples (CLSI, 2006). Reagents that have time-limited stability are studied for shelf life, for consistent performance after loading onto instruments for later use, and for stability during shipment (CLSI, 2009). Studies establishing the performance of calibrator and control materials are needed for tests that rely on such materials.

3.7 Perianalytical Issues

Several aspects of testing are commonly considered along with analytical validation, though they are not formally part of it and often are beyond the control of test developers. These factors can impose limits on the extent to which rigorous analytical validation supports the clinical significance of testing. Conversely, use of analytically validated tests can shed light on factors that should be considered in applying test results for the best clinical effect.

Biological variation of measurands is one such perianalytical factor (Fraser and Hyltoft Petersen, 1993; Westgard et al., 1994; Model, 2012). Targeting cancer-related drugs and genomic tests to specific kinds (e.g., histological types) of tumors is still widely practiced and helpful partly because it can lessen biological variability that would otherwise obscure treatment effects and complicate clinical testing requirements. However, developers rarely account for other biologically relevant factors, such as whether the tumor specimen is obtained from a primary or metastatic site. Though the patient's treatment history prior to providing the specimen is often an element in candidacy for a therapy, effects of previous treatment on test results and on best use of the test are seldom considered. The minimum amount of tumor that must be tested in order to obtain repeated sampling results that are consistent (or well characterized for their heterogeneity) often receives modest attention. If therapeutic effects are shown to depend on these distinctions, then further refinements in design and success criteria for analytical validation studies might ensue.

Preanalytical factors affect the state of the specimen during its acquisition or storage and are important for many measurands. Elapsed time and the temperature experienced before and during tissue fixation sometimes attract much attention (Wolff et al., 2007), as do the methods of preservation for other specimen types (Schwochow et al., 2012). Interest also focuses on determinations of tumor content, compared to the amount of nonneoplastic tissue in specimens. For some tests, these determinations motivate preanalytical dissection and enrichment steps aimed at improving the consistency of test results and their clinical value.

3.8 Beyond the *Test Tube*

Two other areas, software and human factors, deserve mention alongside analytical validation. Modern laboratory tests that meet performance specifications rely on properly functioning software, and there are well-practiced approaches to validation and review of software in IVDs. The interesting development especially over the past decade is the extension of software's role far beyond traditional aspects of process control. Software is now an integral part of test development, including the generation, management, and application of knowledge. For many novel tests, software validation requires more than consideration of computer code in a final state. Now and in the future, software validation links at least three contexts: biomarker discovery, translation to clinical laboratory testing, and modification or evolution of the software as new knowledge is acquired. A growing recognition of this need is evident in recent publications that consider the role of software in the development and performance of genomic tests (Institute of Medicine, 2012; McShane et al., 2013a).

Human factors rarely receive more than incidental consideration for analytical validation of IVDs. A few tests carry training requirements for the performance of processes at the laboratory bench according to instructions for use or for interpretative readout of test results once the bench work is completed. With the emergence of test interpretation and treatment paradigms based on in silico knowledge engines, and as laboratorians and clinicians adapt to the new kinds of data presentation and treatment insights that novel tests will provide, one can anticipate that the importance and use of human factor assessments will increase.

3.9 Analytical Validation in the 'omics Era

It is apparent that analytical validation is a key element in any determination that a test is ready for clinical use. Well-established experimental designs and practices routinely guide new tests' analytical validation. Consideration of other closely related issues, as described earlier, helps to improve analytical expectations and performance. With more reliably correct tests, one can expect better biological insights and targeted use of treatments with greater benefit for patients.

However, analytical validation by traditional means can be an expensive process for any test and especially for 'omics tests. This is evident simply from the number of studies that need to be accomplished for a new analytical platform, or even for a new test on an already established platform. For high-dimensional tests, an emerging practice is the resort to selective validation of representative measurands, sometimes supplemented with data from contrived samples, with the expectation that performance for the entire device is acceptable. Can more robust analytical validation be retained in the 'omics era?

It seems reasonable to anticipate that the same technological advances giving rise to the current challenges for analytical validation of tests for predictive medicine will ultimately provide a pathway for adapting and extending that validation. Large test panels, for which single clinical specimens can provide data points across all the analytes, might enable the accumulation of very large sets of useful analytical data beyond the scope of a single intended use (i.e., a use involving a much smaller gene set). The structure of these datasets within and across genetic loci might enable intermediate readouts that inform about bias and imprecision while still allowing frugal use of clinical specimens. Through some modifications of experimental design and data analysis, one might reach a new set of analytical validation protocols providing high confidence about analytical performance characteristics without breaking the bank.

The imminent availability of genomic reference materials (Zook et al., 2014) is a notable step toward new analytical validation tools. Lacking immediate access to widely accepted reference *methods* for high-volume genomic testing, these reference materials provide a new and valuable resource for the evaluation of analytical performance by clinical test systems. The main thing missing is an accepted path (ranging from specimen acquisition through readout of test results) accounting for the analytical challenges posed by biological matrix. If this path can be established, then more robust analytical validation of novel and complex genomic tests supporting predictive medicine should be within reach.

References

Association for Molecular Pathology. 1999. Recommendations for in-house development and operation of molecular diagnostic tests. *Am J Clin Pathol* 111:449–463.

Beckman, R.A., Clark, J., and Chen, C. 2011. Integrating predictive biomarkers and classifiers into oncology clinical development programmes. *Nat Rev Drug Discov* 10:735–748.

Bijwaard, K., Dickey, J.S., Kelm, K., and Težak, Ž. 2014. The first FDA marketing authorizations of next-generation sequencing technology and tests: Challenges, solutions and impact for future assays. *Expert Rev Mol Diagn*. http://informahealthcare.com/eprint/7tpx7UYiE9V4H9U3ZK9V/full (on-line, ahead of print, accessed November 5, 2014).

CLSI. 2003. *Evaluation of the Linearity of Quantitative Measurement Procedures: A Statistical Approach; Approved Guideline*. NCCLS document EP6-A. Wayne, PA: Clinical and Laboratory Standards Institute.

CLSI. 2005a. *Interference Testing in Clinical Chemistry; Approved Guideline*, 2nd ed. CLSI document EP7-A2. Wayne, PA: Clinical and Laboratory Standards Institute.

CLSI. 2005b. *User Verification of Performance for Precision and Trueness; Approved Guideline*, 2nd ed. CLSI document EP15-A2. Wayne, PA: Clinical and Laboratory Standards Institute.

CLSI. 2005c. *Evaluation of Matrix Effects; Approved Guideline*, 2nd ed. CLSI document EP14-A2. Wayne, PA: Clinical and Laboratory Standards Institute.

CLSI. 2006. *Preliminary Evaluation of Quantitative Clinical Laboratory Measurement Procedures; Approved Guideline*, 3rd ed. CLSI document EP10-A3. Wayne, PA: Clinical and Laboratory Standards Institute.

CLSI. 2008a. *Verification and Validation of Multiplex Nucleic Acid Assays; Approved Guideline*. CLSI document MM17-A. Wayne, PA: Clinical and Laboratory Standards Institute.

CLSI. 2008b. *User Protocol for Evaluation of Qualitative Test Performance; Approved Guideline*, 2nd ed. CLSI document EP12-A2. Wayne, PA: Clinical and Laboratory Standards Institute.

CLSI. 2009. *Evaluation of Stability of In Vitro Diagnostic Reagents; Approved Guideline.* CLSI document EP25-A. Wayne, PA: Clinical and Laboratory Standards Institute.

CLSI. 2010. *Method Comparison and Bias Estimation Using Patient Samples; Approved Guideline*, 2nd ed. (Interim Revision). CLSI document EP09-A2-IR. Wayne, PA: Clinical and Laboratory Standards Institute.

CLSI. 2012. *Evaluation of Detection Capability for Clinical Laboratory Measurement Procedures; Approved Guideline*, 2nd ed. CLSI document EP17-A2. Wayne, PA: Clinical and Laboratory Standards Institute.

Fraser, C.G. and Hyltoft Petersen, P. 1993. Desirable standards for laboratory tests if they are to fulfill medical needs. *Clin Chem* 39:1447–1455.

Freidlin, B. and Simon, R. 2005. Adaptive signature design: An adaptive clinical trial design for generating and prospectively testing a gene expression signature for sensitive patients. *Clin Cancer Res* 11:7872–7878.

Institute of Medicine. 2012. *Evolution of Translational Omics: Lessons Learned and the Path Forward*, C.M. Micheel, S. Nass, and G.S. Omenn, eds. Washington, DC: The National Academies Press.

ISO IS 15193. 2009a. In vitro diagnostic medical devices—Measurement of quantities in samples of biological origin—Requirements for content and presentation of reference measurement procedures.

ISO IS 18113-1. 2009b. In vitro diagnostic medical devices—Information supplied by the manufacturer (labelling)—Part 1: Terms, definitions and general requirements.

Janes, H., Pepe, M.S., Bossuyt, P.M., and Barlow, W.E. 2011. Measuring the performance of markers for guiding treatment decisions. *Ann Intern Med* 154:253–259.

Joint Committee for Guides in Metrology. 2008a. *International Vocabulary of Metrology—Basic and General Concepts and Associated Terms (VIM)*, 3rd ed. http://www.iso.org/sites/JCGM/VIM/JCGM_200e.html (accessed November 5, 2014).

Joint Committee for Guides in Metrology. 2008b. Evaluation of measurement data—Guide to the expression of uncertainty in measurement. Annex D.—"True" value, error and uncertainty. http://www.iso.org/sites/JCGM/GUM/JCGM100/C045315e-html/C045315e.html?csnumber=50461 (accessed November 5, 2014).

Kondratovich, M.V. 2012. Precision of IVDMIA (In vitro diagnostic multivariate index assay) with individual analytes. http://edrn.nci.nih.gov/docs/nci-fda-nist-workshop-on-standards-in-molecular-diagnostics/Marina%20Kondratovich.pdf (accessed January 10, 2014).

Linnet, K. and Boyd, J.C. 2006. Selection and analytical evaluation of methods—With statistical techniques. In: *Tietz Textbook of Clinical Chemistry and Molecular Diagnostics*, C.A. Burtis, E.R. Ashwood, and D.E. Bruns eds., pp. 353–407. St. Louis, MO: Elsevier Saunders.

Mansfield, E., Tezak, Z., Altaie, S., Simon, K., and Gutman, S. 2007a. Biomarkers for pharmacogenetic and pharmacogenomic studies: Locking down analytical performance. *Drug Discov Today Technol* 4:17–20.

Mansfield, E., Tezak, Z., Altaie, S., Simon, K., and Gutman, S. 2007b. Biomarkers for pharmacogenetic and pharmacogenomic studies: Special issues in analytical performance. *Drug Discov Today Technol* 4:21–24.

MAQC Consortium. 2006. The MicroArray Quality Control (MAQC) project shows inter- and intraplatform reproducibility of gene expression measurements. *Nat Biotechnol* 24:1151–1161.

MAQC Consortium. 2010. The MicroArray Quality Control (MAQC)-II study of common practices for the development and validation of microarray-based predictive models. *Nat Biotechnol* 28:827–838.

McShane, L.M., Cavenaugh, M.M., Lively, T.G. et al. 2013a. Criteria for the use of omics-based predictors in clinical trials. *Nature* 502:317–320.

McShane, L.M., Cavenaugh, M.M., Lively, T.G. et al. 2013b. Criteria for the use of omics-based predictors in clinical trials: Explanation and elaboration. *BMC Med* 11:220–241.

Model, F. 2012. Developing companion in vitro diagnostic tests. http://www.psiweb.org/docs/model_developingcdxivd_final.pdf (accessed March 21, 2013).

NCCLS. 2004. *Evaluation of Precision Performance of Quantitative Measurement Methods; Approved Guideline*, 2nd ed. NCCLS document EP5-A2. Wayne, PA: Clinical and Laboratory Standards Institute.

Pennello, G.A. 2013. Analytical and clinical evaluation of biomarkers assays: When are biomarkers ready for prime time? *Clin Trials* 10:666–676.

Pont-Kingdon, T., Gedge F., Wooderchak-Donahue, W. et al. 2012. Design and validation of clinical DNA sequencing assays. *Arch Pathol Lab Med* 136:41–46.

Rehm, H.L., Bale, S.J., Bayrak-Toydemir, P. et al. 2013. ACMG clinical laboratory standards for next-generation sequencing. *Genet Med* 15:733–747.

Schwochow, D., Serieys, L.E.K., Wayne, R.K., and Thalmann, O. 2012. Efficient recovery of whole blood RNA—A comparison of commercial RNA extraction protocols for high-throughput applications in wildlife species. *BMC Biotechnol* 12:33–44.

Slikker, W. 2010. Of genomics and bioinformatics. *Pharmacogenomics J* 10:245–246.

Težak, Ž., Kondratovich, M.V., and Mansfield, E. 2010. US FDA and personalized medicine: In vitro diagnostic regulatory perspective. *Per Med* 7:517–530.

U.S. Food and Drug Administration. 1997. Guidance document for the submission of tumor associated antigen premarket notifications, [510(k)], to FDA. http://www.fda.gov/downloads/MedicalDevices/DeviceRegulationandGuidance/GuidanceDocuments/ucm094124.pdf (accessed November 5, 2014).

U.S. Food and Drug Administration. 2009. Master files. Introduction to master files for devices (MAFs). http://www.fda.gov/MedicalDevices/DeviceRegulationandGuidance/HowtoMarketYourDevice/PremarketSubmissions/PremarketApprovalPMA/ucm142714.htm (accessed November 5, 2014).

U.S. Food and Drug Administration. 2011a. MicroArray Quality Control (MAQC). http://www.fda.gov/ScienceResearch/BioinformaticsTools/MicroarrayQualityControlProject/ (accessed November 5, 2014).

U.S. Food and Drug Administration. 2011b. Class II special controls guidance document: Ovarian adnexal mass assessment score test system. http://www.fda.gov/MedicalDevices/DeviceRegulationandGuidance/GuidanceDocuments/ucm237299.htm (accessed November 5, 2014).

U.S. Food and Drug Administration. 2012. Summary of safety and effectiveness. *therascreen*® KRAS RGQ PCR Kit. http://www.accessdata.fda.gov/cdrh_docs/pdf11/P110030b.pdf (accessed November 5, 2014).

U.S. Food and Drug Administration. 2013. Evaluation of automatic class III designation for MiSeqDx Platform. http://www.accessdata.fda.gov/cdrh_docs/reviews/K123989.pdf (accessed November 5, 2014).

U.S. Food and Drug Administration. 2014a. Blood glucose monitoring test systems for prescription point-of-care use. http://www.fda.gov/downloads/MedicalDevices/DeviceRegulationandGuidance/GuidanceDocuments/UCM380325.pdf (accessed November 5, 2014).

U.S. Food and Drug Administration. 2014b. 510(k) Premarket approval (PMA). http://www.accessdata.fda.gov/scripts/cdrh/cfdocs/cfPMA/pma.cfm?IVDProducts=on (accessed November 5, 2014).

U.S. Food and Drug Administration. 2014c. Medical devices. OIR guidance. http://www.fda.gov/MedicalDevices/DeviceRegulationandGuidance/GuidanceDocuments/ucm070274.htm (accessed November 5, 2014).

Westgard, J.O. 1999. The need for a system of quality standards for modern quality management. *Scand J Clin Lab Invest* 59:483–486.

Westgard, J.O. and Darcy, T. 2004. The truth about quality: Medical usefulness and analytical reliability of laboratory tests. *Clin Chim Acta* 346:3–11.

Westgard, J.O., Seehafer, J.J., and Barry, P.L. 1994. Allowable imprecision for laboratory tests based on clinical and analytical test outcome criteria. *Clin Chem* 40:1909–1914.

White, H.E., Matejtschuk, P., Rigsby, P. et al. 2010. Establishment of the first World Health Organization International Genetic Reference Panel for quantitation of *BCR-ABL* mRNA. *Blood* 116:e111–e117.

Wolff, A.C., Hammond, M.E.H., Schwartz, J.N. et al. 2007. American Society of Clinical Oncology/College of American Pathologists Guideline Recommendations for human epidermal growth factor receptor 2 testing in breast cancer. *Arch Pathol Lab Med* 131:18–43.

Zook, J.M., Chapman, B., Wang, J. et al. 2014. Integrating human sequence data sets provides a resource of benchmark SNP and indel genotype calls. *Nat Biotechnol* 32:246–251.

Section II

Early Clinical Trials Using Biomarkers

4

Phase I Dose-Finding Designs and Their Applicability to Targeted Therapies

Takashi Daimon, Akihiro Hirakawa, and Shigeyuki Matsui

CONTENTS

4.1 Introduction

Phase I clinical trials play an important role as a translational bridge between preclinical trials and subsequent phase II and III trials in the development of therapeutics. For serious or life-threatening diseases such as cancer or AIDS, the early-phase clinical trials in these areas may involve first-in-man trials like for other diseases, but with patients who have advanced conditions or in whom an experimental treatment may be the last hope for survival, rather than healthy volunteers.

In oncology phase I trials, the safety of a new agent is evaluated and reported from the viewpoint of toxicity by grade (level of severity). For a cytotoxic agent that damages or kills disease cells by inhibiting cell division but also affects normal cells, causing side effects, toxicity, and efficacy are usually related to the dose of the agent. A presupposition in general is that the dose–toxicity and dose–efficacy relationships will be parallel as monotonically increasing functions of the dose. Thus, the main goal of phase I trials is to find the highest tolerable dose (seemingly with the highest therapeutic effect), called the maximum tolerated dose (MTD). The toxicity associated with such an MTD is called the dose-limiting toxicity (DLT). (Note that in this chapter, DLT may be simply referred to as toxicity, unless otherwise specifically noted.)

There have already been various dose-escalation or dose-finding designs of phase I trials for cytotoxic agents (Le Tourneau et al., 2009). The designs can be classified into *rule-based (or algorithm-based) designs* and *model-based designs* (Rosenberger and Haines, 2002). Rule-based designs are easy to understand and implement, since the decision rule is intuitive and usually requires no modeling of the dose–toxicity relationship, leading to no complicated calculations based on special statistical software. On the other hand, model-based designs allow for clearer quantitative interpretation of results, since the decision rule is based on an assumed model of the dose–toxicity relationship. The rule-based and model-based designs are often referred to as *nonparametric* and *parametric* designs, respectively. Alternatively, they are sometimes referred to as *memoryless designs* and *designs with memory*, respectively (O'Quigley and Zohar, 2006).

In the last decade or so, targeted therapies, including cytostatic and biological agents, endothelin and multikinase inhibitors, immunotherapy, hormone therapy, and targeted radionuclide therapy, have been the focus of cancer clinical trials. These targeted therapies use agents or other substances such as small molecules, monoclonal antibodies, dendritic cells, and labeled radionuclides, to identify and attack specific diseased cells. Unlike cytotoxic agents, these targeted therapies have a mechanism based on drug-receptor (target) theory. The ideal situation is to have a target so specific for the disease that the agent can be delivered repeatedly at doses that completely kill abnormal cells or stop their growth without toxicity to normal cells. If the ideal situation is attained, the targeted therapies may no longer have side effects compared with traditional cytotoxic therapies. With these new targeted therapies, it is hypothesized that the toxicity does not necessarily increase with increasing dose. Efficacy does not necessarily increase monotonically with increasing dose either, but may plateau after it reaches maximal efficacy; a higher dose past this point no longer yields higher efficacy (Hunsberger et al., 2005; Hoering et al., 2011). As a consequence, emphasis will be placed on efficacy, rather than toxicity. In such a case, the early-phase clinical trials can take the form of a phase I trial focusing on efficacy, provided that the therapies are being monitored as not being toxic during the course of the trial. However, at present, there are not many targeted-therapy-specific designs for phase I trials (Le Tourneau et al., 2009).

One practical approach is to design a study that takes the form of a conventional phase I–II or I/II trial that is viewed as a sequential or simultaneous combination of a phase I trial with a phase II trial. Of note, in a phase I–II trial, the patient populations for the phase I and II parts may be different, possibly enriching the latter part with patients who could potentially benefit from the new agent, while in a phase I/II trial, the same patient population may be studied.

One thing that is common to this approach is that designs must promote patient safety, since it is unknown whether the treatment is safe and it is natural that there is no such thing as a risk-free treatment, even if it is expected to be possibly so from preclinical findings. Therefore, our interest here focuses on the optimum dose that produces the highest and acceptable efficacy, provided that toxicity is acceptable in a phase I–II trial, or that results in a joint outcome of the highest and acceptable efficacy together with acceptable toxicity in a phase I/II trial.

The objective of this chapter is to introduce several dose-escalation or dose-finding designs for early-phase clinical trials of targeted therapies. The chapter is structured as follows: In Section 4.2, we give a definition for some doses that we aim at finding in the early-phase clinical trials, with notations used throughout this chapter. In Section 4.3, we outline rule-based and model-based designs of phase I trials incorporating toxicity alone. Then, in Section 4.4, we provide an overview of designs incorporating both toxicity and efficacy, including those developed in the background of the phase I–II or I/II trials for cytotoxic agents and other designs specific to targeted therapies. Although many designs provided in Sections 4.3 and 4.4 were originally developed for cytotoxic agents, they could potentially be used or adapted for targeted therapies. Finally, we conclude with Section 4.5 with some practical considerations in designing early-phase clinical trials for targeted therapies.

4.2 What Is the Optimum Dose?

Suppose that an early-phase clinical trial consists of the set of K ordered doses of an agent, $S = \{d_1, \ldots, d_K\}$, to treat an enrolled patient, and that a total of n patients is planned to be enrolled in the trial. The doses are usually fixed at several levels before the trial. The increments of the doses for succeeding levels are typically defined according to some variation of a Fibonacci sequence.

Let X denote a random variable for the dose that is used to treat a patient, and x denote a real value of X. If S is specified in advance, x takes any one element of this set, that is, $x \in S$. At present, let us consider mainly binary outcomes of toxicity and efficacy. Thus, let Y_T and Y_E denote random variables for binary toxicity and efficacy outcomes. Each observed value takes the value of 1 if the patient experiences the outcome and 0 otherwise. We consider the following probabilities:

$$\Pr\left(Y_T = y_T \mid X = x\right), \quad y_T \in \{0,1\}, \tag{4.1}$$

$$\Pr\left(Y_E = y_E \mid X = x\right), \quad y_E \in \{0,1\}, \tag{4.2}$$

$$\Pr\left(Y_T = y_T, Y_E = y_E \mid X = x\right), \quad y_T, y_E \in \{0,1\}. \tag{4.3}$$

In particular, one's interest will focus on the probabilities of the presence of toxicity, efficacy, and efficacy together with nontoxicity, the last of which is often called *success*. For these probabilities, let us define, for convenience, the following functions for dose x, that is, the dose–toxicity, dose–efficacy and dose–success curves:

$$R(x) = \Pr\left(Y_T = 1 \mid X = x\right), \tag{4.4}$$

$$Q(x) = \Pr(Y_E = 1 \mid X = x), \tag{4.5}$$

$$P(x) = \Pr(Y_T = 0, Y_E = 1 \mid X = x). \tag{4.6}$$

If Y_T and Y_E are assumed to be independent, $P(x)$ can be given by $P(x) = Q(x)\{1 - R(x)\}$.

A main goal of phase I trials, especially for cytotoxic agents, is to find the MTD. Let d_T^* denote the MTD. For a prespecified maximum acceptable (or tolerated) level for the probability of toxicity, denoted as Γ_T, d_T^* is defined as the maximum of dose x that satisfies

$$\Pr\left(Y_T = 1 \mid X = x\right) \le \Gamma_T. \tag{4.7}$$

In phase I oncology trials, Γ_T often ranges from 0.2 to 0.33. However, the MTD may not necessarily be identified, for example, if the maximum dose that can be administered is below the MTD.

In some trials, a goal may be to find the lowest dose that yields a therapeutic benefit to patients. This dose is called the minimum effective dose (MED). Let d_E^* denote the MED, and Γ_E denote a prespecified minimum acceptable level for the probability of efficacy, although such a level cannot be necessarily identified. The MED, d_E^*, is defined as the minimum of dose x that satisfies

$$\Pr(Y_E = 1 \mid X = x) \geq \Gamma_E. \tag{4.8}$$

In particular, in some phase I/II trials for patients with serious diseases and life-threatening illness, due to fatal toxicity, the efficacy outcome cannot be observed or can be censored. In such a case, because one cannot obtain the marginal distribution of the efficacy outcome, the toxicity and efficacy outcomes in each patient can often be reduced to trinary outcomes (Thall and Russell, 1998): nontoxicity and nonefficacy, $(Y_T=0,\ Y_E=0)=(Z=0)$, efficacy without toxicity, $(Y_T=0,\ Y_E=1)=(Z=1)$, and toxicity $(Y_T=1)=(Z=2)$. Then, for a prespecified minimum acceptable success level in the probability of success, denoted as Γ_E', the MED in Equation 4.8 may be instead defined as the minimum of dose x that satisfies

$$\Pr(Z = 1 \mid X = x) = \Pr(Y_T = 0, Y_E = 1 \mid X = x) \geq \Gamma_E'. \tag{4.9}$$

The goal of phase I/II trials is to find the dose with the highest and acceptable efficacy together with acceptable toxicity. Therefore, the optimum dose (OD) may be defined as the dose maximizing the probability of success. In contrast, the goal of phase I–II trials is to find a dose level with the highest and acceptable efficacy in a dose range with acceptable toxicity that was identified in the phase I step.

4.3 Dose-Finding Designs Based on Toxicity Alone

One definition of the MTD is the dose at which the probability of toxicity is equal to the maximum acceptable level, Γ_T, as mentioned earlier. Another definition is the dose just below the lowest dose with unacceptable toxicity probability level, Γ_T', where $\Gamma_T' > \Gamma_T$ (Rosenberger and Haines, 2002). The former and latter definitions are used in model-based and rule-based designs, respectively.

4.3.1 Rule-Based Designs

4.3.1.1 3+3 Design

The 3+3 design remains commonly used in phase I oncology trials (Storer, 1989). A widely used algorithm of this design may be as follows: initially, one treats 3 patients at a dose level. If 0 out of 3 patients experiences toxicity, then one proceeds to the next higher dose level with a cohort of 3 patients.

If 1 out of 3 patients experiences toxicity, then one treats an additional 3 patients at the same dose level. If 1 out of 6 patients experiences toxicity at a dose level, the dose escalates for the next cohort of patients. If at least 2 out of 6 patients experience toxicity, or 2 out of 3 patients experience toxicity in the initial cohort treated at a dose level, then one has exceeded the MTD. Some investigations will, at this point, declare the previous dose level as the MTD. A more common requirement is to have 6 patients treated at the MTD.

The main advantages of this design are that it is safe and easy to implement and, in addition, through the accrual of 3 patients per dose level, it provides additional information about the between-patient variability of pharmacokinetics (PK) and pharmacodynamics (PD). However, the major disadvantages or criticisms of this design, at least for cytotoxic agents, are that a large proportion of patients are treated at low, possibly subtherapeutic dose levels below the recommended dose for phase II trials when the initial dose level chosen is far below the true MTD, and in addition the MTD is poorly estimated (see, e.g., Iasonos et al., 2008).

4.3.1.2 Accelerated Titration Design

Simon et al. (1997) proposed a family of accelerated titration designs as follows: *Design 1* is the 3+3 design described earlier; *Design 2* continues the accelerated phase unless one patient experiences DLT or two patients experience moderate toxicity during their first course of treatment. If so, the escalation phase switches to Design 1 with 40% dose-step increments; *Design 3* has the same algorithm as Design 2, except with double dose steps (100% dose-step increments) in the accelerated phase; *Design 4* has the same algorithm as Design 3, except that it continues the accelerated phase unless one patient experiences DLT or two patients experience moderate toxicity in *any* course of treatment. Designs 2 through 4 have options to use intrapatient dose modification for a patient who remains in the study, to provide the chance of each patient being treated at the potentially active dose.

In addition, a model that incorporates parameters for intra- and interpatient variation in toxicity and cumulative toxicity is used to analyze trial results.

4.3.2 Model-Based Designs

Model-based designs start with assuming a model for the probability of toxicity:

$$R(x) = \Pr\left(Y_T = 1 \mid X = x\right) = \pi_T(x, \theta), \qquad (4.10)$$

where $\pi_T(x, \theta)$ is assumed to be an increasing function of dose x, x takes any element of a set of doses, that is, $S = \{d_1, \ldots, d_K\}$ if specified in advance, and θ is a parameter or parameter vector.

Given the first j enrolled patients' pair data on dose assignment and toxicity outcome, $D_{T,j} = \{(x_l, y_{T,l});\ l = 1,\ldots,j\}$ $(j = 1,\ldots,n)$, the likelihood $L(D_{T,j};\ \theta)$ is obtained:

$$L\left(D_{T,j};\theta\right) = \prod_{l=1}^{j} \left\{\pi_T\left(x,\theta\right)\right\}^{y_{T,l}} \left\{1 - \pi_T\left(x,\theta\right)\right\}^{\left(1-y_{T,l}\right)}. \tag{4.11}$$

The parameter θ is usually estimated using either the maximum likelihood or Bayesian approach. If the former approach is used, some initial dose escalation based on a rule-based design (see Section 4.3.1) is required to maximize the likelihood given by Equation 4.11 on the interior of the parameter space (O'Quigley and Shen, 1996). If the latter approach is used, it is necessary to specify a prior distribution of θ. The procedure of such a Bayesian approach is generally as follows: the prior distribution is updated as $D_{T,j}$ become available from each successive patient or cohort, and then the posterior distribution of θ is obtained by

$$p\left(\theta \mid D_{T,j}\right) = \frac{L\left(D_{T,j};\theta\right)p\left(\theta\right)}{\int L\left(D_{T,j};\theta\right)p\left(\theta\right)d\theta}. \tag{4.12}$$

Given the posterior distribution, the parameter θ is estimated by, for example, $\tilde{\theta}_j = \int \theta p\left(\theta \mid D_{T,j}\right)d\theta$. The probability of toxicity at x can also be estimated by, for example, $\tilde{R}\left(x\right) = \pi_T(x, \tilde{\theta}_j)$. The included patient is usually then treated at or near the defined MTD. When prespecified stopping rules for safety restrictions, the total number of patients in the trial, etc., have been met, the MTD is selected according to predefined decision criteria, based on the data from all of the patients who were treated and evaluated.

4.3.2.1 Continual Reassessment Method

The continual reassessment method (CRM) was originally proposed by O'Quigley et al. (1990) as a Bayesian model-based design, and subsequently studied as a likelihood approach by O'Quigley and Shen (1996). Many of the model-based designs may originate from the CRM. The CRM starts with assuming a simple one-parameter working model, such as the hyperbolic tangent model, logistic model, or the power model, for $\pi_T(x, \theta)$. The term working means that the assumed model does not necessarily fit well at the whole of some dose–toxicity curve, $R(x)$ (see Equation 4.4), but that it only has to fit locally at the MTD of the curve. Thus, the working model is flexible enough to ensure that for any value of Γ_T, there exists a value of θ such that $\pi_T(x, \theta) = \Gamma_T$. The CRM tries to find the MTD, the dose associated with the probability of toxicity that is close to Γ_T.

Late-onset toxicities may also be a serious concern in phase I trials for, for example, radiation therapies or chemopreventive agents. They prevent complete follow-up of the current patient before admitting a new patient. This results in an impractically long trial duration. The time-to-event continual reassessment method, called *TiTE-CRM*, was developed to circumvent the problem when estimating the MTD (Cheung and Chappell, 2000). In this method, patients who have not experienced toxicity are weighted by the amount of time they have been followed as a proportion of the observation window, whereas patients who have experienced toxicity are assigned a full weight. This allows patients to be entered timely and in a staggered fashion.

A comprehensive review on the CRM and related and extended designs was provided by O'Quigley and Conaway (2010).

4.4 Dose-Finding Designs Based on Toxicity and Efficacy

In this section, we describe dose-finding designs based on mainly binary toxicity and efficacy outcomes, classifying them into rule-based and model-based designs. Of these designs, some were developed for phase I–II or I/II trials for conventional cytotoxic agents, but could be used to those for targeted agents. For targeted therapies, an efficacy outcome might be based on the level of a molecular target, or the change in the level of a target that holds clinical promise. Thus, the usefulness of the designs for targeted therapies depends on the validity of the assays to measure the response (target) and patients having the target. Also, an efficacy outcome may be measured on a continuous scale (see Section 4.4.2.3 for further discussion). Thus, to use some of the designs described in Sections 4.4.1 and 4.4.2, one would need to binarize or dichotomize such an efficacy outcome, to indicate whether or not the agent has had the desired effect on the target.

4.4.1 Rule-Based Designs

4.4.1.1 Proportion or Slope Designs

In early-phase clinical trials of some targeted therapies, such as cancer vaccines and other immunotherapies, where no or acceptable toxicity is expected from preclinical trials, one may measure therapeutic effects as biological activity based on inhibition of a specific molecular target, or based on an immune response, and attempt to identify the minimal dose that is active. However, trials to find such a minimal active dose may be feasible but require much larger number of patients than conventional phase I trials through, for example, 3 + 3 designs with the 3–6 patients per dose level (see Simon et al., 2001; Rubinstein and Simon, 2003; Korn et al., 2006).

Hunsberger et al. (2005) proposed two types of designs to find a biologically active dose, although not necessarily the minimal active dose, called the proportion and slope designs. These designs assume that a targeted therapy will not produce significant toxicity. Thus, dose escalation is solely based on the efficacy outcome. However, if significant toxic side effects occur, the dose escalation would be based on toxicity alone with a rule-based design, for example, the 3 + 3 design (Hunsberger et al., 2005).

The proportion designs ensure that if the true target efficacy rate is low, there will be a high probability of escalating the dose, and if the true efficacy rate is high, there will be a low probability of escalating the dose. The designs mimic the 3 + 3 design. They presented two sets of the designs. The first design, called the *Proportion [4/6]*, is based on distinguishing between efficacy rates of $p_0 = 0.3$ and $p_1 = 0.8$. This means that one wishes to continue to escalate the dose if the true efficacy rate at a dose level is close to 0.3 but to stop escalating the dose if the true efficacy rate is close to 0.8. The second design, called the *Proportion [5/6]*, distinguishes between $p_0 = 0.4$ and $p_1 = 0.9$.

The slope designs continue to escalate the dose as long as the true efficacy rate is increasing and stop escalating the dose when the efficacy rate reaches a plateau or decreases. Specifically, the dose escalation is based on the estimated slope parameter of simple regression using the dose level as the independent variable and the corresponding efficacy rate as the dependent variable. Only the three or four highest dose levels are used to calculate the slope. Escalation stops when the estimated slope parameter <0 (as long as at least one patient experiences efficacy). The dose with the highest efficacy rate is the dose recommended for use in subsequent trials. If two or more dose levels have the highest efficacy rate, the highest dose level is chosen. The authors presented three different designs according to the cohort size and the number of dose levels used to calculate the slope: three patients per cohort with the four highest dose levels, denoted as *Slope 3P/4L*; six patients per cohort with the four highest dose levels, *Slope 6P/4L*; and six patients per cohort with the three highest dose levels *Slope 6P/3L*.

4.4.1.2 Two-Step Designs

A seamless phase I–II design for a targeted agent's trials was proposed by Hoering et al. (2011). This design is composed of two steps: the first step uses a rule-based design for the phase I trial to only assess toxicity and find the MTD, and the second step uses a modified phase II selection design for two or three dose levels at and below the MTD to determine efficacy and evaluate each dose level for both efficacy and toxicity.

Yin et al. (2012) also proposed a two-stage dose-finding design, where in stage 1, the MTD, which will be the upper bound of admissible dose levels, is found by using the designs focusing on toxicity alone (see Section 4.3) and in stage 2, the most effective dose, which has the highest efficacy rate, is found within the admissible dose levels. In particular, to estimate the efficacy probability at each dose level, the authors succeeded in modeling a possible late-onset efficacy by redistributing the mass of the censored observation and estimating the fractional contribution for a censored efficacy outcome.

4.4.1.3 Odds Ratio Trade-Off Designs

A Bayesian design for phase I/II trials without specifying any parametric functional form for the dose–outcome curves was proposed by Yin et al. (2006). They assume a monotonically increasing dose–toxicity curve $R(x)$, but do not impose the monotonic constraint for the dose–efficacy relationship $Q(x)$. They used the following global cross-ratio model to consider jointly modeling the bivariate toxicity and efficacy outcomes:

$$\theta_k = \frac{\Pr(Y_T = 0, Y_E = 0 \mid X = d_k)\Pr(Y_T = 1, Y_E = 1 \mid X = d_k)}{\Pr(Y_T = 0, Y_E = 1 \mid X = d_k)\Pr(Y_T = 1, Y_E = 0 \mid X = d_k)}, \tag{4.13}$$

which quantifies the association between the toxicity and efficacy outcomes. The probability $\Pr(Y_T = y_T, Y_E = y_E \mid X = d_k)$ can be obtained from θ_k and the marginal probabilities $R(d_k)$ and $Q(d_k)$.

They define a set of acceptable doses, D_A, which satisfy $\Pr(R(d_k) < \Gamma_T) > \gamma_T$ and $\Pr(Q(d_k) > \Gamma_E) > \gamma_E$, where γ_T and γ_E are prespecified probability cutoffs. In addition, to facilitate the dose selection, they use the toxicity-efficacy odds ratio contour, where a possible value of $(Q(d_k), R(d_k))$ for the optimum dose d_k is located closest to the lower-right corner (1, 0) in the 2-dimensional efficacy and toxicity domain. The algorithm of this design is similar to the trade-off-based algorithm proposed by Thall and Cook (2004) (see Section 4.4.2).

4.4.1.4 Other Designs and Related Topics

Phase I/II trial designs that combine a modification of the up-and-down rule, called directed walk designs, with smoothed shape-constrained fitting techniques for dose–outcome curves were proposed by Hardwick et al. (2003). A Bayesian design using utility weight value that represents preferences over the consequences of de-escalating the dose, keeping the same dose or escalating the dose, was presented by Loke et al. (2006).

Polley and Cheung (2008) dealt with the design problem of early-phase dose-finding clinical trials with monotone biologic endpoints. They proposed a two-stage design using stepwise testing to identify the MED, aiming to reduce the potential sample size requirement by shutting down unpromising doses in a futility interim analysis. Messer et al. (2010) considered a toxicity-evaluation design for phase I/II cancer immunotherapy trials. This design is based on safety hypothesis testing and an algorithm like the 3+3 design.

4.4.2 Model-Based Designs

The model-based designs start with assuming a model for the bivariate probabilities of binary toxicity and efficacy outcomes, Y_T and Y_E:

$$\Pr(Y_T = y_T, Y_E = y_E \mid X = x) = \pi_{y_T, y_E}(x, \theta), y_T, y_E \in \{0,1\}, \tag{4.14}$$

where θ is a parameter vector. Much of the model-based designs incorporating toxicity and efficacy are based on Bayesian approaches. One reason is to estimate large numbers of parameters for the limited sample sizes of early-phase trials. In the Bayesian approach, given the first j included patients' data, $D_{TE,j} = \{(x_l, y_{T,l}, y_{E,l}); l = 1, \ldots, j\}$ $(j = 1, \ldots, n)$, the likelihood $L(D_{TE,j}; \theta)$ is obtained according to forms of the assumed model, and then the prior distribution of θ is updated to the posterior.

Since the phase I–II or I/II trial focuses on efficacy as well as toxicity, acceptable doses may be required to satisfy

$$\Pr\left(\pi_T(x, \theta) \le \Gamma_T \mid D_{TE,j}\right) \ge \gamma_T, \tag{4.15}$$

$$\Pr\left(\pi_E(x, \theta) \le \Gamma_E \mid D_{TE,j}\right) \ge \gamma_E, \tag{4.16}$$

where γ_T and γ_E are prespecified probability cutoffs, $\pi_T(x, \theta) = \pi_{1,0}(x, \theta) + \pi_{1,1}(x, \theta)$, and $\pi_E(x, \theta) = \pi_{0,1}(x, 0) + \pi_{1,1}(x, \theta)$. Equation 4.16 may be instead replaced by

$$\Pr\left(\pi_{0,1}(x, \theta) \ge \Gamma'_E \mid D_{TE,j}\right) \ge \gamma'_E, \tag{4.17}$$

where γ_E^* is a prespecified probability cutoff. Of the acceptable doses satisfying the aforementioned requirements, the OD may be defined as the dose maximizing the posterior probability of success: $\Pr(\pi_{0,1}(x, \theta) > \Gamma'_E \mid D_{TE,j})$. Such dose is used to treat every enrolled patient. If it does not exist, the trial will be stopped.

4.4.2.1 Repeated SPRT Designs

A new class of designs that can be used in dose-finding studies in HIV was proposed by O'Quigley et al. (2001). To determine the OD that maximizes $\Pr(Y_T = 0, Y_E = 1 \mid X = x)$, they considered the dose–success curve, $P(x) = Q'(x)\{1 - R(x)\}$, where $R(x)$ and $Q'(x)$ are the dose–toxicity curve and dose–efficacy curve given nontoxicity. For estimation of these curves, they presented an approach: first, the likelihood CRM (O'Quigley and Shen, 1996) is used to target some low toxicity rate; second, accumulating information at tried dose levels resulting in success is used to conduct the repeated sequential probability ratio test (SPRT) of H_0: $P(d_k) = p_0$ against H_1: $P(d_k) = p_1$ at increasing dose levels, where p_0 and p_1 ($>p_0$) denote the values for $P(d_k)$ that are considered to be unsatisfactory or satisfactory, respectively. The type I and type II errors are respectively fixed at $\alpha=\Pr(H_1|H_0)$ and $\beta=\Pr(H_0|H_1)$. After inclusion of the first j patients, we calculate

$$s_j(d_k)=r\left[\sum_{l\le j} y_{E,l} I(x_l=d_k, y_{T,l}=0)-j\left\{\log\frac{p_0^*}{p_1^*}-r\right\}\right], \tag{4.18}$$

where $r=\log[\{p_0(1-p_1)\}/\{p_1(1-p_0)\}]$. If $s_j(d_k)>\log\{\beta/(1-\alpha)\}$, then H_1 is accepted and the therapy is determined to be promising at level d_k. If $s_j(d_k)<\log\{(1-\beta)/\alpha\}$, then H_0 is accepted and the therapy is not sufficiently effective at level d_k. This leads to removal of level d_k and lower levels. The target toxicity probability level has now increased to $\Gamma_T+\Delta\Gamma_T$ until a prespecified maximum target level, where $\Delta\Gamma_T$ is a prespecified increment. The trial then continues at level d_{k+1}.

4.4.2.2 Trade-Off Designs

Thall and Russell (1998) captured the patients' toxicity and efficacy outcomes, that is, Y_T and Y_E, by a trinary ordinal outcome Z (see Section 4.2). They assume a proportional odds model for $\pi_z(x, \theta)$, $z \in \{0, 1, 2\}$, since in general, $\pi_0(x, \theta)$ and $\pi_2(x, \theta)$ are assumed to be decreasing and increasing functions of x, respectively. The design considers a dose to be acceptable if it satisfies Equations 4.15 and 4.17.

An improved version of this design was subsequently proposed by Thall and Cook (2004). They used the following model to formulate the bivariate probabilities of Y_T and Y_E, in terms of $\pi_T(x, \theta)$ and $\pi_E(x, \theta)$:

$$\pi_T(x,\theta)=\pi_{1,0}(x,\theta)+\pi_{1,1}(x,\theta)=\text{logit}^{-1}\{\eta_T(x,\theta)\}, \tag{4.19}$$

$$\pi_E(x,\theta)=\pi_{0,1}(x,\theta)+\pi_{1,1}(x,\theta)=\text{logit}^{-1}\{\eta_E(x,\theta)\}, \tag{4.20}$$

where $\eta_T(x, \theta)=\theta_1+\theta_2 x$ and $\eta_E(x, \theta)=\theta_3+\theta_4 x+\theta_5 x^2$. That is, the toxicity is assumed to be monotonic in x, but the efficacy is assumed to be quadratically nonmonotonic in x. For the association between Y_T and Y_E, they use the following Gumbel model (suppressing x and θ):

$$\pi_{y_T,y_E}=\pi_T^{y_T}(1-\pi_T)^{1-y_T}\pi_E^{y_E}(1-\pi_E)^{1-y_E}$$
$$+(-1)^{y_T+y_E}\pi_T(1-\pi_T)\pi_E(1-\pi_E)\frac{\exp(\rho)-1}{\exp(\rho)+1}, \tag{4.21}$$

where ρ is an association parameter. If Y_T and Y_E are independent, ρ is equal to zero. Therefore, the model has a vector of six parameters, $\theta = (\theta_1, \theta_2, \theta_3, \theta_4, \theta_5, \rho)^T$.

A set of efficacy-toxicity trade-off contours that partition the 2-dimensional outcome probability domain of possible values of (π_E, π_T) is used to treat successive patient cohorts at acceptable doses and find the OD, instead of directly using Equations 4.15 and 4.16. Thall et al. (2008) extended this design by accounting for patient's covariates and dose–covariate interactions.

A simple modified version of the design of Thall and Russell (1998), called the trivariate or trinary outcome CRM (TriCRM), was proposed by Zhang et al. (2006). They use the continuation-ratio model, but dose assignment is based on criteria that are different from the aforementioned designs. Mandrekar et al. (2007) provided a generalization of the TriCRM design for two-agent combination. Mandrekar et al. (2010) wrote a review on these designs for a single or two-agent combination.

4.4.2.3 Other Designs and Related Topics

The Bayesian utility-based phase I/II design incorporating bivariate both ordinal toxicity and efficacy outcomes was proposed by Houede et al. (2010) to select the optimal dose combination of a biological agent and a chemotherapeutic agent. In some situations, efficacy will be continuous rather than binary or categorical, whereas it will often be appropriate to represent toxicity as a binary outcome. In general, dichotomizing or categorizing a continuous outcome leads to loss of information. To solve this problem, there exist several Bayesian approaches to jointly model continuous efficacy and binary toxicity (see, e.g., Bekele and Shen, 2005; Zhou et al., 2006; Hirakawa, 2012). There exists a Bayesian design that jointly models toxicity and efficacy as time-to-event outcomes (see Yuan and Yin, 2009).

A dose-schedule-finding design to find a combination of dose and treatment schedule under bivariate binary outcomes of toxicity and efficacy was presented by Li et al. (2008). An excellent review on several Bayesian early-phase trial designs that were tailored to accommodate specific complexities of the treatment regimen and patient outcomes in clinical settings was provided by Thall (2010).

For a combination of two or more agents, a few dose-finding designs based on both efficacy and toxicity have been developed (Huang et al., 2007; Houede, 2010; Whitehead et al., 2011; Hirakawa, 2012).

4.5 Concluding Remarks

Even if nonmonotonicity of the dose–efficacy relationship for a target agent is recognized, dose-finding designs based solely on toxicity, particularly rule-based designs, have been widely used in oncology. Parulekar and Eisenhauer (2004) have investigated methods of dose escalation and determination of the recommended phase II dose employed in 60 previous single-agent phase I trials for a total of 31 targeted agents, including small molecules, antibodies, and antisense oligodeoxynucleotides. Thirty-six of the 60 trials determined the dose for phase II trials based solely on toxicity, and only 8 trials took into consideration the PK measurements, while the remaining 16 determined the dose based on other factors (including those without description of the factors) in dose determination. As one example from the 16 trials, Cunningham et al. (2000) evaluated several efficacy outcomes, including PK measurements, tumor responses, and markers, in addition to toxicity outcomes, in a phase I trial of c-Raf kinase antisense oligonucleotide ISIS 5132 in 34 advanced cancer patients with 16 different tumor types. They reported that one patient with ovarian carcinoma had a significant response with a 95% reduction in CA-125 level that is a well-known tumor marker for ovarian and uterine cancers. This is one of the limited examples of phase I trials for targeted therapies that evaluated multiple efficacy outcomes in dose determination. Takimoto (2009) argued that, although determination of the MTD in phase I trials still provides valuable information for future drug development, the final dose selection should be made after a thorough review of the entirety of PK, PD, biomarkers, and biological and clinical activities.

While measurement of the efficacy on molecular targets seems logical and useful in phase I trials, there are several practical barriers as follows: (1) the difficulty of defining the appropriate measure for the therapeutic effects for a specific drug; (2) the lack of reliable assays and the difficulty in obtaining the required tumor specimens; and (3) the lack of clear evidence linking minimum levels of target expression to drug effect. See Parulekar and Eisenhauer (2004) and Korn (2004) for further discussion about these issues. If these barriers can be overcome and the molecular target has a prospect of predicting clinical outcomes as surrogates for clinical benefit, it might allow us to enrich an early-phase trial, selecting patients, rather than taking all comers as with conventional phase I trials. Eisenhauer (2000) also provided a discussion about using alternative endpoints in phase I trials when they are previously validated in either mouse or man. She suggested that ideally the trial could be designed to search for the maximum target-inhibiting dose (MTID) and the more traditional MTD. If the MTID and MTD are found to be similar at the end of the study, selection of the recommended phase II dose is straightforward. If they are substantially different, it may be most appropriate to select the dose with maximum target effect, provided that toxicity is acceptable, for further evaluation.

Even when efficacy outcomes were taken into consideration in selecting the recommended dose for phase II trials at the end of the phase I trial, these outcomes were not necessarily incorporated in dose escalation/de-escalation for individual patients in the course of the phase I trial, such as in the study of Cunningham et al. (2010). One of the major reasons behind this may be related to the lack of well-understood dose-finding designs that are easy to implement. With respect to a decision tree for escalating and de-escalating the dose based on efficacy and toxicity outcomes, Meany et al. (2010) employed a rather complex decision tree based on an outcome of maximum target inhibition as the primary endpoint, in addition to toxicity outcomes, in a pediatric phase I trial. Notably, another issue is how to select an optimal one among many possible decision trees when planning phase I trials using a decision tree.

To address the issues regarding endpoints and other considerations in phase I trials for target agents, the NDDO Research Foundation has established the Methodology for the Development of Innovative Cancer Therapies (MDICT). The scientific presentations and discussions of the MDICT task force were summarized in Booth et al. (2008). The MDICT task force recommended the phase I algorithm for target agents including toxicity and efficacy endpoints. See Booth et al. (2008) for further details about this algorithm.

References

Bekele, B.N. and Shen, Y. (2005). A Bayesian approach to jointly modeling toxicity and biomarker expression in a phase I/II dose-finding trial. *Biometrics* 61, 344–354.

Booth, C.M., Calvert, A.H., Giaccone, G., Labbezoo, M.W., Seymour, L.K., Eisenhauer, E.A., and on behalf of the Task Force on Methodology for the Development of Innovative Cancer Therapies. (2008). Endpoints and other considerations I phase I studies of targeted anticancer therapy: Recommendations from the task force on Methodology for the Development of Innovative Cancer Therapies (MDICT). *Eur J Cancer* 44, 19–24.

Cheung, Y.K. and Chappell, R. (2000). Sequential designs for phase I clinical trials with late-onset toxicities. *Biometrics* 56, 1177–1182.

Cunningham, C.C., Holmlund, J.T., Schiller, J.H. et al. (2000). A phase I trial of c-raf kinase antisense oligonucleotide ISIS 5132 administered as a continuous intravenous infusion in patients with advanced cancer. *Clin Cancer Res* 6, 1626–1631.

Eisenhauer, E.A. (2000). Phase I and II evaluation of novel anticancer agents; are response and toxicity the right endpoints? *Onkologie* 23, 2–6.

Hardwick, J., Meyer, M.C., and Stout, Q.F. (2003). Directed walk designs for dose response problems with competing failure modes. *Biometrics* 59, 229–236.

Hirakawa, A. (2012). An adaptive dose-finding approach for correlated bivariate binary and continuous outcomes in phase I oncology trials. *Stat Med* 31, 516–532.

Hoering, A., LeBlanc, M., and Crowley, J. (2011). Seamless phase I-II trial design for assessing toxicity and efficacy for targeted agents. *Clin Cancer Res* 17, 640–646.

Houede, N., Thall, P.F., Nguyen, H., Paoletti, X., and Kramar, A. (2010). Utility-based optimization of combination therapy using ordinal toxicity and efficacy in phase I/II trials. *Biometrics* 66, 532–540.

Huang, X., Biswas, S., Oki, Y., Issa, J.-P., and Berry, D.A. (2007). A parallel phase I/II clinical trial design for combination therapies. *Biometrics* 63, 429–436.

Hunsberger, S., Rubinstein, L.V., Dancey, J., and Korn, E.L. (2005). Dose escalation trial designs based on a molecularly targeted endpoint. *Stat Med* 24, 2171–2181.

Iasonos, A., Wilton, A.S., Riedel, E.R., Seshan, V.E., and Spriggs, D.R. (2008). A comprehensive comparison of the continual reassessment method to the standard 3 + 3 dose escalation scheme in phase I dose-finding studies. *Clin Trials* 5, 465–477.

Korn, E.L. (2004). Nontoxicity endpoints in phase I trial designs for targeted, non-cytotoxic agents. *J Natl Cancer Inst* 96, 977–978.

Korn, E.L., Rubinstein, L.V., Hunsberger, S.A. et al. (2006). Clinical trial designs for cytostatic agents and agents directed at novel molecular targets. In *Novel Anticancer Agents: Strategies for Discovery and Clinical Testing* (eds., Adjei, A.A. and Buolamwini, J.K.), pp. 365–378. London, U.K.: Academic Press.

Le Tourneau, C., Lee, J.J., and Siu, L.L. (2009). Dose escalation methods in phase I cancer clinical trials. *J Natl Cancer Inst* 101, 708–720.

Li, Y., Bekele, B.N., Ji, Y., and Cook, J.D. (2008). Dose-schedule finding in phase I/II clinical trials using a Bayesian isotonic transformation. *Stat Med* 27, 4895–4913.

Loke, Y.-C., Tan, S.-B., Cai, Y.Y., and Machin, D. (2006). A Bayesian dose finding design for dual endpoint phase I trials. *Stat Med* 25, 3–22.

Mandrekar, S.J., Cui, Y., and Sargent, D.J. (2007). An adaptive phase I design for identifying a biologically optimal dose for dual agent drug combinations. *Stat Med* 26, 2317–2330.

Mandrekar, S.J., Qin, R., and Sargent, D.J. (2010). Model-based phase I designs incorporating toxicity and efficacy for single and dual agent drug combinations: Methods and challenges. *Stat Med* 29, 1077–1083.

Meany, H., Balis, F.M., Aikin, A. et al. (2010). Pediatric phase I trial design using maximum target inhibition as the primary endpoint. *J Natl Cancer Inst* 102, 909–912.

Messer, K., Natarajan, L., Ball, E.D., and Lane, T.A. (2010). Toxicity-evaluation designs for phase I/II cancer immunotherapy trials. *Stat Med* 29, 712–720.

O'Quigley, J. and Conaway, M. (2010). Continual reassessment method and related dose-finding designs. *Stat Sci* 25, 202–216.

O'Quigley, J., Hughes, M.D., and Fenton, T. (2001). Dose-finding designs for HIV studies. *Biometrics* 57, 1018–1029.

O'Quigley, J., Pepe, M., and Fisher, L. (1990). Continual reassessment method: A practical design for phase 1 clinical trials in cancer. *Biometrics* 46, 33–48.

O'Quigley, J. and Shen, L.Z. (1996). Continual reassessment method: A likelihood approach. *Biometrics* 52, 673–684.

O'Quigley, J. and Zohar, S. (2006). Experimental designs for phase I and phase I/II dose-finding studies. *Br J Cancer* 94, 609–613.

Parulekar, W.R. and Eisenhauer, E.A. (2004). Phase I trial design for solid tumor studies of targeted, non-cytotoxic agents: Theory and practice. *J Natl Cancer Inst* 96, 990–997.

Polley, M.-Y. and Cheung, Y.K. (2008). Two-stage designs for dose-finding trials with a biologic endpoint using stepwise tests. *Biometrics* 64, 232–241.

Rosenberger, W.F. and Haines, L.M. (2002). Competing designs for phase I clinical trials: A review. *Stat Med* 21, 2757–2770.

Rubinstein, L.V. and Simon, R.M. (2003). Phase I clinical trial design. In *Handbook of Anticancer Drug Development* (eds., D.R. Budman, A.H. Calvert, E.K. Rowinsky), pp. 297–308. Philadelphia, PA: Lippincott Williams & Wilkins.

Simon, R.M., Freidlin, B., Rubinstein, L. et al. (1997). Accelerated titration designs for phase I clinical trials in oncology. *J Natl Cancer Inst* 89, 1138–1147.

Simon, R.M., Steinberg, S.M., Hamilton, M. et al. (2001). Clinical trial designs for the early clinical development of therapeutic cancer vaccines. *J Clin Oncol* 19, 1848–1854.

Storer, B.E. (1989). Design and analysis of phase I clinical trials. *Biometrics* 45, 925–937.

Takimoto, C.H. (2009). Maximum tolerated dose: Clinical endpoint for a bygone era? *Targ Oncol* 4, 143–147.

Thall, P.F. (2010). Bayesian models and decision algorithms for complex early phase clinical trials. *Stat Sci* 25, 227–244.

Thall, P.F. and Cook, J.D. (2004). Dose-finding based on efficacy-toxicity tradeoffs. *Biometrics* 60, 684–693.

Thall, P.F., Nguyen, H.Q., and Estey, E.H. (2008). Patient-specific dose finding based on bivariate outcomes and covariates. *Biometrics* 64, 1126–1136.

Thall, P.F. and Russell, K.E. (1998). A strategy for dose-finding and safety monitoring based on efficacy and adverse outcomes in phase I/II clinical trials. *Biometrics* 54, 251–264.

Whitehead, J., Thygesen, H., and Whitehead, A. (2011). Bayesian procedures for phase I/II clinical trials investigating the safety and efficacy of drug combinations. *Stat Med* 30, 1952–1970.

Yin, G., Li, Y., and Ji, Y. (2006). Bayesian dose-finding in phase I/II clinical trials using toxicity and efficacy odds ratios. *Biometrics* 62, 777–787.

Yin, G., Zheng, S., and Xu, J. (2012). Two-stage dose finding for cytostatic agents in phase I oncology trials. *Stat Med* 32, 644–660.

Yuan, Y. and Yin, G. (2009). Bayesian dose finding by jointly modelling toxicity and efficacy as time-to-event outcomes. *J Roy Stat Soc Ser C* 58, 719–736.

Zhang, W., Sargent, D.J., and Mandrekar, S. (2006). An adaptive dose-finding design incorporating both toxicity and efficacy. *Stat Med* 25, 2365–2383.

5

An Overview of Phase II Clinical Trial Designs with Biomarkers

Lisa McShane and Sally Hunsberger

CONTENTS

5.1 Introduction

Phase II trials aim to gather information on the clinical activity of a new agent in order to determine whether the agent should proceed to phase III trials for further development. Numerous phase II trial designs are used in oncology (Simon 1989; Rubinstein et al. 2005, 2009; Green et al. 2012). Increasingly phase II clinical trials of new cancer therapies are incorporating biomarkers that are thought to be potentially informative for the likelihood that a patient will benefit from the therapy under investigation (i.e., predictive biomarkers) (McShane et al. 2009). The strength of preliminary evidence for potential predictive biomarkers may vary widely from study to study, and this is generally reflected in the choice of phase II design. At the time a phase II trial is initiated, there might be reasonable confidence in what biomarker is likely to be predictive, but there could be uncertainty about the most appropriate form of the biomarker (e.g., gene mutation, gene amplification, gene expression, or protein expression), and the assay might still be research grade. It may be acceptable to use such a biomarker in a phase II setting with the understanding that the phase II trial provides an opportunity to establish activity of the therapy and to refine the biomarker or discover new biomarkers that might ultimately be helpful for guiding use of the therapy in clinical practice.

Several phase II designs incorporating biomarkers have been proposed. The designs vary in the amount of information required about the biomarker, the number of biomarkers used, the use of randomization, the choice of endpoint, the assumptions required, and the objectives that will be accomplished by conducting the trial. Biomarkers may also be embedded in phase II trials for exploratory purposes, for example, to better understand the mechanism of action of a drug, but such exploratory objectives are not the main focus here. Readers are referred elsewhere for additional discussion that includes exploratory uses of biomarkers in phase II trials (McShane et al. 2009) and for an introduction to some basic strategies for designs that do not necessarily involve biomarkers (Rubinstein et al. 2009).

This chapter is organized according to whether the trial design uses randomization or not and by whether the design relies on single or multiple biomarkers. For simplicity of discussion, it is assumed that the biomarkers of interest are binary. We comment on this assumption briefly before we launch into discussion of specific trial designs incorporating biomarkers. Although the examples in this chapter focus on oncology trials, we comment in the final section on generalizations of these designs and their application outside of the medical specialty of oncology.

5.2 Biomarker Measurement

The biomarker and the assay used to measure it may undergo multiple refinements as the experimental therapeutic proceeds through the development process toward clinical use. In a phase II trial, the biomarker assay should satisfy some clinically acceptable minimum robustness and reproducibility requirements so that the trial patient population is meaningfully defined. The biomarker, and any cut-points applied to continuous biomarkers, might only be tentative and based on data from preclinical studies or possibly very preliminary efficacy results or pharmacokinetic and pharmacodynamic data from phase I studies. The goal in phase II trials is to strike a balance between enriching the trial population sufficiently to increase the odds of seeing a treatment effect, if there is one, and not unduly restricting the patient population to the point of permanently excluding a significant portion of patients who might benefit from the experimental agent.

Many biomarkers are measured by a process that has some underlying continuous measurement scale, for example, percent stained cells measured by an immunohistochemical assay, quantitation of protein by mass spectrometry, or gene expression quantified by reverse transcription polymerase chain reaction. If trial eligibility will be dependent on the value of the single continuous biomarker, it will usually be necessary to apply a cut-point to that biomarker value to produce a binary result for trial eligibility determination, and eventually to determine which patients should receive the drug when it is used in clinical practice. In some situations, a panel, or profile, of biomarkers may be believed to be informative for identification of which patients are likely to benefit from a new therapy. The component biomarkers in the panel may be combined into a decision algorithm or prediction model that yields a binary result indicating which patients should receive the new therapy. Due to the inherent binary nature of the decisions regarding which patients to include in a phase II trial or which patients to offer a new therapy when it reaches clinical use, and for simplicity of discussion, the remainder of this chapter focuses on binary biomarkers. For discussion of considerations in the development and validation of continuous genomic signatures in clinical trials, see Chapter 17.

5.3 Nonrandomized Single-Arm Trials with a Single Biomarker and Single Experimental Agent

Historically, many phase II clinical trials of new therapeutic agents in oncology have been single-arm trials with objective tumor response as an endpoint (Simon 1989). Objective response rate is a meaningful measure of activity for traditional anticancer agents that are cytotoxic. Some newer anticancer agents have novel mechanisms of action that target specific biological pathways to inhibit tumor growth, that is, the agents are cytostatic, and traditional tumor shrinkage endpoints may not adequately capture their effects. It is possible for agents or agent combinations to have both cytotoxic and growth inhibitory effects (Kummar 2006). Alternative endpoints such as progression-free survival (PFS) or overall survival (OS) are needed for phase II trials if agent effects are not primarily tumor shrinkage (Rubinstein et al. 2011). Due to the challenges in reliably assessing PFS, it is often dichotomized in phase II trial designs (e.g., patient free of progression at 3 months or alive at 6 months). When using a time-to-event endpoint in a single-arm trial, it can be more difficult to set an appropriate benchmark for the purpose of establishing convincing evidence of agent activity. If the trials results are interpreted in subgroups defined by biomarkers, then the challenges are even greater. In these situations, it can be difficult to select endpoints that provide convincing evidence of tumor activity. We elaborate on these issues later.

When biological understanding of the mechanism of action of an experimental agent provides strong evidence that the agent will be active only in tumors with particular characteristics defined by a biomarker, then it is appropriate for early phase II trials to be restricted to patients whose tumors possess that biomarker (biomarker-positive). If a single-arm, single-agent trial is conducted in a biomarker-positive population, one must be careful in setting a benchmark for the endpoint due to the potential for prognostic effects of the biomarker, particularly if the trial endpoint is PFS. Historical response rates and progression rates most likely apply to unselected populations, and there is the potential that tumors that are positive for the biomarker will have different response or progression rates even in the context of standard therapies or no therapy. This would imply that different benchmark rates for the endpoint would apply to establish evidence of activity in a single-arm trial conducted only in the biomarker-positive subgroup. For example, consider a situation in which a biomarker with 50% prevalence is prognostic in the setting of standard therapy, with median PFS of 6 months in the biomarker-negative subgroup and 11 months in the biomarker-positive subgroup, or 8 months for the unselected patient population. If a new targeted agent is studied in the biomarker-positive subgroup only and results in median PFS of 11 months, it would appear to offer a 38% prolongation in median PFS compared to historical experience in the unselected population when in reality it offered no benefit over standard therapy in the targeted biomarker-positive subgroup.

If there is uncertainty about whether the activity of a novel agent will be limited to the subpopulation of tumors that possess a particular biomarker, or there is uncertainty about the best way to measure the biomarker, a single-arm trial might be conducted in an unselected population. If it turns out that the benefit of the agent is limited to the biomarker-positive subgroup, then a standard single-arm trial in an unselected population may fail to find an effect because the benefit in the biomarker-positive subgroup is diluted by the lack of benefit in the biomarker-negative subgroups. To address this concern when there is at least some evidence suggesting that a biomarker might be associated with benefit from the experimental agent, it can be useful to stratify on a candidate biomarker so that sufficient patients are accrued to allow one to draw some meaningful conclusion within each biomarker subgroup. Two phase II trials could be run in parallel, one in each biomarker-defined subgroup, or the trials could be coordinated to accrue from the same stream of patients with allowance for early termination of accrual in the biomarker-negative subgroup if early results do not look promising in that subgroup.

A biomarker-adaptive parallel Simon two-stage design (Simon 1989) has been proposed for evaluation of a targeted agent that is expected to have different activity (response rate) in biomarker-positive and biomarker-negative subgroups (Jones and Holmgren 2007). As summarized in McShane et al. (2009), the adaptive parallel two-stage design (Figure 5.1) starts as two

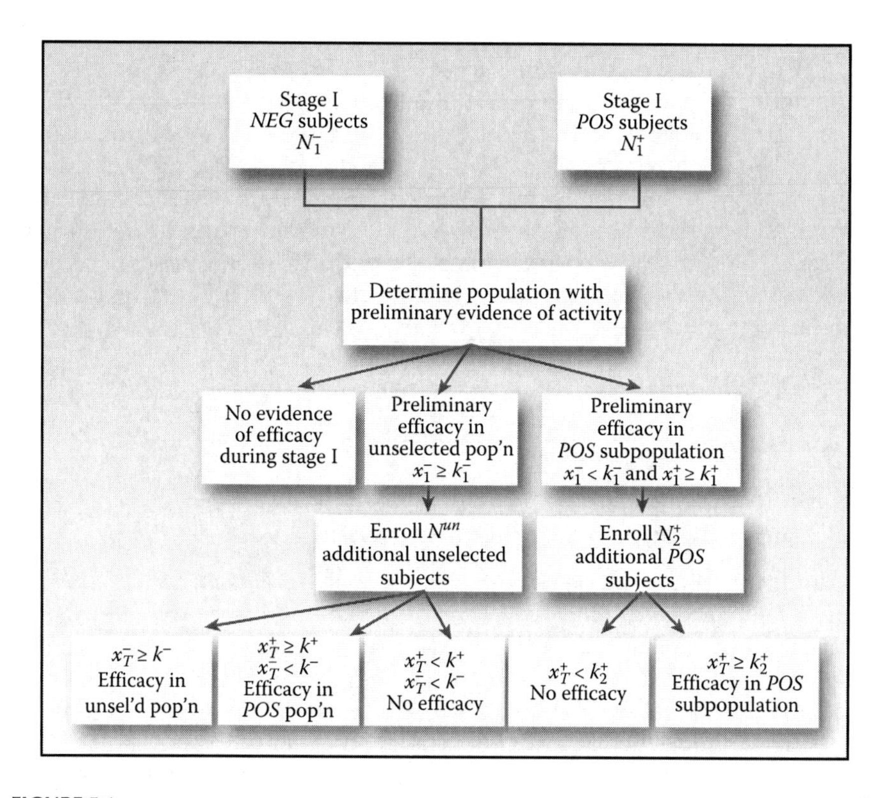

FIGURE 5.1
Schema of adaptive parallel two-stage phase II design. (Reprinted from *Contemp. Clin. Trials*, 28, Jones, C.L and Holmgren E., An adaptive Simon two-stage design for phase 2 studies of targeted therapies, 654–661, 2007, with permission from Elsevier; From McShane, L.M. et al., *Clin. Cancer Res.*, 15, 1898, 2009.)

parallel studies, one conducted in N_1^- biomarker-negative subjects and the other conducted in N_1^+ biomarker-positive subjects. The design continues enrolling N^{un} unselected subjects during the second stage if the number of responses to the drug in the biomarker-negative group in the first stage, X_1^-, meets or exceeds a cutoff of k_1^-. The design enrolls N_2^+ additional biomarker-positive subjects during the second stage and no further biomarker-negative subjects if the number of responses in the biomarker-negative group fails to attain the cutoff k_1^-, while the number of responses in the biomarker-positive group in the first stage, X_1^+, meets or exceeds a cutoff of k_1^+. A total of N^+ and N^- biomarker-positive and biomarker-negative subjects, respectively, will have been enrolled by the end of the second stage. A total of X_T^+ (biomarker-positive group) and X_T^- (biomarker-negative group) responders will have been observed. To make final conclusions regarding efficacy, total responses X_T^+ and X_T^- are then compared against cutoffs k^+ and k^- if unselected patients continued to be enrolled during the second stage, or X_T^+ is compared against the cutoff k_2^+ if only biomarker-positive subjects were enrolled in the second stage. The trial stage- and subgroup-specific samples sizes $N_1^-, N_1^+, N^{un}, N_2^+$ and cutoffs $k_1^-, k_1^+, k^-, k^+, k_2^+$ are determined so that they control the probability of correct conclusions in the biomarker-positive and unselected patient groups. The adaptive design can result in a reduction of expected sample size compared to the nonadaptive two parallel designs. Both the adaptive and nonadaptive designs require careful choice of appropriate benchmark response rates in each of the biomarker-defined subgroups for reasons already discussed for the standard single-arm trial in an enriched patient population.

5.4 Randomized Two-Arm Trials with a Single Biomarker and a Single Experimental Agent

Randomized trials may be preferred for a variety of reasons when evaluating a new targeted agent restricted to a biomarker-positive population (Rubinstein et al. 2005, 2009, 2011). Already mentioned was the difficulty in specifying benchmarks for endpoints in single-arm trials in subpopulations. Another situation in which a single-arm trial would be hard to interpret is when the new targeted agent is given together with an existing agent known to have activity. With uncertainty about the contribution of the existing agent to the overall tumor response in the presence of the experimental agent and restricted to the biomarker-positive subgroup, it can be very difficult to define an appropriate benchmark response rate or progression-free survival rate for a single-arm trial. In order to keep the phase II sample sizes manageable and complete studies in a reasonable timeframe, two differences between randomized phase III studies and randomized phase II designs are (1) the endpoint will typically not be a definitive clinical benefit endpoint like OS but instead be an early measure of clinical activity like response rate or PFS, and (2) the type 1 error rate (alpha level, significance level) will typically be larger than the 0.05 used in a phase III trial.

Freidlin and colleagues (2012) proposed a novel randomized phase II design that can be used to guide decisions regarding the design of a phase III trial for further development of an investigational agent that is linked to a biomarker. Four possible recommendations can result from use of the proposed phase II design: (1) conduct a phase III trial with a biomarker-enrichment design, (2) conduct a randomized phase III trial with a biomarker-stratified design, (3) conduct a randomized phase III design without using the biomarker, and (4) drop consideration of the investigational agent. Descriptions of the biomarker-enrichment design and biomarker-stratified design and other designs along with an extensive discussion of the relative advantages and disadvantages of the various phase III design options are provided by Freidlin et al. (2010) and in Chapters 8 through 10 and 16 of this book.

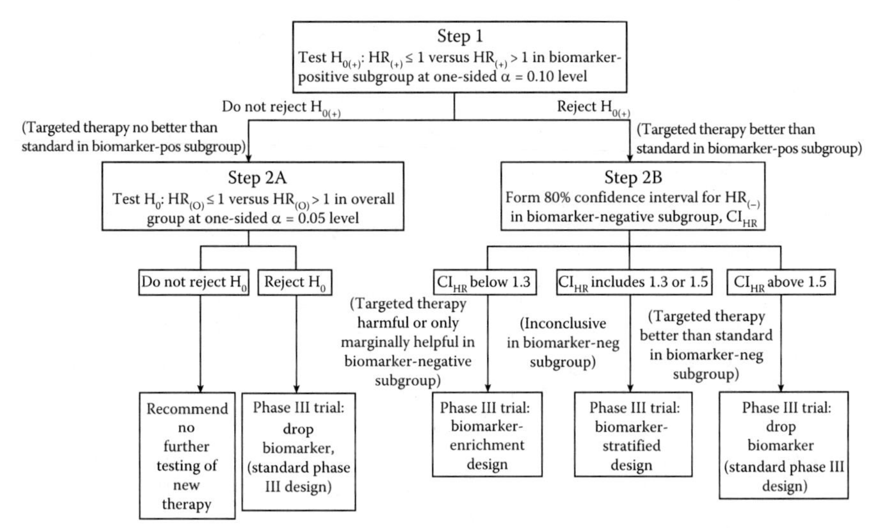

FIGURE 5.2
Schema of phase II randomized design for selection of phase III biomarker-based design. (From Freidlin, B. et al., *J. Clin. Oncol.*, 30, 3304, 2012.)

A schema of the Freidlin et al. (2012) design is presented in Figure 5.2. The design is described assuming a PFS endpoint, but other endpoints could be used. Briefly, step 1 is to test the null hypothesis that PFS is equal in the two treatment arms (new versus control) in the biomarker-positive subgroup when enough events are observed in that subgroup to have at least 90% power to detect a specified treatment effect using a one-sided 0.10 level test (e.g., 56 events are required to have 90% power to detect a doubling of hazard ratio). If step 1 does not reject, then the null hypothesis that PFS is the same in the entire group of randomized patients is tested at a one-sided 0.05 level of significance (step 2A). If this test in step 2A does not reject, then the recommendation is to terminate development of the agent. If the test in step 2A does reject, then it is concluded that the new agent potentially has some activity in the entire population and should be taken forward into a phase III randomized trial dropping the biomarker. If the test in step 1 rejects, then the design proceeds to step 2B in which a two-sided 80% confidence interval is formed for the hazard ratio in the biomarker-negative subgroup (hazard in control group divided by hazard in experimental group). If that confidence interval falls entirely below 1.3, then it is concluded that the new agent is no more than minimally effective in the biomarker-negative subgroup, and a biomarker-enrichment design is recommended for the phase III trial. If the confidence interval falls entirely above 1.5, then it is concluded that there is some evidence that the agent has activity in the entire population and a randomized phase III trial dropping the biomarker is recommended. Sample size estimates for the design ranged from approximately 70–140 patients per biomarker subgroup under an accrual stopping rule that ensures adequate number of patients are accrued within each biomarker subgroup. These estimates were obtained assuming median PFS under standard treatment was 6 months, and the biomarker-positivity rate was between 20% and 67%.

Table 5.1 displays the operating characteristics of the Freidlin et al. (2012) design under a variety of combinations of marker prevalence and treatment effects within each of the biomarker-defined subgroups. When the biomarker prevalence ranges from 20% to 67%, the design reliably (≥87% chance) directs the investigator to no further testing of the experimental agent when the truth is that it offers no benefit in either subgroup. When the hazard ratio is at 1.5 in favor of the new agent in both biomarker subgroups, the design has only 10%–22% chance of recommending no further testing of the agent and will rarely (≤3% chance) recommend an enrichment design for phase III. The most challenging situation is one in which the new agent is slightly inferior to the control therapy in the biomarker-negative subgroup. If the hazard ratio is 1.75 in favor of the new agent in the biomarker-positive subgroup and 0.75 modestly in favor of the control therapy in the biomarker-negative subgroup, then the chance that the design directs the investigator to an enrichment design for phase III drops to 66%–73% when biomarker prevalence is 50%–67%, and the chance that a biomarker-stratified design is recommended is 15%–20%. This behavior is a reflection of the fact that the number of patients will be fairly small in the biomarker-negative subgroup when the biomarker prevalence is high. By continuing on to use of a biomarker-stratified design in phase III, a decision can be made more confidently about whether to abandon the new agent for the biomarker-negative subgroup.

5.5 Nonrandomized Multiarm Trials with Multiple Biomarkers and Multiple Experimental Agents

A natural extension of the single-arm trial conducted in a biomarker-positive subgroup is a nonrandomized multiarm trial that can serve as a screening platform for experimental agents. All patients are accrued through a central system and are tested for a panel of biomarkers for which experimental targeted agents are available. On the basis of the biomarker findings in a patient's tumor, the patient is directed to a therapy arm delivering an appropriate targeted therapy (Figure 5.3). This design is not intended to definitively evaluate the predictive ability of the biomarkers; the main goal is to determine whether the agents can demonstrate activity in biomarker-defined

TABLE 5.1

Simulated Probabilities of Four Decision Outcomes of Randomized Phase II Biomarker Design under Different Scenarios

	Scenario						Probabilities of Recommendations for Trial Design for Future Phase III Testing			
	Biomarker-Positive Subgroup			Biomarker-Negative Subgroup						
Number	Expt. Tx. Median PFS	Control Median PFS	Hazard Ratio	Expt. Tx. Median PFS	Control Median PFS	Hazard Ratio	Enrichment Design	Biomarker-Stratified	No Biomarker	No Further Testing
							Prevalence of biomarker positive = 20%			
1.	4	4	1.0	4	4	1.0	0.06	0.04	0.03	0.87
2.	8	4	2.0	4	4	1.0	0.53	0.36	0.01	0.10
3.	6	4	1.5	6	4	1.5	0.01	0.52	0.38	0.10
4.	7	4	1.75	7	4	1.75	<0.01	0.51	0.48	0.01
5.	8	4	2.0	6	4	1.5	0.02	0.79	0.18	0.02
6.	8	4	2.0	5	4	1.25	0.13	0.76	0.06	0.06
7.	7	4	1.75	3	4	0.75	0.76	0.02	<0.01	0.22
8.	6	6	1.0	4	4	1.0	0.06	0.04	0.02	0.87
							Prevalence of biomarker positive = 33%			
1.	4	4	1.0	4	4	1.0	0.06	0.05	0.03	0.87
2.	8	4	2.0	4	4	1.0	0.50	0.40	0.01	0.09
3.	6	4	1.5	6	4	1.5	0.01	0.52	0.34	0.14
4.	7	4	1.75	7	4	1.75	<0.01	0.54	0.44	0.02
5.	8	4	2.0	6	4	1.5	0.02	0.79	0.17	0.03
6.	8	4	2.0	5	4	1.25	0.13	0.76	0.06	0.06
7.	7	4	1.75	3	4	0.75	0.75	0.04	<0.01	0.22
8.	6	6	1.0	4	4	1.0	0.06	0.05	0.02	0.88

(Continued)

TABLE 5.1 (*Continued*)

Simulated Probabilities of Four Decision Outcomes of Randomized Phase II Biomarker Design under Different Scenarios

	Scenario						Probabilities of Recommendations for Trial Design for Future Phase III Testing			
	Biomarker-Positive Subgroup			Biomarker-Negative Subgroup						
Number	Expt. Tx. Median PFS	Control Median PFS	Hazard Ratio	Expt. Tx. Median PFS	Control Median PFS	Hazard Ratio	Enrichment Design	Biomarker-Stratified	No Biomarker	No Further Testing
							Prevalence of biomarker positive = 50%			
1.	4	4	1.0	4	4	1.0	0.04	0.06	0.02	0.88
2.	8	4	2.0	4	4	1.0	0.38	0.53	<0.01	0.08
3.	6	4	1.5	6	4	1.5	0.02	0.52	0.23	0.22
4.	7	4	1.75	7	4	1.75	0.01	0.60	0.33	0.06
5.	8	4	2.0	6	4	1.5	0.03	0.79	0.14	0.04
6.	8	4	2.0	5	4	1.25	0.12	0.77	0.05	0.07
7.	7	4	1.75	3	4	0.75	0.66	0.15	<0.01	0.20
8.	6	6	1.0	4	4	1.0	0.04	0.06	0.02	0.88
							Prevalence of biomarker positive = 67%			
1.	4	4	1.0	4	4	1.0	0.04	0.06	0.02	0.88
2.	8	4	2.0	4	4	1.0	0.38	0.61	<0.01	0.01
3.	6	4	1.5	6	4	1.5	0.03	0.68	0.16	0.14
4.	7	4	1.75	7	4	1.75	0.01	0.71	0.25	0.02
5.	8	4	2.0	6	4	1.5	0.03	0.85	0.11	0.01
6.	8	4	2.0	5	4	1.25	0.13	0.83	0.03	0.010
7.	7	4	1.75	3	4	0.75	0.73	0.20	<0.01	0.06
8.	6	6	1.0	4	4	1.0	0.04	0.06	0.01	0.89

Source: Freidlin, B. et al., *J. Clin. Oncol.*, 30, 3304, 2012.
Note: Simulations are based on 50,000 replications.

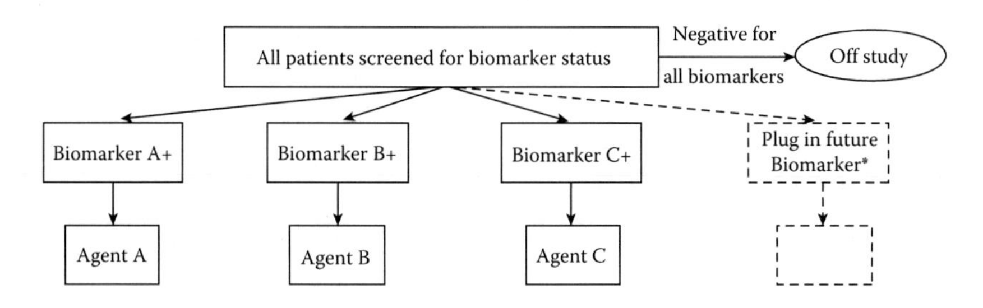

FIGURE 5.3
Schema of nonrandomized multiarm signal-finding trial with multiple biomarkers and multiple experimental agents. *This design allows for adding new biomarker-defined subgroups and corresponding targeted experimental agents during the course of the trial.

subgroups where preliminary understanding of the mechanism of action of the drug suggests there is greatest likelihood of their having activity. It may be a single biomarker that is associated with each targeted agent, or a collection of biomarkers might be used to test for activation of a particular pathway that is targeted by one of the experimental agents. Formal combination of biomarkers into a mathematical classifier to select therapy is also possible. The details of constructing such classifiers are covered elsewhere in this book (see Chapters 12, 14, and 15). All of the issues concerning choice of endpoint and choice of benchmark for establishing activity in the possible presence of prognostic effects also apply here as they did in the case of a single-arm single biomarker trial.

A nonrandomized multiarm trial such as just described can function as multiple independent single-arm trials, and viewed this way, no statistical adjustment to control overall type I error should be necessary. However, in some situations, there might be relationships between the biomarkers or between the agents. Some adaptive designs have been proposed to *borrow information* between arms. Such adaptive approaches generally require modeling assumptions, and larger sample sizes may be needed to protect against misspecification of models and achieve robust results. Readers are referred to Chapters 6, 7, and 16 for a discussion of adaptive designs.

A logistical issue that may arise in these multiarm, multiple biomarker trials is how to allocate treatment to patients whose tumors possess more than one of the biomarkers that determine eligibility for the investigational agents included in the trial. If the percent overlap in biomarker prevalence between any two arms is very small, this should not present much of a problem because the influence on the results should be minimal regardless of the arm to which a patient with more than one biomarker is assigned. If the overlap is substantial, then a decision has to be made to either randomly assign the patient (with either equal or weighted allocation) to one of the arms or to prioritize the arms by some deterministic rule. If patients who are positive for more than one marker have substantially different outcome than patients who are positive for only a single marker, then the study arm-specific results must be interpreted with care to acknowledge that the patients with overlapping biomarkers are over- or underrepresented; these situations may warrant considering patients whose tumors are positive for more than one marker to belong to a different biological group than those whose tumors are positive for only a single marker and potentially modifying therapy choice accordingly.

5.6 Randomized Multiarm Trials with Multiple Biomarkers and Multiple Experimental Agents

A natural extension of a randomized trial conducted in a biomarker-positive subgroup is a randomized multiarm trial with multiple biomarkers that can serve as a screening platform for experimental agents. All patients are accrued through a central system and are tested for a panel of biomarkers for which experimental targeted agents are available. On the basis of the biomarker findings in a patient's tumor, the patient is directed to a particular randomization that includes an arm containing a targeted therapy directed at that biomarker (Figure 5.4). As in the case of the nonrandomized multiarm trial with a multiple biomarkers discussed in the previous section, it may be a single biomarker that is associated with each targeted agent, or a collection of biomarkers, possibly combined into a mathematical classifier, might be used to test for activation of a particular pathway that is targeted by one of the experimental agents. An important advantage of a randomized design compared to a nonrandomized design is that it avoids problems of confounding by biomarker prognostic effects and eliminates the difficulty of specifying an outcome benchmark for establishing activity in a single arm. Randomization is also generally advisable when evaluating combinations of agents unless one can confidently rule out the possibility of any of the

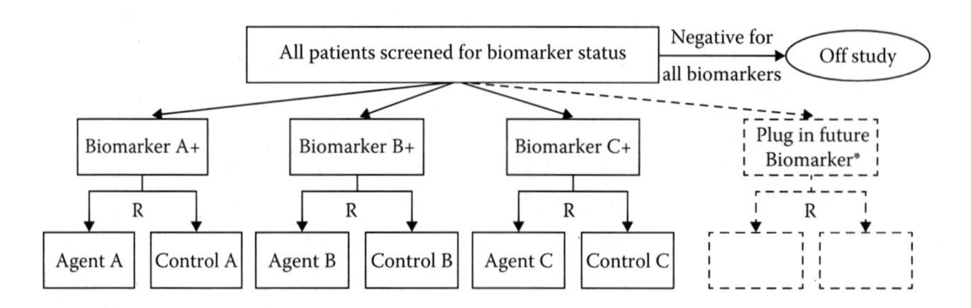

FIGURE 5.4
Schema of multiarm randomized trial with multiple biomarkers and multiple experimental agents (R denotes randomization). *This design allows for adding new biomarker-defined subgroups and corresponding targeted experimental agents during the course of the trial.

individual agents having activity when used alone (Rubinstein et al. 2011). The price paid for these protections is that a substantially larger sample size is generally required to conduct a randomized clinical trial compared to a nonrandomized trial (with reliable historical controls).

There can be considerable flexibility in the nature of the randomization within each biomarker subgroup. Within each biomarker subgroup, there could be a simple randomization between a targeted agent and a control treatment, or one could randomize between multiple agents each targeting that biomarker. If the patients on the trial have exhausted all standard treatment options, then for each targeted agent the matched control arm could be a randomization to any of the other treatment arms if it is believed that the agents could have potentially beneficial off-target effects and the toxicities are minimal. The design within each biomarker subgroup could be a phase II selection design, in which there is randomization to multiple agents targeting that biomarker, or it could be a phase II screening design in which one or more experimental agents is randomized against a standard therapy (Rubinstein et al. 2005, 2009). Multiarm trials with several experimental arms and a shared control arm can offer substantial efficiency advantages in both phase II and phase III trials (Freidlin et al. 2008). The idea of a shared control arm should not be misinterpreted to mean that the same patients can serve as controls for all patients receiving any biomarker-targeted therapy. The control patients must be matched on biomarker characteristics to those of the patients on the targeted therapy arm to which it is paired in order to avoid confounding biomarker prognostic effects with treatment effects. In addition, no statistical adjustment to control overall type I error across biomarker subgroups should be necessary for the reasons cited previously for nonrandomized multiarm biomarker-based trials.

Some percentage of patients who are screened for a trial involving multiple biomarkers will be negative for all biomarkers. These patients can either be declared ineligible for the trial or they could be randomized to one of the agents in the trial if they have exhausted all standard treatment options and if it is believed that the agents could have potentially beneficial off-target effects and the toxicities are minimal. If there is a standard therapy available for these patients, they could be assigned to a common standard therapy control arm. This would allow for assessment of prognostic effects of the markers by comparing outcome for marker-positive patients randomized to control within their biomarker subgroup to outcome for biomarker-negative patients who received that same control therapy. Outcome for these patients who are negative for all biomarkers would not be included in the primary statistical comparisons of treatment effect within each biomarker subgroup. As previously discussed for the nonrandomized multiarm trials with multiple biomarkers, decisions have to be made regarding how to assign therapy for patients who are positive for more than one biomarker, and this may affect interpretation of the study results.

5.7 Randomized Phase II/III Trials with Biomarkers

A primary goal of a phase II trial is to screen experimental agents to establish preliminary evidence of efficacy and decide whether it is worthwhile to proceed to a definitive phase III trial. Phase II/III trials have been proposed as a means to seamlessly proceed from a phase II trial to a phase III trial when an experimental agent shows an effect on an intermediate endpoint that serves as the phase II endpoint (Hunsberger et al. 2009; Korn et al. 2012). Usually the intermediate endpoint is an endpoint such as PFS or tumor response that can be observed sooner than the definitive phase III endpoint (e.g., OS). However, it is also possible to use the same endpoint for the phase II intermediate analysis as for the definitive phase III analysis.

The full sample size for a phase II/III trial is calculated using the definitive phase III endpoint. An intermediate analysis is performed after a specified number of events for the phase II endpoint have been observed on the study. Usually accrual is allowed to continue in the period between the time that the specified number of phase II events is reached and the time that the intermediate analysis results become available. In situations where the phase II endpoint is the same as the phase III endpoint, or when accrual is rapid and there is concern about substantially overaccruing patients should the phase II analysis result in a recommendation to terminate the study, it may be advisable to temporarily suspend accrual until completion of the phase II analysis. If the comparison based on the intermediate endpoint meets specified criteria (i.e., consistent with promise of the experimental agent), then accrual to the trial continues to the full sample size. If the study continues to full accrual, then patients who were accrued to the phase II trial continue to be followed for observation of the definitive phase III clinical endpoint along with the additional patients (Figure 5.5). No adjustment to the type I error for the phase III analysis is needed for the phase II/III design because the interim analysis of the phase II endpoint allows only for early stopping when there is evidence for futility and not for superiority. To protect against premature stopping and the possibility of missing an effective agent, one typically allows a fairly generous type I error for the phase II analysis (e.g., $\alpha = 0.10$) and chooses a phase II sample size (for the intermediate analysis) that provides high power to detect a moderate-size treatment effect on the intermediate endpoint.

Important issues to consider in the specification of the phase II intermediate analysis are the choice of endpoint and target effect size. Tumor response may be an appropriate endpoint when the experimental agent is expected to have as its primary mode of action be tumor shrinkage, but some targeted agents are not expected to produce substantial tumor shrinkage; rather, they may be expected to hit a molecular target and halt or slow disease progression, but not result in robust tumor shrinkage. In this case, progression-free

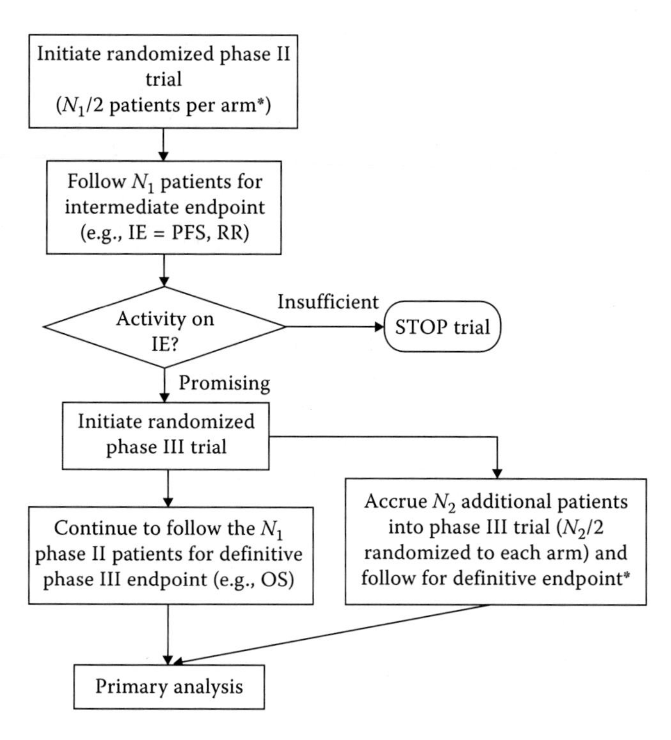

FIGURE 5.5
Schema of phase II/III design. *The sample sizes N_1 and N_2 are the numbers of patients needed to observe the numbers of events required for the phase II and III analyses.

survival would be a better intermediate endpoint. If there is sufficient confidence that the mechanism of action of the targeted agent operates through a biomarker, then it may be reasonable to use the biomarker as an endpoint in the phase II portion of the trial, possibly in combination with some evidence for delayed tumor progression. With a biomarker, however, specification of an appropriate target treatment effect size for the phase II intermediate analysis may be challenging because it may not be clear what magnitude of effect on the phase II endpoint translates to an effect on the definitive phase III endpoint.

The phase II/III trial design can be used with multiple experimental agents where each agent is compared to the control arm when the interim analysis is conducted. Only experimental arms that pass the criteria when compared to the control arm move forward to the phase III component of the study. A question that arises for multiarm trials such as these is whether type I error should be adjusted to account for the fact that there are multiple comparisons of experimental arms with the control arm. A reasonable guideline is that if the experimental arms are substantially different and could just as likely have been evaluated in separate trials, then adjustment for multiple comparisons is not necessary. In contrast, if the experimental arms are related (e.g., varying dose or schedule of same agent, or alternate formulations of an agent), then a multiple comparisons adjustment should be applied (Freidlin et al. 2008; Korn et al. 2012).

Parallel phase II/III designs can also be used to study multiple biomarkers and targeted agents. Separate randomized phase II/III study designs are followed for each group of patients defined by a particular biomarker. Within a biomarker-defined subgroup, patients are randomized to either standard of care or to an experimental agent targeted to that biomarker. This type of design is appealing when there is a common screening protocol that can be used to assign patients to different biomarker subgroups. An example of a multiple biomarker phase II/III design is a *master protocol* under development for investigation of several targeted therapies for squamous cell lung cancer (Ledford 2013; Ong 2013).

5.8 Summary and Generalizations

A wide variety of options for phase II designs incorporating biomarkers are available. Several of the basic options used in oncology have been discussed in this chapter, and hybrid designs incorporating several of these basic features can also be used. Increasingly, multiphase, multiple-biomarker trial designs that concurrently evaluate experimental treatments and biomarkers used to guide treatment selection, while transitioning seamlessly from early phase trials to confirmatory phase III trials, are being proposed (Kaplan et al. 2013). To extend these designs to medical settings other than oncology, one must decide on what are the meaningful clinical endpoints in those other settings. These other settings might include chronic or relapsing and remitting diseases, infectious diseases, or rare diseases (Korn et al. 2013) that present additional challenges and opportunities for innovative trial design and analysis strategies (Peace 2009). Important considerations in other disease settings include where and when to measure the biomarkers. In oncology, one usually has the opportunity to measure biomarkers in the patient's tumor at diagnosis or recurrence, or assess germline DNA variants or circulating protein biomarkers in patient blood or other bodily fluids, including serial collection. A myriad of other biomarkers may be of relevance to treatment of cancer and other medical conditions, for example, presence and type of infectious agent or biomarkers of inflammatory or immune response. Better understanding of disease biology and appropriate use of biomarkers will lead to more rational, informative, and effective phase II trials, and a more efficient drug development process.

References

Freidlin, B., E.L. Korn, R. Gray et al. 2008. Multi-arm clinical trials of new agents: Some design considerations. *Clin Cancer Res* 14:4368–4371.

Freidlin, B., L.M. McShane, E.L. Korn. 2010. Randomized clinical trials with biomarkers: Design issues. *J Natl Cancer Inst* 102:152–160.

Freidlin, B., L.M. McShane, M.-Y.C. Polley et al. 2012. Randomized phase II trial designs with biomarkers. *J Clin Oncol* 30:3304–3309.

Green, S., J. Benedetti, A. Smith, J. Crowley. 2012. *Clinical Trials in Oncology*, 3rd ed. Boca Raton, FL: Chapman & Hall/CRC.

Hunsberger, S., Y. Zhao, R. Simon. 2009. A comparison of phase II study strategies. *Clin Cancer Res* 15:5950–5955.

Jones, C.L., E. Holmgren. 2007. An adaptive Simon two-stage design for phase 2 studies of targeted therapies. *Contemp Clin Trials* 28:654–661.

Kaplan, R., T. Maughan, A. Crook et al. 2013. Evaluating many treatments and biomarkers in oncology: A new design. *J Clin Oncol* 31(36):4562–4568.

Korn, E.L., B. Freidlin, J.S. Abrams et al. 2012. Design issues in randomized phase II/III trials. *J Clin Oncol* 30:667–671.

Korn, E.L., L.M. McShane, B. Freidlin. 2013. Statistical challenges in the evaluation of treatments for small patient populations. *Sci Transl Med* 5:178sr3.

Kummar, S., M. Gutierrez, J.H. Doroshow et al. 2006. Drug development in oncology: Classical cytotoxics and molecularly targeted agents. *Br J Clin Pharmacol* 62:15–26.

Ledford, H. 2013. 'Master protocol' aims to revamp cancer trials. *Nature* 498:146.

McShane, L.M., S. Hunsberger, A.A. Adjei. 2009. Effective incorporation of biomarkers into Phase II trials. *Clin Cancer Res* 15:1898–1905.

Ong, M.B.H. (November 15, 2013). "Master Protocol" to rely on biomarkers in testing multiple lung cancer agents. *The Cancer Letter*, p. 1. Retrieved February 21, 2014, from http://www.cancerletter.com/articles/20131115/CL39-43.pdf.

Peace, K.E. 2009. *Design and Analysis of Clinical Trials with Time-to-Event endpoints.* Boca Raton, FL: Chapman & Hall/CRC.

Rubinstein, L.V., J. Crowley, P. Ivy et al. 2009. Randomized phase II designs. *Clin Cancer Res* 15:1883–1890.

Rubinstein, L.V., E.L. Korn, B. Freidlin et al. 2005. Design issues of randomized phase II trials and a proposal for phase II screening trials. *J Clin Oncol* 23:7199–7206.

Rubinstein, L.V., M. LeBlanc, M.A. Smith. 2011. More randomization in phase II trials: Necessary but not sufficient. *J Natl Cancer Inst* 103:1075–1077.

Simon, R. 1989. Optimal two-stage designs for phase II clinical trials. *Contr Clin Trials* 10:1–10.

6

Bayesian Adaptive Methods for Clinical Trials of Targeted Agents

Peter Thall

CONTENTS

6.1 Introduction

This chapter provides an overview of Bayesian concepts and methods for design and conduct of clinical trials of treatment regimens, including targeted agents. A targeted treatment regimen may consist of one agent, a combination of agents, or a sequence of agents given over multiple stages, and it also may specify the dose, schedule, or schedule–dose combinations of each agent. The illustrations include Bayesian dose-finding based on time to toxicity, dose-finding based on both toxicity and efficacy, and randomized trials to evaluate effects of multiple targeted regimens on efficacy or an event time such as progression-free survival (PFS) or overall survival (OS) time.

Patient-specific or subgroup-specific decision rules are defined in terms of a vector, $\mathbf{Z}=(Z_1,\ldots, Z_p)$, of binary or quantitative biomarkers such as gene or protein expressions, and possibly a vector, $\mathbf{X}=(X_1,\ldots, X_q)$, of conventional prognostic variables such as performance status or number of prior therapies. The decision rules are refined repeatedly during trial conduct using updated posteriors as new patient data are acquired, hence are sequentially adaptive between patients.

Denote the set of agents being evaluated by $\mathcal{T}=\{\tau_1,\ldots, \tau_J\}$. Each design's final conclusion is not a single optimal element or subset of $\mathcal{T}$ to be given to all patients. Rather, a design selects or recommends *individualized* treatment combinations that choose a subset of $\mathcal{T}$ tailored to a given patient's $(\mathbf{Z}, \mathbf{X})$. An individualized treatment regimen of targeted agents is a function, ρ, from the set of all $(\mathbf{Z}, \mathbf{X})$ to the set of all 2^J subsets of $\mathcal{T}$, with $\rho(\mathbf{Z}, \mathbf{X})=\varphi$, the empty set, corresponding to *Do not treat this patient* (DNT). Each set $\rho(\mathbf{Z}, \mathbf{X})$ includes τ_js that are *targeted* at one or more gene or protein biomarkers in $\mathbf{Z}$. In this sense, the designs and rules are adaptive within patients. For example, temporarily ignoring $\mathbf{X}$, if $\tau=\{\tau_1, \tau_2, \tau_3\}$, with τ_3 conventional therapy, and $\mathbf{Z}=(Z_1, Z_2)$ are two indicators of particular cancer cell surface markers, the optimal regimen may be $\rho(0, 0)=\{\tau_3\}$, $\rho(1, 0)=\{\tau_1, \tau_3\}$, $\rho(0, 1)=\{\tau_2, \tau_3\}$, or $\rho(1, 1)=\{\tau_1, \tau_2, \tau_3\}$. Alternatively, if no conventional therapy exists for the disease, then $\mathcal{T}=\{\tau_1, \tau_2\}$ and $\rho(0, 0)=\varphi$, no treatment. An example is well-differentiated liposarcoma, with τ_1 targeting estrogen receptor–positive disease $(Z_1=1)$ and τ_2 targeting androgen receptor–positive disease $(Z_2=1)$. If it is certain that (1) each τ_j can only benefit patients with $Z_j=1$, (2) there are no other agents with established efficacy, and (3) toxicity is negligible, then an optimal regimen would be $\rho(1, 1)=\{\tau_1, \tau_2\}$, $\rho(1, 0)=\tau_1$, $\rho(0, 1)=\tau_2$, $\rho(0, 0)=\varphi$. If any of these three assumptions are not true, then one or more clinical trials to evaluate τ_1 and τ_2 must be conducted. In early phase I or I–II evaluation, each τ_j may be extended, for example, to a set $\{\tau_j(d_1),\ldots, \tau_j(d_5)\}$ of the agent given at five possible doses, and a further elaboration could involve two or more administration modes or schedules of τ_j (Braun et al., 2007; Thall et al., 2013).

While a great deal of science motivates the use of $\mathbf{Z}$, in clinical practice it is often important to include common, well-understood prognostic covariates, $\mathbf{X}$. For example, an agent τ_1 may target an overexpressed protein represented by Z_1 with the aim to disrupt a signaling pathway leading to cancer cell growth. If τ_1 also causes immunosuppression and a patient has received $X_1=2$ previous immunosuppressive therapies, then potential adverse effects of τ_1 in that patient must be considered along with its potential benefits. Statistical formalisms and genomic/proteomic data notwithstanding, physicians have been choosing individualized treatment regimens based on patient prognostic variables for thousands of years.

To provide a concrete frame of reference, many of the designs discussed here will refer to the problem of clinically evaluating a new molecule, M, targeting the KRAS pathway in patients with locally advanced non-small-cell lung cancer (NSCLC). The patients have approximate median

DFS time 8 months with standard therapy comprising chemotherapy with carboplatin + paclitaxel and radiation therapy (chemoradiation, C). Each component of C is given at an established dose/schedule. The two patient subgroups are KRAS+ ($Z = 1$, abnormal expression, caused by a mutated KRAS gene) and KRAS− ($Z = 0$, normal KRAS gene expression or *wild type*). Two treatments are considered, C and $C + M$.

6.2 Design Issues for Trials of Targeted Agents

In developing a targeted anticancer therapy, conventionally it is first demonstrated that a molecule designed to activate or deactivate a particular target can kill cancer cells *in vitro*, then that it can shrink tumors or extend survival in rodents that have been given the targeted cancer. Such results are not sufficient to imply that the agent will be either safe or effective in humans, or what the best dose or schedule of the agent, or possibly a combination including the agent may be. This can be assessed only by giving the agent to humans who have the disease and observing their outcomes in a clinical trial. While this empirical point is obvious to biostatisticians and clinical oncologists, it is often missed by laboratory-based researchers who may be overly optimistic based on preclinical data. Because many new targeted agents turn out to be ineffective in humans, researchers should be prepared for failure, not just success. Because many new agents are not as safe as anticipated and may have severe adverse effects, formal safety monitoring/stopping rules are essential to protect patients enrolled in clinical trials. For targeted agents showing substantive antidisease effects in humans, this may not be due to the precise mechanism initially believed, but rather to antidisease effects in patients not having the targeted gene or protein abnormality. Trial designs must anticipate such unexpected outcomes.

As new targeted agents flood the clinical trial arena, it is essential to utilize resources efficiently. A major feasibility issue is the time required to evaluate $\mathbf{Z}$ for each newly enrolled patient since it is undesirable to delay therapy unduly. It is also important to harvest as much useful information per patient as possible. In addition to OS time, a patient's actual clinical outcome often is a vector of longitudinal and event time variables. In treatment of solid tumors, these often include some combination of ordinal severities of different types of toxicity (cf. Bekele and Thall, 2003), time to toxicity (Cheung and Chappell, 2000; Yuan and Yin, 2009), and an ordinal response, such as PD (progressive disease), SD (stable disease), PR (partial response), and CR (complete response) for solid tumors. These variables are often evaluated repeatedly, subject to informative discontinuation of follow-up due to patient dropout or the decision by the attending physician that toxicity or PD precludes further treatment (cf. Wang et al., 2012). In chemotherapy of acute leukemia or lymphoma, typical outcomes include the times to infection, CR, or resistant disease (Thall et al., 2002) and, among patients who initially achieve a CR, subsequent DFS time (Shen and Thall, 1998). In stem cell transplant (SCT), common outcomes include the times to engraftment, disease recurrence, infection, graft-versus-host-disease, or death. SCT trial data also routinely include longitudinal counts of a variety of blood cells defined in terms of their surface biomarkers. In such settings, the common practice in trial design of characterizing patient outcome as either one binary *response* or one right-censored event time wastes a great deal of useful information. Ignoring covariates, multiple outcomes, longitudinal data, or adaptive treatment decisions made by physicians may lead to misleading conclusions about treatment effects (cf. Hernan et al., 2000; Wahed and Thall, 2013). With complex outcomes and treatment–biomarker interactions, *treatment effect* becomes a high-dimensional object, and conventional statistical methods become inadequate. Utilizing all or most of the available information is very challenging, very time consuming, and typically leads to complex statistical models and trial designs (cf. Thall and Wathen, 2005; Thall et al., 2007; Saville et al., 2009; Zhao et al., 2011).

Bayesian models and posterior decision criteria provide a practical paradigm to account for multiple sources of variability, borrow strength between related subgroups, and construct designs with multiple, sequentially adaptive decision rules (cf. Thall et al., 1995). Such decision rules may (1) select an optimal treatment regimen or a set of regimens; (2) terminate one or more regimens, or the entire trial, due to excessive toxicity or poor efficacy; (3) change sample size based on updated estimates of design or model parameters; or (4) change randomization probabilities adaptively within subgroups to favor empirically more successful regimes (cf. Thall and Wathen, 2005, 2007). With targeted agents, each of these decisions may be made differently for individual patients or subgroups depending on $(\mathbf{Z}, \mathbf{X})$. Optimizing each patient's regimen as a function of $(\mathbf{Z}, \mathbf{X})$ is the ultimate goal of individualized, targeted treatment. Since the combination of decision rules used in a trial may be quite complex, in practice it is necessary to use computer simulation of the trial as a design tool to calibrate fixed prior or hyperprior parameters, and design parameters, to ensure that the design has good frequentist properties.

In clinical research, false negative conclusions may be far more destructive errors than false positives. Despite the deeply ingrained requirement to control type I error in conventional clinical trials, a false positive conclusion almost certainly will be discovered if an ineffective or unsafe new treatment receives regulatory approval and subsequently is used to treat patients. How detrimental this is to patients during this later, so-called *phase IV* evaluation process depends on what other treatments are available. Because the medical research community avidly seeks therapeutic improvements, any treatment advanced by a false positive must compete with promising new treatments, and often with previous *standard* treatments. In contrast, a putatively ineffective new agent that actually could provide substantive benefit is unlikely to be explored further or given to future patients. One prominent cause of false negatives is that, because immense resources are spent on large-scale trials of very few agents, many new agents simply are not evaluated clinically. A less obvious problem is the common failure to do a good job of optimizing a new agent's dose and schedule. If an ineffective or suboptimal dose or schedule is chosen in a small early-phase trial, this may cripple a new agent's ability to hit its target, and subsequent evaluation of the agent's long-term antidisease effects may be doomed to failure (cf. Thall, 2012; Section 2).

In trials of targeted agents, these problems are more severe. Because many regime–biomarker interaction parameters must be estimated, the risks of incorrect decisions are much greater. Rather than two $C+M$ and C treatment effect parameters to be evaluated and compared, the NSCLC trial has four effects on each outcome, corresponding to $(\rho, Z)=(C+M, 1)$, $(C+M, 0)$, $(C, 1)$, $(C, 0)$, and the effect of M must be evaluated in each of the two biomarker subgroups. With J targeted agents and p binary biomarkers, there are $J \times p$ agent–biomarker interactions, and potentially 2^J regimens. Since even moderately large J and p produce intractably large numbers of targeted regimens and parameters to be evaluated, inevitably clinical trial strategies must include practical, reliable methods for dimension reduction that select agents, biomarkers, and agent–biomarker combinations to evaluate.

6.3 Dose-Finding Trials

6.3.1 A Phase I Trial with KRAS+ Patients

An optimal dose of M, when combined with C, may be determined in several ways, depending on clinical outcomes, ethics, and feasibility. A 24-patient phase I trial was designed to choose an *optimal* dose, d^{opt}, from four levels, based on toxicity. Toxicity was defined to include grade 4 esophagitis, esophageal perforation, dermatitis, or nausea/vomiting; and grade 3 or 4 nonhematological toxicities including anorexia, fatigue, infection, and pneumonitis, occurring within 70 days from the start of therapy. With $C+M$, most of the risk of toxicity may be attributed to C. Due to logistical difficulties with the long, 70-day toxicity evaluation period, the TiTE-CRM (Cheung and Chappell, 2000; Section 6.3.2.3) was used, with target toxicity probability 0.60. This unusually high target was chosen because there is a baseline rate of .35 with C and, as in most toxicity-based phase I trials, it was believed that a dose associated with this higher toxicity rate would also provide higher efficacy in terms of longer DFS. Accrual was restricted to KRAS+ patients, motivated by the belief that it would be unethical to include KRAS− patients since they do not have the biomarker targeted by M and thus should not be exposed to potential toxicity of M before d^{opt} has been determined. The plan was to conduct a subsequent randomized trial of C versus $C+M(d^{opt})$ including both KRAS+ and KRAS– patients, where $M(d^{opt})$ is M given at the d^{opt} determined in phase I. Excluding KRAS– patients from phase I implies that it is more desirable to deprive KRAS– patients of potential benefit of M as a trade-off for excluding the additional risk of toxicity, due to M and beyond that of C, before d^{opt} has been determined. At the same time, it was believed that, given the d^{opt} for M for which the probability of toxicity with $C+M(d^{opt})$ was closest to 0.60, it would be ethical to randomize patients between C and $C+M(d^{opt})$.

6.3.2 A Phase I Trial with KRAS+ and KRAS– Patients

It could be argued that, given the 8-month median DFS with C, potential improvement in DFS due to adding M is a desirable trade-off for the risk of toxicity in KRAS– patients in phase I. If both KRAS+ and KRAS– patients are included in phase I, one may consider the possibility that these two subgroups may have different toxicity rates and hence different d^{opt} values. The following phase I design accommodates this.

Define G subgroups in terms of $(\mathbf{Z}, \mathbf{X})$, indexed by $g=0, 1,\ldots, G-1$ with $g=0$ the baseline subgroup. The goal is to determine d_g^{opt} for each g. Denote the numerically standardized doses by $\mathbf{D}=\{d_1,\ldots, d_m\}$. Let T = time to toxicity, T^o = observed time to toxicity or right-censoring, and $\delta=I(T^o=T)$, so (T^o, δ) is the observed outcome. Let T^* be a fixed reference time, specified by the physician, and denote $\pi(d, g, \theta)=\Pr(T \le T^* | d, g, \theta)$, the probability of toxicity by T^* for a patient in subgroup g given dose $d \in D$, where θ is the model parameter vector. In the NSLC trial, $m=4$ doses and $T^*=70$ days. One might use $Z=I(\text{KRAS+})$, $X_1=I(\text{good PS})$, and $X_2=0$, 1, or 2 previous treatments to determine $G=12$ subgroups. Since it is not feasible to reliably determine $G=2\times 2\times 3=12$ optimal doses with $N_{max}=24$, either a larger N_{max} is needed or G must be reduced. One may obtain $G=4$ by collapsing (X_1, X_2) into $X_{1,2}=I[X_1=1 \text{ and } X_2=0]$, an indicator of favorable prognosis. In practice, a design's reliability should be investigated for several (G, N_{max}) pairs by computer simulation during the design process. The trade-off between practical limitations on N_{max} and the desire to investigate larger G or $\mathbf{Z}$ is central to trial design for individualized therapy and targeted agents.

The pdf and survivor function of $[T|d, g, \theta]$ are $f(t|d, g, \theta)$ and $\mathbf{F}(t|d, g, \theta)=\Pr(T\ge t|d, g, \theta)$ for $t>0$, so $\pi(d, g, \theta)=1-\mathbf{F}(T^*|d, g, \theta)$. The distribution of T may be chosen based on prior knowledge about the form of the toxicity hazard function over $[0, T^*]$. Some practical choices are a Weibull, which has a monotone increasing, decreasing, or constant (exponential) hazard, a gamma, or a lognormal, which may have a nonmonotone hazard. Model choice depends on flexibility, tractability, and robustness, and should be studied by computer simulation. A linear term characterizing how T varies with (d, g) is

$$\eta(d,g,\theta) = \mu + \alpha d + \sum_{g=1}^{G-1} (\beta_g + d\gamma_g),$$

with $\theta = (\mu, \alpha, \beta_1, \ldots, \beta_{G-1}, \gamma_1, \ldots, \gamma_{G-1})$, so $\dim(\theta) = 2G$. For the lognormal, $\eta(d, g, \theta)$ is the mean of $\log(T)$, for the exponential or Weibull $\eta(d, g, \theta)$ acts on the log hazard domain, etc. The baseline subgroup ($g = 0$) dose effect is α and, in each subgroup $g \geq 1$, $\mu + \beta_g$ is the main effect and $\alpha + \gamma_g$ is the dose effect, so γ_g is the dose–subgroup interaction. It is essential to include the γ_gs since, if in fact $\gamma_g^{true} \neq 0$, then assuming a model without the γ_gs can lead to erroneous conclusions and a design with poor performance. Each patient's data are (T^o, δ, d, g), and the likelihood is the usual form for right-censored event time data,

$$L(T^o, \delta | d, g, \theta) = \{f(T^o | d, g, \theta)\}^{\delta} \{F(T^o | d, g, \theta)\}^{1-\delta}.$$

For n patients, $data_n = \left\{\left(T_i^o, \delta_i, d_{[i]}, g_i\right),\ \ i = 1, \ldots, n\right\}$, the likelihood is $L_n = \Pi_i L\left(T_i^o, \delta_i | d_{[i]}, g_i, \theta\right)$, and given prior $p\left(\theta \mid \tilde{\theta}\right)$, the posterior is $p(\theta | data_n) \propto L_n \times p\left(\theta \mid \tilde{\theta}\right)$, computed by Monte Carlo Markov chain methods (Robert and Cassella, 1999).

For priors, one may assume $\mu \sim N\left(\tilde{\mu}, \tilde{\sigma}_\mu^2\right), \alpha \sim N_0\left(\tilde{\alpha}, \tilde{\alpha}_\alpha^2\right)$, a normal truncated below at 0 to ensure that $\alpha > 0$, $\beta_1, \ldots, \beta_{G-1} \sim iid\ N\left(\tilde{\beta}, \tilde{\sigma}_\beta^2\right)$ and $\gamma_1, \ldots, \gamma_{G-1} \sim iid\ N\left(\tilde{\gamma}, \tilde{\sigma}_\gamma^2\right)$, with the additional constraints that all $\alpha + \gamma_g > 0$. In the lognormal case where $\log(T) \sim N(\eta(d, g, \theta), \sigma_T^2)$, the variance σ_T^2 may have an inverse gamma or uniform prior. There are several strategies for establishing $\tilde{\theta}$ (cf. Thall and Cook, 2004; Thall et al., 2011). One approach is to elicit prior means of $\pi(d_r, g, \theta)$ for all mG pairs of (d_r, g), use nonlinear least-squares or pseudo-sampling (Thall and Nguyen, 2012) to solve for the hyperparameter means, and calibrate the hyperparameter variances during the computer simulation to obtain $\tilde{\theta}$ that gives sensible priors for the $\pi(d_r, g, \theta)$s, and a design with good operating characteristics (OCs). Prior effective sample size (Morita et al., 2008, 2010) may be used as a tool in this process.

Generalizing the TiTE-CRM, given a fixed target π^*, each $d^{opt}(g) = d^{opt}(g, data)$ may be defined as the dose minimizing $|\pi^* - \pi(d_r, g, data)|$, where $\pi(d_r, g, data) = E\{\pi(d_r, g, \theta) | data\}$, $r = 1, \ldots, m$. If desired, different subgroup-specific fixed targets $\pi^*(g)$, $g = 0, 1, \ldots, G-1$ may be specified. For example, in the NSCLC trial with $G = 4$ based on $Z = \{+1, -1\}$ and $X_{1,2}$, one may use $\pi_g^* = 0.35$ in the two subgroups with $X_{1,2} = 1$ and $\pi_g^* = 0.50$ in the two subgroups with $X_{1,2} = 0$. The simplest model ignores $\mathbf{X}$ and has $G = 2$, so $\theta = (\mu, \alpha, \beta_1, \gamma_1)$.

The trial may be conducted as follows. In subgroup g, treat the first three patients enrolled at that subgroup's specified starting dose, and for each patient thereafter give the dose $d^{opt}(g, data_n)$ based on the current posterior using $data_n$ from all subgroups. One also may impose the constraint that, within each subgroup, an untried dose level may not be skipped when escalating. In subgroup g, if the lowest dose is unacceptably toxic, formally $\Pr\left\{\pi(d, g, \theta) > \pi_g^* \mid data_n\right\} > p_{g,U}$, then accrual to that subgroup is terminated with no dose selected; otherwise, at the end of the trial, $d^{opt}(data_{g,N_{max}})$ is chosen.

6.3.3 A Phase I–II Trial with KRAS+ and KRAS− Patients

A Bayesian phase I–II method that bases dose-finding on $\mathbf{Y} = (Y_E, Y_T)$, where Y_T indicates toxicity and Y_E indicates efficacy, accounting for prognostic covariates $\mathbf{X}$, was proposed by Thall et al. (2008). This may be extended to include a binary biomarker, Z, as follows. For a patient with covariates $(Z, \mathbf{X})$ treated with dose d, let $\pi_k(d, Z, \mathbf{X}, \theta) = \Pr(Y_k = 1 | d, Z, \mathbf{X}, \theta)$, $k = E, T$, with $\pi(d, Z, \mathbf{X}, \theta) = (\pi_E(d, Z, \mathbf{X}, \theta), \pi_T(d, Z, \mathbf{X}, \theta))$. Denote these for brevity by π_E, π_T, and π when no meaning is lost. The method requires an informative prior on $\mathbf{X}$ effect parameters, obtained from historical data. In contrast, noninformative priors on any effects associated with either Z or d should be used. Rather than choosing one best dose, the trial data are used to select optimal $(Z, \mathbf{X})$-specific doses.

The data from the trial's first n patients are $D_n = \{(Y_i, Z_i, X_i, d_{[i]}), i = 1,\ldots, n\}$. Denote the historical data by $H = \{(Y_i, X_i, \tau_{[i]}), i = 1,\ldots, n_H\}$, where $\{\tau_1,\ldots, \tau_m\}$ are historical treatments and $\tau_{[i]}$ is the ith patient's treatment. Unsubscripted τ denotes either a dose or historical treatment. Denote $\mathbf{X}^+ = (Z, \mathbf{X})$. The following Bayesian model provides a basis for using $\boldsymbol{H}$ to learn about covariate effects and, during the trial, account for joint effects of $(d, \mathbf{X}^+)$ on π based on $D_n^H = D_n \cup H$. For a patient with covariates $\mathbf{X}^+ = (Z, \mathbf{X})$ treated with τ, let $\pi_{a,b}(\tau, \mathbf{X}^+, \theta) = \Pr(Y_E = a, Y_T = b | \tau, \mathbf{X}^+, \theta)$, for $a, b \in \{0, 1\}$, with $\pi_k(\tau, \mathbf{X}^+, \theta) = \Pr(Y_k = 1 | \tau, \mathbf{X}^+, \theta)$ for $k = E, T$. For link function φ, denote the linear terms $\eta_k = \varphi(\pi_k)$. A model is determined by the marginals $\pi_E = \varphi^{-1}(\eta_E)$ and $\pi_T = \varphi^{-1}(\eta_T)$ and one association parameter, ψ. For a bivariate model, one may use Gumbel–Morgenstern copula to obtain

$$\pi_{a,b} = \pi_E^a \left(1 - \pi_E\right)^{1-a} \pi_T^b \left(1 - \pi_T\right)^{1-b} + \left(-1\right)^{a+b} \psi \pi_E \left(1 - \pi_E\right) \pi_T \left(1 - \pi_T\right), \quad (6.1)$$

with $-1 \le \upsilon \le 1$. For fitting H, the linear terms are

$$\eta_k\left(T_r, \mathbf{X}, \theta\right) = \mu_{k,r} + \beta_k X + \xi_{k,r} X, \quad \text{for } r = 1,\ldots, m_H \quad \text{and} \quad k = E, T. \quad (6.2)$$

The covariate main effects are $\boldsymbol{\beta}_k = (\beta_{k,1},\ldots, \beta_{k,q})$, interactions between $\mathbf{X}$ and historical treatment τ_r are $\boldsymbol{\xi}_{k,r} = (\xi_{k,r,1},\ldots, \xi_{k,r,q})$, and the m_H historical treatment main effects are $\mu_k = (\mu_{k,1},\ldots, \mu_{k,mH})$. For the trial data, the linear terms are

$$\eta_k\left(d, X^+, \theta\right) = \phi_k\left(d, \alpha_k\right) + \beta_k^+ X^+ + d\gamma_k^+ X^+, \quad \text{for } k = E,\ T. \tag{6.3}$$

For each k, covariate main effects are $\beta_k^+ = \left(\beta_{k,Z}, \beta_k\right)$, and dose–covariate interactions are $\gamma_k^+ = \left(\gamma_{k,Z}, \gamma_k\right)$. A key assumption required by the method is that the covariates **X** are prognostic both historically and in the trial, and moreover that the posterior distribution of their main effects obtained from H will be a valid prior for their main effects in each $\pi_k(d, Z, \mathbf{X}, \theta)$. Main dose effects on π_E and π_T are characterized by $\varphi_E(d, \alpha_E)$ and $\varphi_T(d, \alpha_T)$, which should be formulated to reflect the application. For cytotoxic agents, $\varphi_T(x, \alpha_T) = \alpha_{T,0} + \alpha_{T,1}x$ with $\Pr(\alpha_{T,1} > 0) = 1$ ensures $\pi_T(d, \mathbf{Z}, \theta)$ increases in d, while π_k nonmonotone in d may be appropriate for biological agents.

The likelihood for the current trial data is

$$L(D_n \mid \theta) = \prod_{i=1}^{n}\prod_{a=0}^{1}\prod_{b=0}^{1}\left\{\pi_{a,b}\left(d_{[i]}, Z_i, \theta\right)\right\}1^{\{\mathbf{Y}_i=(a,b)\}}.$$

and the posterior based on D_n^H is

$$p\left(\alpha, \gamma^+, \beta^+, \psi \mid D_n^H\right) \alpha\, L(D_n \mid \theta)\, p\left(\alpha, \gamma^+\right) p(\beta, \psi \mid H). \tag{6.4}$$

To determine a prior for the model used in trial conduct, one starts by fitting $\boldsymbol{H}$ to obtain an informative posterior $p(\boldsymbol{\mu}, \boldsymbol{\beta}, \boldsymbol{\xi}, \psi \mid \boldsymbol{H})$. The marginal posterior $p(\beta, \psi \mid \boldsymbol{H})$ for the prognostic covariates is used as an informative prior on $(\boldsymbol{\beta}, \psi)$ at the start of the trial. Since nothing is known about effects $\boldsymbol{\alpha}$, $\boldsymbol{\gamma}$ of the experimental agent, and $\beta_{k,Z}$, $\gamma_{k,Z}$ are biomarker effects, their priors all should be noninformative. For prior means, set $E(\boldsymbol{\gamma}^+) = 0$, and obtain prior $E(\boldsymbol{\alpha})$ by eliciting means of $\pi_E(d_j, X^+, \boldsymbol{\theta})$ and $\pi_T(d_j, X^+, \boldsymbol{\theta})$ at several values of d_j and solving for $E(\boldsymbol{\alpha})$, using one of the least squares or pseudo-sampling methods noted earlier. As before, prior variances may be calibrated to control the ESS of the priors on $p\{\pi_k(d_j, X^+, \boldsymbol{\theta})\}$ for all $k = E, T$ and d_j, and obtain a design with good operating characteristics.

During the trial, $(Z, \mathbf{X})$-specific doses are chosen adaptively using quantities computed from the posterior, $p(\boldsymbol{\alpha}, \boldsymbol{\gamma}^+, \boldsymbol{\beta}^+, \psi \mid D_n^H)$. To account for both d and X^+, two decision criteria are used. The first determines whether d is *acceptable* for given $(Z, \mathbf{X})$. The second is the *desirability* of each d given (Z, X), using a function quantifying trade-off between π_E and π_T. Constructing covariate-specific acceptability bounds from elicited values, while straightforward, is somewhat involved. Several possible geometric methods may be used to define the desirability $\varsigma_n(d, Z, X)$ of d for a patient with biomarker Z and prognostic covariates **X**, based on efficacy-toxicity trade-offs. Detailed explanations are given in Thall et al. (2008). Given $\boldsymbol{D}_n$, the set $A_n(\mathbf{X}^+)$ of acceptable doses for a patient with covariates $\mathbf{X}^+ = (Z, \mathbf{X})$ consists of all d satisfying

$$\Pr\left[\pi_E\left(d,X^+,\theta\right) < \underline{\pi}_E\left(X^+\right) \mid D_n^H\right] < p_E \quad \text{and}$$

$$\Pr\left[\pi_T\left(d,X^+,\theta\right) > \overline{\pi}_T\left(X^+\right) \mid D_n^H\right] < p_T. \tag{6.5}$$

The cutoffs p_T and p_E should be calibrated to obtain good OCs. During the trial, $A_n(\mathbf{X}^+)$ changes adaptively for each $\mathbf{X}^+ = (Z, \mathbf{X}_{1,2})$, and if $A_n(\mathbf{X}^+)$ is empty, no dose is acceptable for that patient. To conduct the trial, $A_n(\mathbf{X}^+)$ is computed for each new patient, and the following decision rules are applied. If $A_n(\mathbf{X}^+)$ is empty, the patient is not treated. If $A_n(\mathbf{X}^+)$ consists of a single dose, then that dose is used by default. If two or more dose are acceptable, then the dose maximizing $\varsigma_n(d, Z, X_{1,2})$ is given.

As an illustration, using $(Z, X_{1,2})$ from the NSCLC trial, suppose the doses of M are {100, 200, 300, 400, 500} mg/m^2. A possible set of optimal doses if the agent is active in both biomarker subgroups, the KRAS+ patients need less of the agent to obtain the same antidisease effect, and good prognosis patients can tolerate a higher dose, is as follows:

Z	$X_{1,2}$	$d^{opt}(Z, X_{1,2})$
KRAS+	Good	400
KRAS+	Poor	200
KRAS–	Good	500
KRAS–	Poor	300

Using $d^{opt}(Z, X_{1,2})$ is an individualized version of targeted agent M when administered in combination with C.

6.4 General Structure for Learning, Refining, and Confirming

It is useful to think about the process of developing and clinically evaluating new treatment regimens as having *learning* and *confirmation* stages (cf. Sheiner, 1997). In the conventional paradigm, one may consider phases I and II learning and phase III confirmation. A sequence of trials of targeted agents is more complex, with more stages that may overlap. Learning what belongs in $\mathbf{Z}$ via genomics/proteomics, *discovery*, is not the same thing as using $\mathbf{Z}$ to learn about effects of ρ on clinical outcomes, although they certainly are related. A possible multistage strategy for the process of clinical evaluation is as follows. In practice, each ρ must include a small number of elements of $\mathcal{T}$ in order to be therapeutically feasible. For example, a five-agent combination may be suggested by $\mathbf{Z}$, but new five-agent dose combinations are very difficult to ethically and feasibly evaluate for safety in humans.

Delivery optimization: Based on early safety and possibly efficacy, determine or optimize dose or dose schedule, for each $\tau \in \mathcal{T}$, possibly certain two-agent or three-agent combinations, possibly combined with standard therapy, such as $C+M$ in the NSCLC example.

Randomized comparative evaluation: Following delivery optimization of all $\rho(\mathbf{Z})$ to be studied, use group sequential (GS) decision making to comparatively evaluate the regimens using *weeding, selection,* and *confirmation. Weeding* is a process of dropping agents, subgroups, or agent–subgroup combinations due to either low efficacy or excessive toxicity. Adaptive *futility* rules are used to do this. *Selection* is a process of choosing a feasibly small set of ρ that are promising within specific $\mathbf{Z}$ subgroups. *Confirmation* aims to obtain conclusions regarding effects of single or multiagent regimens within specific $\mathbf{Z}$ subgroups that will motivate final decisions or actions, such as promulgating conclusions about what $\mathbf{Z}$ and $\rho(\mathbf{Z})$ are a reliable basis for clinical practice. One may think of weeding as dropping the lower end and selection as moving forward the upper end of an ordered set of treatment regimens, in subgroup $\mathbf{Z}$, based on a treatment effect parameter $\theta(\rho, Z)$, where the ordering may vary substantially with $\mathbf{Z}$. A Bayesian subgroup-specific futility rule stops assignment of ρ in subgroup Z if $\theta(\rho, \mathbf{Z})$ is likely to be substantively smaller than $\theta(\rho', \mathbf{Z})$ for at least one $\rho' \neq \rho$, according to some posterior criterion. Similarly, ρ may be selected in subgroup Z if, *a posteriori*, $\theta(\rho, \mathbf{Z})$ is likely to be larger than most $\theta(\rho', \mathbf{Z})$ for $\rho' \neq \rho$.

6.5 Two-Arm Trials with Biomarker Subgroups

6.5.1 Two-Arm NSCLC Trial

Comparing $C+M$ to C while accounting for one binary Z illustrates a simple 2×2 case. Given an individualized dose function for M, such as $d^{opt}(Z, X_{1,2})$ in the previous illustration, consider the question of whether $C+M$ improves T=PFS time compared to C. Denote the indicator of $C+M$ by ρ. To simplify the discussion, we suppress the fact that ρ and M are functions of $(Z, \mathbf{X})$, and only consider effects of Z. Suppose the distribution of $[T|\rho, Z, \theta]$ has been determined by goodness-of-fit analyses of historical data and assume that the model's linear term takes the form

$$\eta(\rho, Z, \theta) = \theta_0 + \theta_1\rho + \theta_2 Z + \theta_{12}\rho Z. \tag{6.6}$$

For example, denoting $\mu_{\tau,Z} = E\,(T|\tau, Z, \theta)$, under an exponential distribution $\eta(\tau, Z, \theta) = \log(\mu_{\tau,Z})$, under a lognormal $\eta(\tau, Z, \theta) = E\{\log(T)|\tau, Z, \theta\}$, and so on. For $Z=0$, the effect of adding the optimized targeted agent M to C is θ_1, while for $Z=1$ this effect is $\theta_1+\theta_{12}$, and θ_{12} is the *RAS-M* interaction. Assume that the parameters are defined so that larger θ_1 or θ_{12} corresponds to superiority (longer mean PFS time) with $C+M$ compared to M. The assumption that M will have no effect in KRAS− patients says $\theta_1=0$. Under this assumption, one would conduct a randomized trial comparing $C+M$ to C in KRAS+ patients only. However, if in fact M is effective in KRAS− patients ($\theta_1>0$), excluding KRAS− patients would guarantee a false negative in this subgroup. The further assumption that $C+M$ will provide a substantive improvement over C in KRAS+ patients ($\theta_{12}>\delta$ for large $\delta>0$) implies that only $C+M$ should be given to KRAS+ patients, and a randomized clinical trial should not be conducted since giving C alone would be unethical. Such assumptions replace clinical evaluation of a targeted agent in humans by subjective inferences based on preclinical data in rodents or cell lines. Many laboratory-based scientists have precisely this sort of belief about a targeted agent that they have developed in laboratory experiments.

6.5.2 Designs That Deal with Biomarker–Subgroup Interactions

Maitournam and Simon (2005) compared a conventional randomized trial design, an untargeted design, to a targeted design restricted to patients who are biomarker positive ($Z=1$), and showed that the relative power of the two approaches depends on the biomarker prevalence, $\Pr(Z=1)$, the magnitudes of the treatment effects in the two subgroups, and reliability of evaluation of Z, that is, assay sensitivity and specificity. For multiple biomarkers, $\mathbf{Z}$, that all are putatively associated with sensitivity to a targeted agent, Freidlin and Simon (2005b) proposed a two-stage design where a *biomarker-positive* classifier is developed in stage 1 and two tests for the effect of M are done in stage 2, one overall and the other in the biomarker sensitive subgroup. In the survival time setting with one biomarker, Karuri and Simon (2012) proposed a logically similar two-stage Bayesian design, with point mass distributions on comparative treatment effects. Prior to stage 2, the design drops subgroups, either both or only biomarker-negative patients, if the stage 1 data show it is likely that there is no treatment effect in the subgroup. Adaptive signature designs are discussed in Chapter 18 (Freidlin and Simon).

Much of the literature on frequentist designs is devoted to the technical problem of determining design parameters given prespecified GS test size and power. Song and Choi (2007) applied closed testing to obtain a two-stage procedure wherein a test of overall effect is carried out and, if the global null is rejected, a test is then carried out in a subgroup of interest, allowing treatment–subgroup interaction. For binary outcomes, Tang and Zhao (2013) randomized patients between two treatment arms in two stages using unbalanced randomization with probabilities chosen to minimize the expected overall number of failures, given specified size and power, also accounting for classification error in Z.

6.5.3 Two-Arm Bayesian Designs with Biomarker–Subgroup Interactions

A Bayesian randomized trial to compare $C+M$ to C in two subgroups defined by Z may be conducted as follows. All of the following rules may be applied group-sequentially. The monitoring schedule and sample size are very important since they play central roles in determining the design's OCs, along with the decision rules. Futility rules are applied throughout the trial, but superiority rules are applied only in the latter portion of the trial. Given a minimum desired improvement δ_1 in mean DFS from adding M to C, a futility rule stops accrual to subgroup Z if

$$\Pr\{\mu_{C+M,Z} > \mu_{C,Z} + \delta_1 \,|\, data_n\} < p_{L,z}, \tag{6.7}$$

for small lower decision cutoff $p_{L,Z}$. Since patient safety is never a secondary concern in an ethical clinical trial, similar stopping rules for adverse events can be constructed and applied throughout the trial (cf. Thall et al., 1995). For example, if $\pi_{\rho,Z}$ denotes the probability of toxicity with $\rho = C+M$ or C in subgroup Z, and $\bar{\pi}$ is a fixed upper limit based on clinical experience or historical data, then accrual should be stopped in subgroup Z if

$$\Pr\{\pi_{\rho,Z} > \bar{\pi} \,|\, data_n\} > p_{U,Z,tox} \tag{6.8}$$

One may declare $C+M$ promising compared to C in subgroup Z if

$$\Pr(\mu_{C+M,Z} > \mu_{C,Z} + \delta_2 \,|\, data_n) > p_{U,Z}, \tag{6.9}$$

for slightly larger $\delta_2 > \delta_1$, using upper decision cutoff $p_{U,Z}$. The same sort of criterion may be used to confirm that $C+M$ is superior to C in subgroup Z for substantially larger $\delta_3 > \delta_2$. Given a monitoring schedule, the cutoffs of these one-sided decision rules and sample size should be calibrated via computer simulation to obtain desired overall type I error and power, and possibly also each within-subgroup false negative rate. If desired, a symmetric two-sided version of this procedure could be defined by including similar rules with the roles of C and $C+M$ reversed. Rules of this sort may be replaced by analogous Bayesian rules based on predictive probabilities (cf. Anderson, 1999) or Bayes factors (cf. Spiegelhalter et al., 2004).

If no standard therapy exists and one wishes to evaluate two targeted agents, $\tau = \{\tau_1, \tau_2\}$, with corresponding biomarker indicators $\mathbf{Z} = (Z_1, Z_2)$, then there are four biomarker subgroups, $\mathbf{Z} = (1, 1), (1, 0), (0, 1)$, and $(0, 0)$. A modified version of the above design with symmetric rules randomizes patients between τ_1 and τ_2, and uses futility rules to stop accrual to τ_j in subgroup $\mathbf{Z}$ if

$$\Pr\{\mu_{t_j,\mathbf{z}} > \mu_0 + \delta_1 \,|\, data_n\} < p_{L,Z}, \tag{6.10}$$

where μ_0 is the historical mean DFS. There are eight such futility rules, one for each combination of agent τ_j and biomarker signature $\mathbf{Z}$. Weeding out unpromising τ_j – **Z** combinations is important so that the remaining combinations may be enriched. If neither τ_1 nor τ_2 is stopped due to futility in subgroup **Z**, then τ_1 may be declared superior to τ_2 in this subgroup if

$$\Pr\{\mu_{\tau_1,\mathbf{Z}} > \mu_{\tau_2,\mathbf{Z}} + \delta_3 \mid data_n\} > p_{U,Z}, \tag{6.11}$$

with the symmetric subgroup-specific rule used to declare τ_2 superior to τ_1. An elaboration of this design might also include the combination $\tau_1 + \tau_2$ for a three-arm trial, and thus require a more complex model and three pairwise comparative rules of the form (6.11), or possibly posterior probabilities of the form $\Pr\{\mu_{\tau_1+\tau_2,Z} > \max\{\mu_{\tau_1,Z}, \mu_{\tau_2,Z}\} + \delta_S \mid data_n\}$. A very different design is motivated by the assumption that τ_j can benefit only patients with $Z_j = 1$ for each $j = 1, 2$. This design would not randomize, but rather would use $\tau_1 + \tau_2$ to treat all patients with $(Z_1, Z_2) = (1, 1)$, τ_1 to treat all patients with $(Z_1, Z_2) = (1, 0)$, and τ_2 to treat all patients with $(Z_1, Z_2) = (0, 1)$.

The decision cutoffs may be elaborated as parametric functions that vary with sample size to facilitate optimization with regard to expected sample size for given overall type I and type II error rates. For a Bayesian two-arm trial to compare survival or PFS time with adaptive model selection, Wathen and Thall (2008) use the boundary functions $p_U(data_n) = a_U - b_U(N^+(data_n)/N)^{c_U}$ and $p_L(data_n) = a_L + b_L(N^+(data_n)/N)^{c_L}$, where $N^+(data_n)$ is the number of events observed through n patients, and $p_L(data_n) \leq p_U(data_n)$. To adapt their decision rules to accommodate biomarker subgroups, denote $p_{\tau_1>\tau_2,Z,\delta,n} = Pr(\mu_{\tau_1,Z} > \mu_{\tau_2,Z} + \delta \mid data_n)$ and $p_{\tau_2>\tau_1,Z,\delta,n}$ similarly. Decision rules may be defined as follows, where δ_1 is a minimal $|\mu_{\tau_1,Z} - \mu_{\tau_2,Z}|$ effect and δ_2 is a larger, clinically meaningful effect.

1. *Futility*: If $\max\{p_{\tau_1>\tau_2,Z,\delta_1,n}, p_{\tau_2>\tau_2,Z,\delta_1,n}\} < p_L(data_n)$, then stop accrual in subgroup Z and conclude there is no meaningful $\tau_1 - \tau_2$ effect in this subgroup.
2. *Superiority*: If $p_{\tau_1>\tau_2,Z,\delta_2,n} > p_U(data_n) > p_{\tau_2>\tau_1,Z,\delta_2,n}$, then stop accrual in subgroup Z and conclude $\tau_1 > \tau_2$ in this subgroup.

Otherwise, continue accrual in subgroup Z. If accrual is stopped in one or more subgroups, the overall sample size should not be reduced, so that the remaining subgroups are enriched. In practice, the rules are applied group-sequentially at successive points where $N^+(data_n)$ equals prespecified values. As suggested earlier, with four or more subgroups, it may be useful to only apply the futility rules initially and apply superiority rules for larger n.

6.5.4 Potential Consequences of Ignoring Subgroups

Most conventional clinical trial designs implicitly assume homogeneity by ignoring subgroups. Statistical models and methods that ignore subgroups produce decisions based on treatment effect estimates that actually are averages across subgroups. A simple example of the consequences of ignoring patient heterogeneity in the single-arm, phase II setting of an experimental treatment E versus historical control C was given by Wathen et al. (2008). Denote the probability of response with treatment $\tau = E$ or C in subgroup $Z=0$ or 1 by $\pi_{\tau,Z}$. Under a Bayesian model with logit $\{\pi_{\tau,Z}\} = \eta_{\tau,Z}$ of the form (6.6), accrual is stopped in subgroup Z if $\Pr(\pi_{E,Z} > \pi_{C,Z} + \delta_Z \mid data) < p_Z$. A simulation study was conducted of a 100 patient trial with $\Pr(Z=0) = \Pr(Z=1) = 0.50$, and prior means 0.25 for both $\pi_{E,0}$ and $\pi_{C,0}$, and 0.45 for both $\pi_{E,1}$ and $\pi_{C,1}$. These correspond to historical response rates of 25% and 45% in the two subgroups. The targeted improvements were $\delta_0 = \delta_1 = 0.15$, and the decision cutoffs p_0, p_1 were calibrated to ensure within-subgroup incorrect stopping probabilities 0.10 for $Z=1$ if $\pi_{E,1}^{true} = 0.45 + 0.15 = 0.60$, and also 0.10 for $Z=0$ if $\pi_{E,0}^{true} = 0.25 + 0.15 = 0.40$. Comparison of this design to the analogous design that ignores Z and uses null mean $\pi_E = (0.25 + 0.45)/2 = 0.35$ showed that, in the treatment–subgroup interaction case where $\pi_{E,1}^{true} = 0.60$ (E gives improvement 0.15 over C if $Z=1$) and $\pi_{E,1}^{true} = 0.25$ (E gives no improvement over C if $Z=0$), the design ignoring subgroups stopped the trial and rejected E with probability 0.42. This implies a false negative probability of 0.42 if $Z=1$ and a false positive probability of $1 - 0.42 = 0.58$ if $Z=0$ in this case. In practical terms, with this treatment–subgroup interaction, one could do about as well as a design that ignores subgroups by not bothering to conduct a clinical trial and simply flipping a coin. Similar results hold for randomized trials and also were found by Thall et al. (2008) in the phase I–II dose-finding setting for dose–covariate interactions. The general point is extremely important. If there is in fact a treatment–subgroup interaction, then ignoring subgroups can produce extremely unreliable conclusions. This is particularly problematic for trials of multiple targeted agents since a vector of J binary biomarkers implies up to 2^J subgroups, although they are far from being disjoint.

6.6 Randomized Discontinuation Designs

The randomized discontinuation design (RDD; Kopec et al., 1993; Rosner et al., 2002) for targeted agents that aim to achieve SD or better categorizes patient outcome Y_s at each of $s=1$ or 2 stages of therapy as R (response), SD, or PD (progressive disease). All patients are given the targeted agent, τ, in stage 1. If $Y_1 = R$, then τ is given in stage 2; if $Y_1 = \text{PD}$, then the patient is taken off study; if $Y_1 = \text{SD}$, then the patient is randomized between τ and placebo (discontinuation). In practice, PD also includes toxicity that precludes further treatment with τ. This is an example of an *enrichment* design in the sense that patients more likely to benefit from τ are more likely to be kept on the agent for stage 2. Rosner et al. (2002) presented the RDD in the context of cytostatic agents, where SD or better, $SD^+ = $ (SD or R), is considered success. Freidlin and Simon (2005) found that, compared to a conventional randomized design, the RDD design has substantial power loss for comparing τ to placebo in terms of $\Pr(Y_2 = \text{PD})$. The RDD is an elaboration of a simple single-arm phase IIA activity trial for τ based on stage 1 of therapy alone (cf. Gehan, 1961; Thall and Sung, 1998) that includes an additional second stage of therapy where treatment is chosen adaptively using Y_1. In this sense, the RDD is a randomized comparison of the two-stage dynamic treatment regimens $\rho_1 = (\tau^{(1)}, \tau^{(2)})$ and $\rho_2 = (\tau^{(1)}, DNT^{(2)})$, where $\tau^{(1)}$ means *give* τ *in stage 1*, $\tau^{(2)}$ means *give* τ *in stage 2 if* Y_1 *was* SD^+, and $DNT^{(2)}$ means *do not treat or give placebo in stage 2 if* Y_1 *was* SD^+. The RDD randomizes patients between ρ_1 and ρ_2. An elaboration might also specify salvage treatments for PD, and treatments for toxicity.

Some Bayesian extensions of the RDD are as follows. If the clinical payoff for comparing the two regimens is Y_2, then, denoting $\pi_{2,\tau} = \Pr(Y_2 = SD^+ | Y_1 = SD, \tau \text{ in stage 2})$ and $\pi_{2,\text{DNT}} = \Pr(Y_2 = SD^+ | Y_1 = SD, \text{DNT in stage 2})$, a large value of $\Pr(\rho_1 > \rho_2 | data) = \Pr(\pi_{2,\tau} > \pi_{2,\text{DNT}} | data\}$, say above 0.95 or 0.99, would lead to the conclusion that giving τ is better than not treating the patient in stage 2 if SD is seen with τ in stage 1. Values of $\Pr(\rho_1 > \rho_2 | data)$ near 0.50 correspond to no difference, and values near 0 to ρ_2 being superior. It may be useful to add a Bayesian futility rule that stops the trial early if

$$\Pr\left\{\pi_{1,\tau} > \pi_1^* \mid data_n\right\} < p_{1,L} \tag{6.12}$$

where

$\pi_{1,\tau} = \Pr(Y_1 = SD^+ | \tau \text{ in stage 1})$

π_1^* is a fixed minimum stage 1 activity level in terms of SD^+, say 0.20

To accommodate competing targeted agents, say τ_1 and τ_2, a generalization of the RDD might randomize patients between τ_1 and τ_2 for stage 1. If τ_1 is given in stage 1, then the stage 2 adaptive rule might be to give τ_2 if $Y_1 = \text{PD}$; randomize between τ_1 and τ_2 if $Y_1 = \text{SD}$; and repeat τ_1 in stage 2 if $Y_1 = R$. The two regimens being compared are $\rho_1 = (\tau_1, \tau_2)$ and $\rho_2 = (\tau_2, \tau_1)$, where ρ_1 says to start with τ_1 in stage 1, repeat τ_1 in stage 2 if $Y_1 = SD^+$, and switch to τ_2 in stage 2 if $Y_1 = \text{PD}$. The regimen ρ_2 is obtained by switching the roles of τ_1 and τ_2. Schematically, ρ_1 may be expressed as $(\tau_1, Y_1 = \text{PD} \rightarrow \tau_2, Y_1 = SD^+ \longrightarrow \tau_1)$. Bayesian comparison of ρ_1 and ρ_2 may be done as for the 2 regimens in the RDD, given earlier. For $J > 2$ agents, however, there would be $J(J-1)/2$ such two-stage regimens, so even for $J = 3$ there are 6 regimens. For $J \geq 3$, stage 1 futility rules of the form (6.12) become very important. For example, dropping τ_1 due to stage 1 futility would eliminate both (τ_1, τ_2) and (τ_1, τ_3), and thus allow more patients to be randomized to the remaining four regimes. This may be thought as *between patient enrichment* of multistage targeted regimens.

6.7 Multiple Agents and Multiple Targets

None of the aforementioned extensions of the RDD account for **Z**, and elaborations that do so unavoidably are much more complicated. For example, subgroup-specific stage 1 futility rules might be used, based on $\pi_{1,\tau_j(Z)} = \Pr\left(Y_1 = SD^+ \mid \tau_j, Z\right)$ for each τ_j and biomarker subgroup **Z**. More generally, when either $\mathbf{Z}=(Z_1,\ldots, Z_p)$ has $p>1$ entries or $\tau=\{\tau_1,\ldots, \tau_J\}$ has $J>1$ targeted agents, practical issues of discovery, delivery optimization, and obtaining reliable comparative evaluations are much more difficult. Ignore known prognostic covariates **X** for simplicity. Even with $p=2$ targets and $J=2$ targeted agents, where putatively τ_j targets Z_j for each $j=1, 2$ the NSCLC trial has four biomarker-defined subgroups {(0, 0), (1, 0), (0, 1), (1, 1)} for (Z_1, Z_2), and four possible treatment combinations, $\{C, C+\tau_1, C+\tau_2, C+\tau_1+\tau_2\}$. It is tempting to simply randomize patients with $(Z_1, Z_2)=(1, 1)$ between C and $C+\tau_1+\tau_2$, patients with $(Z_1, Z_2)=(1, 0)$ between C and $C+\tau_1$, patients with $(Z_1, Z_2)=(0, 1)$ between C and $C+\tau_2$, and use C to treat all patients with $(Z_1, Z_2)=(0, 0)$, controlling the sample sizes in the four treatment combination in some fashion. This strategy is motivated by the assumption that each τ_j has potential antidisease activity only in patients with $Z_j=1$, which often is incorrect. A simpler strategy is to only include two arms, C and $C+\tau_1+\tau_2$. While this may seem very appealing, it cannot discover whether, for example, an observed improvement of $C+\tau_1+\tau_2$ over C in mean PFS could be achieved with $C+\tau_1$, that is, τ_2 provides no additional clinical benefit. Moreover, the issues of toxicity and determining acceptable doses for combinations must be addressed. Even for $p=2$, optimizing dose pairs is well known to be an extremely complex and difficult problem in single-arm phase I trials, and very little work has been done for $p\geq 3$. Recall the example in the 2×2 case of huge false positive and false negative error rates if homogeneity of treatment effect across Z is assumed but in fact there are substantial τ–Z interactions.

Inevitably, some strategy for dimension reduction must be devised. Michiels et al. (2011) propose permutation tests for a confirmatory two-arm trial based on survival time under a Weibull distribution with multiple biomarkers, where treatment–biomarker interactions are of interest, controlling the overall type I error for multiple tests. Tests are obtained by computing an overall biomarker score $\mathbf{wZ}=w_1Z_1+\cdots+w_J Z_J$ for each patient and permuting **Z** among the patients within each treatment group. This sort of approach works if $Z_1,\ldots, Z_J$ all go in the same direction, that is, larger Z_j corresponds to the hypothesis that τ_j has greater antidisease effect. With K targeted agents, $\tau_1,\ldots, \tau_K$, after applying weeding rules to drop unpromising τ_j–**Z** combinations, one may focus attention on the most promising combinations in terms of the posteriors of $\mu_{\tau j,\, \mathbf{Z}}$ and select a small subset for further evaluation. For example, one may rank order these based on $E(\mu_{\tau j},\, _{\mathbf{Z}}|data_n)$ or $\Pr(\mu_{\tau j,\, \mathbf{Z}}>\mu^*|data_n)$ for fixed μ^* and select the largest m, where m is a small, feasible number to evaluate. A comparative rule might select τ_j for further evaluation in subgroup **Z** if

$$\Pr(\mu_{\tau j,\mathbf{Z}} > \min_{r,\mathbf{Z}}\{\mu_{\tau r,\mathbf{Z}}\} \,|\, data_n) > p_{U,\mathbf{Z}}. \tag{6.13}$$

If ranking is the objective, then an advantage of the Bayesian approach is that the posteriors of the ranks themselves may be computed (cf. Laird and Louis, 1989). In terms of the means, for $j = 1, \ldots, K$, the rank of τ_j in subgroup **Z** is

$$R(\tau_j, \mathbf{Z}) = \sum_{l=1}^{K} I\left(\mu_{\tau_j,\mathbf{Z}} \geq \mu_{\tau_l,\mathbf{Z}}\right)$$

One may base decisions, similar to those given earlier in terms of parameters, on the joint posterior of $R(\tau_1, \mathbf{Z}), \ldots, R(\tau_K, \mathbf{Z})$.

For targeted regimens $\tau_1, \ldots, \tau_K$ with J biomarker subgroups, assume a model with linear terms $\eta = \{\eta_{\tau_r,j}, r = 1,2,\ j = 1, \ldots, J\}$, where each real-valued $\eta_{\tau_r,j} = \text{link}(\mu_{\tau_r,j})$ for mean outcome $\mu_{\tau_r,j}$ of treatment τ_r in subgroup j. If it is realistic to assume that these effects are exchangeable across subgroups within each treatment, one may assume the level 1 priors $\eta_{\tau_r,1}, \ldots, \eta_{\tau_r,j} \sim iid\ N\left(\tilde{\mu}_{\tau_r}, \tilde{\sigma}^2_{\tau_r}\right)$ for each $r = 1, \ldots, K$. For treatment τ_r, the deviation of treatment effect from the overall mean due to subgroup j is $\Delta_{j(r)} = \mu_{\tau_r,j} - \tilde{\mu}_{\tau_r}$, so $\Delta_{1(r)}, \ldots, \Delta_{K(r)} \sim iid\ N\left(0, \tilde{\sigma}^2_{\tau_r}\right)$ for each r. This model is saturated, with KJ parameters $\boldsymbol{\eta}$ and $2K$ fixed hyperparameters, $\tilde{\theta} = \left(\tilde{\mu}_{\tau 1}, \ldots, \tilde{\mu}_{\tau K}, \tilde{\sigma}^2_{\tau 1}, \ldots, \tilde{\sigma}^2_{\tau K}\right)$. If one further assumes a hierarchical model with level 2 priors (hyperpriors) $\tilde{\mu}_{\tau 1}, \ldots, \tilde{\mu}_{\tau K}, \sim iid\ N(a, b)$ and $\tilde{\sigma}^2_{\tau 1}, \ldots, \tilde{\sigma}^2_{\tau K}, \sim \text{uniform}\left[0, U_{\sigma^2}\right]$, then there are three fixed level 2 hyperparameters, $\varphi = (a, b, U_{\sigma 2})$, regardless of K and J. This model shrinks the estimated posterior mean treatment effects toward each other and shrinks the subgroup effects toward each other within treatments.

A futility rule to stop accrual in subgroup j may take the form

$$\Pr\{\max_{r \neq r'} | \eta_{\tau_r,j} \quad \eta_{\tau_{r'},j} | < \delta_1 \,|\, data_n\} < p_L. \tag{6.14}$$

Identifying a substantive treatment–subgroup effect might be done relative to a historical value η^H based on $\Pr(\eta_{\tau_r,j} > \eta^H + \delta_2 \,|\, data) > p_U$. A similar rule using only the trial data would be $\Pr(\eta_{\tau_r,j} > \max\{\eta_{\tau_m,l} : (m,l) \neq (r,j)\} + \delta_2 \,|\, data)$. The overall effect of τ_r is $\bar{\eta}_r = \sum_j w_j \eta_{r,j}$, where w_j is the probability of subgroup j. A comparison of overall treatment effects between τ_r and $\tau_{r'}$ could be based on $\Pr\left(|\bar{\eta}_r - \bar{\eta}_{r'}| > \delta_2 \,|\, data\right) > p_U$. The fact that there are $K(K-1)/2$ such pairwise comparisons would create the usual multiplicity issues. With all of these rules, however, shrinkage of posteriors among biomarker subgroups or treatment arms may help to control the overall false positive rates.

A final point pertains to uncertainty about **Z**, which can take at least two forms. The first pertains to whether a particular Z_j should have been included in a given gene or protein signature **Z**, or was included erroneously. It is very undesirable to treat a patient with an agent targeting an element of **Z** that was included erroneously or, alternatively, to fail to use an agent targeting a protein that should have been included but was either not discovered or excluded erroneously. All of the methods discussed here could be elaborated by including a vector $\mathbf{p}_Z$ where each entry $p(Z_j)$ is the probability that Z_j is correct, for example, using a beta prior if Z_j is binary. Such indexes of uncertainty might be obtained from previous genomic discovery studies. The second source of uncertainty assumes that **Z** is qualitatively correct, but pertains to whether each entry of a particular patient's $\mathbf{Z}_i$ was measured with error, specifically whether each binary $Z_{i,j}$ was incorrectly scored as a false positive or false negative, or continuous $Z_{i,j}$ is actually $Z_{i,j}^{true} + \epsilon_{i,j}$ where $\epsilon_{i,j}$ is, say, Gaussian measurement error. Given that some **Z** is assumed to be qualitatively correct, each patient's $\mathbf{Z}_i$ could have an associated probability distribution $q(\mathbf{Z}_i)$ to account for possible misclassification or measurement error, and here a Bayesian hierarchical model assuming that patients are exchangeable would be appropriate.

Acknowledgment

This research was partially supported by NIH grant RO1 CA 83932.

References

Andersen J.D. Use of predictive probabilities in phase II and phase III clinical trials. *J Biopharm Stat* 9(1): 67–79, 1999.

Bekele B.N. and P.F. Thall. Dose-finding based on multiple toxicities in a soft tissue sarcoma trial. *J Am Stat Assoc* 99: 26–35, 2004.

Braun T.M., P.F. Thall, H.Q. Nguyen, and M. de Lima. Simultaneously optimizing dose and schedule of a new cytotoxic agent. *Clin Trials* 4: 113–124, 2007.

Cheung Y.K. and R. Chappell. Sequential designs for phase I clinical trials with late-onset toxicities. *Biometrics* 56: 1177–1182, 2000.

Freidlin B. and R. Simon. Evaluation of randomized discontinuation design. *J Clin Oncol* 23: 50948, 2005a.

Freidlin B. and R. Simon. Adaptive signature design: An adaptive clinical trial design for generating and prospectively testing a gene expression signature for sensitive patients. *Clin Cancer Res* 11(21): 7872–7878, 2005b.

Gehan E.H. The determination of the number of patients required in a preliminary and a follow-up trial of a new chemotherapeutic agent. *J Chronic Dis* 13: 346353, 1961.

Hernan M.A., B. Brumback, and J.M. Robins. Marginal structural models to estimate the causal effect of zidovudine on the survival of HIV-positive men. *Epidemiology* 11: 561–570, 2000.

Karuri S.W. and R. Simon. A two-stage Bayesian design for co-development of new drugs and companion diagnostics. *Stat Med* 31: 901–914, 2012.

Kopec J.A., M. Abrahamowicz, and J.M. Esdaile. Randomized discontinuation trials: Utility and efficiency. *J Clin Epidemiol* 46: 95971, 1993.

Laird N. and T.A. Louis. Empirical Bayes ranking methods. *J Educ Stat* 14: 29–46, 1989.

Maitournam A. and R. Simon. On the efficiency of targeted clinical trials. *Stat Med* 24: 329–339, 2005.

Michiels S., R.E. Potthoff, and S.L. George. Multiple testing of treatment-effect-modifying biomarkers in a randomized clinical trial with a survival endpoint. *Stat Med* 30: 1502–1518, 2011.

Morita S., P.F. Thall, and P. Mueller. Determining the effective sample size of a parametric prior. *Biometrics* 64: 595–602, 2008.

Morita S., P.F. Thall, and P. Mueller. Evaluating the impact of prior assumptions in Bayesian biostatistics. *Stat Biosci* 2: 1–17, 2010.

Robert C.P. and G. Cassella. *Monte Carlo Statistical Methods*. New York: Springer, 1999.

Rosner G.L., W. Stadler, and M.J. Ratain. Randomized discontinuation design: Application to cytostatic antineoplastic agents. *J Clin Oncol* 20: 447884, 2002.

Saville B., H. Ah, and G. Koch. A robust method for comparing two treatments in a confirmatory clinical trial via multivariate time-to-event methods that jointly incorporate information from longitudinal and time-to-event data. *Stat Med* 29: 75–85, 2009.

Sheiner L.B. Learning versus confirming in clinical drug development. *Clin Pharmacol Ther* 61: 27591, 1997.

Shen Y. and P.F. Thall. Parametric likelihoods for multiple non-fatal competing risks and death. *Stat Med* 17: 999–1016, 1998.

Song Y. and Y.H. Choi. A method for testing a prespecified subgroup in clinical trials. *Stat Med* 26: 3535–3549, 2007.

Spiegelalter D.J., K.R. Abrams, and J.P. Myles. *Bayesian Approaches to Clinical Trials and Health-Care Evaluation*. Chichester, U.K.: John Wiley & Sons, 2004.

Tang L. and X-H. Zhao. A general framework for marker design with optimal allocation to assess clinical utility. *Stat Med* 32: 620–630, 2013.

Thall P.F. Bayesian adaptive dose-finding based on efficacy and toxicity. *J Stat Res* 14: 187–202, 2012.

Thall P.F. and J.D. Cook. Dose-finding based on efficacy-toxicity trade-offs. *Biometrics* 60: 684–693, 2004.

Thall P.F. and H.Q. Nguyen. Adaptive randomization to improve utility-based dose-finding with bivariate ordinal outcomes. *J Biopharm Stat* 22: 785–801, 2012.

Thall P.F., H.Q. Nguyen, T.M. Braun, and M. Qazilbash. Using joint utilities of the times to response and toxicity to adaptively optimize schedule-dose regimes. *Biometrics* 69(3): 673–682, 2013.

Thall P.F., H.Q. Nguyen, and E.H. Estey. Patient-specific dose-finding based on bivariate outcomes and covariates. *Biometrics* 64: 1126–1136, 2008.

Thall P.F., R. Simon, and E.H. Estey. Bayesian sequential monitoring designs for single-arm clinical trials with multiple outcomes. *Stat Med* 14: 357–379, 1995.

Thall P.F. and H.-G. Sung. Some extensions and applications of a Bayesian strategy for monitoring multiple outcomes in clinical trials. *Stat Med* 17: 1563–1580, 1998.

Thall P.F., H.-G. Sung, and E.H. Estey. Selecting therapeutic strategies based on efficacy and death in multi-course clinical trials. *J Am Stat Assoc* 97: 29–39, 2002.

Thall P.F., A. Szabo, H.Q. Nguyen, C.M. Amlie-Lefond, and O.O. Zaidat. Optimizing the concentration and bolus of a drug delivered by continuous infusion. *Biometrics* 67: 1638–1646, 2011.

Thall P.F. and J.K. Wathen. Covariate-adjusted adaptive randomization in a sarcoma trial with multi-stage treatments. *Stat Med* 24: 1947–1964, 2005.

Thall P.F. and J.K. Wathen. Practical Bayesian adaptive randomization in clinical trials. *Eur J Canc* 43: 860–867, 2007.

Thall P.F., L.H. Wooten, C.J. Logothetis, R. Millikan, and N.M. Tannir. Bayesian and frequentist two-stage treatment strategies based on sequential failure times subject to interval censoring. *Stat Med* 26: 4687–4702, 2007.

Wahed A. and P.F. Thall. Evaluating joint effects of induction-salvage treatment regimes on overall survival in acute leukemia. *J R Stat Soc Ser C* 62: 67–83, 2013.

Wang L., A. Rotnitzky, X. Lin, R. Millikan, and P.F. Thall. Evaluation of viable dynamic treatment regimes in a sequentially randomized trial of advanced prostate cancer. *J Am Stat Assoc* 107: 493–508, (with discussion, pp. 509–517; rejoinder, pp. 518–520), 2012.

Wathen J.K. and P.F. Thall. Bayesian adaptive model selection for optimizing group sequential clinical trials. *Stat Med* 27: 5586–5604, 2008.

Wathen J.K., P.F. Thall, J.D. Cook, and E.H. Estey. Accounting for patient heterogeneity in phase II clinical trials. *Stat Med* 27: 2802–2815, 2008.

Yuan Y. and G. Yin. Bayesian dose-finding by jointly modeling toxicity and efficacy as time-to-event outcomes. *J R Stat Soc Ser C* 58: 719–736, 2009.

Zhao Y., D. Zeng, M.A. Socinski, and M.R. Kosorok. Reinforcement learning strategies for clinical trials in nonsmall cell lung cancer. *Biometrics* 67: 14221433, 2011.

7

Outcome-Adaptive Randomization in Early Clinical Trials

Edward Korn and Boris Freidlin

CONTENTS

7.1 Introduction

Random treatment assignment in randomized clinical trials helps to remove any bias due to systematic pretreatment differences in patient populations and allows an inference concerning the causal relationship between the treatment and outcome. Although the treatment assignment is typically randomized equally among the control and experimental treatments, sometimes patients are preferentially randomized to an experimental treatment as compared to the control treatment, for example, in a 2:1 fashion, to make the trial more attractive to patients. In outcome-adaptive randomization (also known as response-adaptive randomization), the randomization ratio is not fixed throughout the trial, but changes based on the accruing outcome data. In particular, the assignment probability to an experimental treatment arm increases as the accruing outcome data suggest that the experimental treatment is better than the control treatment (whether or not it is truly better). Outcome-adaptive randomization has intuitive appeal in that, on average, a higher proportion of patients will be treated on better treatment arms, if there are such (Cornfield et al. 1969; Zelen 1969).

In theory, outcome-adaptive randomization could be used in definitive phase III trials as well as in earlier phase II trials. In practice, because of implementation issues with long-term definitive outcome measures and potential bias due to changing patient populations over time (discussed later), the use of outcome-adaptive randomization has been confined to earlier trials, and that is the focus of this chapter. Outcome-adaptive randomization is typically implemented in a Bayesian framework, that is, accruing outcome data updating prior distributions for treatment-arm outcome distributions. For example, 20 trials conducted at the M.D. Anderson Cancer Center in 2000–2005 used outcome-adaptive randomization implemented with Bayesian methodology (Biswas et al. 2009). However, there is nothing inherently Bayesian about randomizing a higher proportion of patients to treatment arms that appear to be doing better. In addition, regardless of whether or not a Bayesian approach is used to implement outcome-adaptive randomization, one can still assess frequentist operating characteristics of using outcome-adaptive randomization (Berry 2006). In fact, in the early clinical trial setting, the frequentist type 1 error of recommending an inactive therapy for further definitive testing is of critical importance, as well as the type 2 error of not recommending an active therapy for further testing.

In this chapter, we will compare outcome-adaptive randomization (called adaptive randomization for simplicity) to fixed randomization in the early clinical trials setting. To focus on the type of randomization, we will try to ensure that all the trial designs have the same operating characteristics and the same interim monitoring rules. We begin in the next section by comparing trial designs with fixed unbalanced randomization (e.g., 2:1 randomization in favor of the experimental treatment). Although this type of randomization is not adaptive, it demonstrates the main inefficiency caused by adaptive randomization. This is followed in Section 7.3 by a presentation of the properties of adaptive randomization studied via simulation. Section 7.4 examines adaptive randomization in the setting of multiarm trials, where there are multiple experimental arms to be compared to the control treatment arm. In Section 7.5, we discuss two trials that used adaptive randomization within biomarker-defined subgroups, the ISPY-2 trial and the BATTLE trial. Section 7.6 discusses two potentially problematic issues with adaptive randomization. We end the chapter with our conclusions concerning adaptive randomization in light of the results presented here.

7.2 Fixed Unbalanced Randomization

We focus on comparing a standard treatment versus an experimental treatment. If one is interested in getting trial results (for guiding development of the experimental agent) as quickly as possible and the most information about between-arm treatment difference, then a standard equal (1:1) randomization is generally the best (assuming the accrual rate is independent of the trial design) (Brittain and Schlesselman 1982). There remains the question of (1) how inefficient other randomization ratios are, and (2) how the average outcome of the patients treated in the trial (e.g., the average response rate) differs based on the randomization ratio used in the trial. In this section, we address these questions by simulating trials where more patients are randomized to the experimental arm than the control arm, but with the probability (>1/2) that a patient is randomized to the experimental arm being fixed throughout the trial.

Table 7.1 considers a trial designed to detect an improvement in response rate from 20% for the control treatment to 40% for the experimental treatment. The operating characteristics of the trial designs (using a normal approximation to the difference in proportions) are set at typical randomized phase II levels (Rubinstein et al. 2005): the type I error (probability of declaring the experimental treatment better than the control when it is not) has been set at 10%, and the power (probability of declaring the experimental treatment better than the control when it has a 40% response rate and the control has a 20% response rate) has been set at 90%. The trial with a balanced (1:1) randomization requires a total of 132 patients, and the trial with a 2:1 randomization ratio requires a total of 153 patients (top row of Table 7.1). Another way to say this is that the information about the treatment effect obtained from 66 patients in each treatment arm is the same as obtained with 102 patients in the experimental arm and 51 in the control arm. Although the high randomization ratios (4:1, 9:1) are uncommon in fixed randomization designs, they are used in the adaptive randomization designs discussed in the next section.

The sample size of the trial is not the only consideration when considering unequal randomization. Three parameters that can be used to evaluate the relative merits of such designs for the patients accrued on the trial are the expected number of responders, the expected number of nonresponders, and the probability that a patient will be a responder. As these parameters depend on the true response rates in the treatment arms, they are shown for a number of alternatives in Table 7.1. Consider the trial-design alternative effect (40% versus 20% response rate), which is bolded in Table 7.1. The 1:1 randomization trial has, on average, 39.6 responders, 92.4 nonresponders, and a 30.0% chance of response for participants. The 2:1 randomization has 51.0 responders, 102.0 nonresponders, and a 33.3% response probability, and the even higher randomization ratios (4:1, 9:1) having larger numbers of responders, larger number of nonresponders, and higher average response probabilities. Having a larger number of responders and a higher response probability is a good thing, but having a larger number of nonresponders and a larger overall sample size is not. Under the null hypothesis, the unbalanced randomization ratios have no

TABLE 7.1

Average Proportion of Responders ($P(R)$), Number of Responders ($\#R$), and Number of Nonresponders ($\#NR$) for Various Randomized Phase II Trial Designs Using Fixed Unbalanced Randomization (One-Sided Type 1 Error = 10%, Power = 90% at 20% versus 40% Response Rates, Results Based on 500,000 Simulations)

Response Rates by Treatment Arm		***K*:1 Randomization Ratio [Total Sample Size of the Trial]**											
		1:1 [$n = 132$]			**2:1 [$n = 153$]**			**4:1 [$n = 210$]**			**9:1 [$n = 380$]**		
C[a]	E[a]	$P(R)$	$\#R$	$\#NR$	$P(R)$	$\#R$	$\#NR$	$P(R)$	$\#R$	$\#NR$	$P(R)$	$\#R$	$\#NR$
0.2	0.2	20.0%	26.4	105.6	20.0%	30.6	122.4	20.0%	42.0	168.0	20.0%	76.0	304.0
0.2	0.3	25.0%	33.0	99.0	26.6%	40.8	112.2	28.0%	58.8	151.2	29.0%	110.2	269.8
0.2	**0.4**	**30.0%**	**39.6**	**92.4**	**33.3%**	**51.0**	**102.0**	**36.0%**	**75.6**	**134.4**	**38.0%**	**144.4**	**235.6**
0.2	0.5	35.0%	46.2	85.8	40.0%	61.2	91.8	44.0%	92.4	117.6	47.0%	178.6	201.4

Note: Characteristics of trial designs corresponding to the trial alternative hypothesis are in the bolded row.

[a] C = control arm, E = experimental treatment arm.

benefits, while retaining the drawback of a larger trial size. Note that since experimental treatments frequently have additional toxicities, the large number of patients being assigned the experimental treatments means that the unbalanced randomization is not only leading to slower drug development but is also potentially harming patients.

7.3 Properties of Adaptive Randomization Trials

In this section, we evaluate the operating characteristics of trial designs using adaptive randomization. There are many ways to implement adaptive randomization. We consider the method of Thall and Wathen (2007):

$$\text{Assignment probability to experimental treatment arm} = \frac{[P(E > C)]^a}{[P(E > C)]^a + [1 - P(E > C)]^a} \tag{7.1}$$

where $a = 1/2$ and $P(E > C)$ is the posterior probability that the experimental treatment is better than the control treatment estimated from the data seen so far.

Uniform prior distributions for the response rates are used, so that this is an easy calculation (Thompson 1933). If the response rate is looking better (worse) for E than C, then the posterior probability $P(E > C)$ will be larger (smaller) than 1/2, and then a higher (lower) proportion of patients would be assigned to E than to C. For example, if $P(E > C)$ equaled 0.05, 0.10, 3.3, 0.5, 0.7, 0.9, or 0.95, then patients would be assigned to the experimental treatment with probability 0.19, 0.25, 0.4, 0.5, 0.6, 0.75, or 0.81, respectively.

The estimator (7.1) of the assignment probability can be very unstable at the beginning of the trial because there are little data at that point to estimate $P(E > C)$. One possibility is to have a run-in period with the randomization probability being 1/2 before starting to use (7.1). Another approach that we will use here is the one given by Thall and Wathen (2007): Use formula (7.1) but with $a = n/(2N)$, where n is the current sample size of the trial and N is the maximum sample size of the trial. This approach yields assignment probabilities closer to 1/2 earlier in the trial. For example, if the current estimate of $P(E > C)$ is 0.9, the assignment probability to the experimental treatment arm would be 0.57, 0.63, and 0.70 if the trial was one-quarter, one-half, or three-quarters completed, respectively. In addition, one would want to prevent the assignment probability from becoming too extreme, so we cap the probability of arm assignment at 0.8 (similar results were seen when the cap was 0.9).

Table 7.2 displays the results for the adaptive randomization and the 1:1 and 2:1 fixed randomization using the same phase II operating characteristics as described in Section 7.2. The adaptive approach requires a total of 140 patients as compared to 132 patients for a fixed 1:1 randomization. Under the null hypothesis (response rates = 20% in both arms), the probability of response for a study participant is the same for all designs (20%), but there will be more nonresponders with the adaptive randomization (112.0 versus 105.6) because of the increased sample size. When the new treatment is beneficial, the adaptive randomization provides a slightly higher probability response: 33.2% versus 30% under the design alternative (Table 7.2, row 3, bolded). At the same time, the adaptive design results in higher numbers of nonresponders than 1:1 randomization except when the treatment effect exceeds the design alternative.

In addition to the operating characteristics presented in Table 7.2, one needs to consider extreme cases that can occur with outcome-adaptive randomization. For example, with response rates of 20% versus 30%, the outcome-adaptive randomization treats on average 59.7% of the patients on the better experimental arm (Table 7.2, row 2). However, even though this is true, there is a 5% chance that outcome-adaptive randomization would randomize at least 16 more patients to the inferior control arm in this scenario. (By random chance, unconstrained equal 1:1 randomization would assign at least 16 patients more to the inferior arm about 10% of the time. However, in practice, equal randomization is typically performed using randomized blocks that ensure that practically the same number of patients is assigned to each treatment arm.)

Trials with adaptive randomization frequently have interim monitoring based on the assignment probability (trials without adaptive randomization also frequently have interim monitoring). For example, Faderl et al. (2008) suggest stopping their trial and declaring the experimental treatment better than the control treatment if $P(E>C)>p_{stop}$, where $p_{stop}=0.95$; Giles et al. (2003) use $p_{stop}=0.85$ in a similar manner. These investigators also suggest stopping the trial if $P(E>C)<p_{stop}$, and declaring the control treatment better. However, this type of symmetric inefficacy/futility monitoring is inappropriate for the type of one-sided question we are considering here (Freidlin et al. 2010a). Instead, for simplicity, we will not consider inefficacy/futility monitoring in the simulations. If the trial reaches a maximum sample size without stopping for efficacy, we declare that the experimental treatment does not warrant further study.

Table 7.3 displays the results of the simulations using early stopping for the adaptive randomization and 1:1 fixed randomization. The maximum sample sizes (190 and 208 for fixed randomization and the adaptive design, respectively) and value of p_{stop} (0.984) were chosen so that the trial designs had type I error of 10% and power 90% for the alternative of 20% versus 40% response rates. (This interim monitoring is much more aggressive than would be typically used in a definitive phase III trial, which is why these maximum sample sizes are so much larger than the sample sizes without interim monitoring, 132 and 140.) In terms of probability of response for

TABLE 7.2

Average Proportion of Responders ($P(R)$), Number of Responders (#R), Number of Nonresponders (#NR) and Overall Proportion Treated on the Experimental Arm (E) for Various Randomized Phase II Trial Designs, Some of Which Use Adaptive Randomization[a] (One-Sided Type 1 Error = 10%, Power = 90% at 20% versus 40% Response Rates, Results Based on 500,000 Simulations)

Response Rates by Arm		Fixed Sample Size (1:1) [N=132]			Fixed Sample Size (2:1) [N=153]			Adaptive Randomization [N=140]			
C[b]	E[b]	$P(R)$	#R	#NR	$P(R)$	#R	#NR	$P(R)$	#R	#NR	Overall% Treated on E Arm
0.2	0.2	20.0%	26.4	105.6	20.0%	30.6	122.4	20.0%	28.0	112.0	50.0
0.2	0.3	25.0%	33.0	99.0	26.6%	40.8	112.2	26.0%	36.4	103.6	59.7
0.2	**0.4**	**30.0%**	**39.6**	**92.4**	**33.3%**	**51.0**	**102.0**	**33.2%**	**46.5**	**93.5**	**66.2**
0.2	0.5	35.0%	46.2	85.8	40.0%	61.2	91.8	41.0%	57.4	82.6	69.9

Note: Characteristics of trial designs corresponding to the trial alternative hypothesis are in the bolded row.

[a] Adaptive randomization is using the method of Thall and Wathen (2007) but with no early stopping and randomization-arm probability capped at 80%.

[b] C = control arm, E = experimental treatment arm.

TABLE 7.3

Average Sample Size, Proportion of Responders ($P(R)$), Number of Responders ($\#R$), and Number of Nonresponders ($\#NR$) for Fixed 1:1 and Adaptive Randomized Phase II Trial Design[a] (One-Sided Type 1 Error = 10%, Power = 90% at 20% versus 40% Response Rates, Results Based on 500,000 Simulations)

Response Rates by Treatment Arm		Fixed 1-1 (Maximum Sample Size = 190)				Adaptive Randomization (Maximum Sample Size = 208) Capped at 80% Assignment Probability			
C[b]	E[b]	Average Sample Size	$P(R)$	$\#R$	$\#NR$	Average Sample Size	$P(R)$	$\#R$	$\#NR$
0.2	0.2	177.9	20.3%	35.6	142.3	194.3	20.2%	38.8	155.5
0.2	0.3	135.2	25.9%	33.8	101.4	147.6	26.3%	37.9	109.7
0.2	**0.4**	**78.4**	**31.4%**	**23.6**	**54.8**	**83.7**	**32.1%**	**26.4**	**57.3**
0.2	0.5	43.3	36.6%	15.1	28.2	45.3	37.1%	16.5	28.8

Notes: Trials are stopped early for superiority of the experimental treatment if the $P(E > C) > 0.984$. Characteristics of trial designs corresponding to the trial alternative hypothesis are in the bolded row.

[a] Adaptive randomization is using the method of Thall and Wathen (2007).

[b] C = control arm, E = experimental treatment arm.

a participant, the two designs perform very similarly: the differences are less than 1% across the range of simulated scenarios. When compared by the number of nonresponders, the adaptive design can be nontrivially worse, for example, on average 13 more nonresponders using the adaptive design under the null hypothesis.

7.4 Multiarm Trials

Multiarm trials that have one control arm and multiple experimental arms offer an efficient way to test multiple treatments (Freidlin et al. 2008). Adaptive randomization can be used in mutiarm trials. It has been asserted that the "adaptive randomization light shines brightest in complicated multiarm settings" (Berry 2011) rather than in two-arm trials. This assertion can be checked by simulations (Korn and Freidlin 2011b): Table 7.4 presents simulation results for a trial with three experimental treatment arms and a control arm. For the adaptive randomization, after 20 patients had been equally randomized to the 4 arms, the randomization probability for an arm was taken to be proportional to the posterior mean response rate for that arm (but never less than 10% for an actively accruing arm) using independent uniform prior distributions. (The posterior mean response rate for an arm with x responses seen in the first n patients is simply $(x+1)/(n+2)$.) For both designs, the pairwise type 1 error rates were taken to be 10%, the pairwise powers were taken to be 90%, an experimental arm was stopped early for efficacy if the posterior probability that it had a better response rate than the control arm was >98%, and an experimental arm was stopped early for futility if the posterior probability that it had a better response rate than the control arm was <15%. For the equal randomization design, the (maximum) sample size per arm is set to 53 (to ensure the designated error rates). For the adaptive randomization design, we limited the pairwise sample sizes by $1/n(\text{control})+1/n(\text{expt } i) \geq 2/53$, $i=1, 2, 3$, to help avoid unreasonably large sample sizes. As with the results for two-armed trial designs, outcome-adaptive randomization yields a slightly larger proportion of patients that have a response, a larger number of responders, but at the cost of a larger (and therefore longer) trial and a larger number of nonresponders.

A different type of adaptive randomization for multiarm trials has been proposed that essentially ensures that the number of patients on the control arm will be approximately the same as the number of patients on the experimental arm with the most patients (Trippa et al. 2012). Since much of the inefficiency of standard adaptive randomization comes from the smaller sample size in the control arm as compared to the sample sizes in any treatment arms that are effective, the proposal gains back much of the inefficiency of a standard adaptive randomization. However, there are three

TABLE 7.4

Average Sample Size, Proportion of Responders ($P(R)$), Number of Responders ($\#R$), and Number of Nonresponders for Fixed 1:1:1:1 and Adaptive Randomized Phase II Trial Design[a] (Pairwise One-Sided Type 1 Error = 10%, Power = 90% at 35% versus 65% Response Rates, Results Based on 20,000 Simulations)

Response Rates by Treatment Arm (One Control Arm, Three Experimental Arms)				Fixed 1-1-1-1 Randomization (Maximum Sample Size = 212)				Adaptive Randomization (Maximum Sample Size = 303[b])			
C	*E1*	*E2*	*E3*	Average Sample Size	*P(R)*	*#R*	*#NR*	Average Sample Size	*P(R)*	*#R*	*#NR*
0.35	0.35	0.35	0.35	134.3	35.1%	47.0	87.3	140.9	35.1%	49.3	91.6
0.35	0.35	0.35	0.65	122.6	40.4%	48.6	74.0	130.1	41.0%	52.3	77.8
0.35	0.35	0.65	0.65	108.5	46.4%	49.6	58.9	114.8	47.2%	53.5	61.3
0.35	0.65	0.65	0.65	86.2	55.2%	47.5	38.7	91.7	57.1%	52.1	39.6

[a] Adaptive randomization described in text.

[b] This is the maximum sample size seen in the 20,000 simulations for the global null case (line 1). The 95th percentile of the sample size distribution for this case is 231.

additional considerations worth noting. First, if the trial has only two treatment arms (one experimental arm and the control arm), the proposed adaptive randomization procedure reduces to a 1 – 1 randomization fixed-sample size trial design. The proponents of the new procedure apparently agree that adaptive randomization should not be used in this situation (Trippa et al. 2013). Secondly, since patients will be randomized to the control arm even if it is doing poorly, the design no longer has the attractive feature of placing patients on the trial arms that appear to be doing best.

The third consideration to note with the proposed adaptive randomization is that it, like other outcome-adaptive randomization designs, involves intensive interim analyses of the accruing data. Interim monitoring for futility/inefficacy is a standard part of randomized clinical trial designs in which experimental treatment arms that are not doing sufficiently well as compared to the control treatment arm are dropped during the trial (Freidlin and Korn 2009). In fact, since the proposed adaptive randomization is assigning fewer patients to experimental arms that appear to be doing worse, it can be thought of as a type of intensive futility/inefficacy monitoring. Therefore, a relevant comparison of adaptive randomization and 1:1 randomization should include interim monitoring for the latter (Freidlin and Korn 2013). Table 7.5 displays one such comparison using trial designs with one control arm and three experimental arms, and a total sample size of 140 for all the trial designs; the power and average sample sizes are given for (1) an equal (balanced) randomization fixed sample-size design with no interim monitoring, (2) the adaptive randomization design as described in Trippa et al. (2012), and (3) an equal randomization design incorporating commonly used group sequential futility monitoring. The results in Table 7.5 demonstrate that the proposed adaptive randomization procedure compared to an equal randomization fixed sample-size design has higher power for experimental arms that work and smaller average sample sizes for experimental arms that do not, replicating the results of Trippa et al. (2012). For example, there is a power benefit of 88% versus 80% when there is a single active experimental arm (Table 7.5, row 2). However, compared to an equal randomization with a standard group sequential design, there is no advantage of the adaptive randomization procedure in terms of power or numbers of patients assigned to efficacious treatment arms.

7.5 Multiarm Trials with Randomization within Biomarker-Defined Subgroups

Biomarkers can be used to define subgroups within which different treatment questions can be definitively assessed (Freidlin et al. 2010b). In earlier clinical trials, biomarkers can be used in a more exploratory manner: patients

TABLE 7.5

Empirical Power (Average Sample Size) for Each of Three Experimental Arms (*E*1, *E*2, *E*3) versus a Control Arm (*C*) for Three Experimental Trial Designs[a] (Results Based on 50,000 Simulations)

Response Rates (One Control Arm, Three Experimental Arms)				Equal Randomization Design with Fixed Sample Size and No Interim Monitoring[b]			Adaptive Randomization Design[c]			Equal Randomization Group-Sequential Design with Futility Monitoring[d]		
C	*E*1	*E*2	*E*3	*E*1	*E*2	*E*3	*E*1	*E*2	*E*3	*E*1	*E*2	*E*3
0.1	0.1	0.1	0.1	0.10	0.10	0.11	0.10	0.10	0.10	0.10	0.10	0.10
				(35)	(35)	(35)	(32.7)	(32.5)	(32.6)	(29.9)	(29.9)	(29.9)
0.1	0.3	0.1	0.1	0.80	0.10	0.11	0.88	0.10	0.10	0.88	0.10	0.10
				(35)	(35)	(35)	(45.4)	(25.3)	(25.4)	(45.3)	(23.6)	(23.7)
0.1	0.3	0.3	0.1	0.80	0.81	0.11	0.83	0.83	0.10	0.83	0.83	0.10
				(35)	(35)	(35)	(37.8)	(37.8)	(22.9)	(38.1)	(38.2)	(22.5)
0.1	0.3	0.3	0.3	0.80	0.81	0.80	0.80	0.80	0.80	0.80	0.80	0.80
				(35)	(35)	(35)	(33.5)	(33.5)	(33.4)	(34.4)	(34.4)	(34.4)
0.1	0.5	0.3	0.1	1.0	0.81	0.11	>0.99	0.82	0.10	>0.99	0.82	0.10
				(35)	(35)	(35)	(40.4)	(35.7)	(22.3)	(40.2)	(37.2)	(22.4)

[a] Testing each experimental arm versus the control arm with a chi-squared test with one-sided significance level 0.10 for all designs. Total sample size is 140 for each trial design.

[b] 140 patients are randomly assigned 1:1:1:1 to four arms.

[c] 140 patients are randomly assigned to four arms according to the adaptive randomization design described in Trippa et al. (2012), using (in place of the posterior probability that the hazard ratio is greater than one) the posterior probability that the experimental treatment response rate is higher than the control treatment response rate (assuming a uniform prior distribution). The tuning parameters values were used as recommended in Trippa et al. (2012): η is an increasing linear function with η at the overall sample size equal to 0.25, and $a=3$ and $b=1.75$.

[d] 140 patients are randomly assigned 1:1:1:1 to four arms with potential futility stopping: for each experimental versus control comparison, group sequential stopping for futility is performed after (20, 30, 40, 50, 60) patients are enrolled on the corresponding two arms using a (−1, −0.5, −0.1, 0.1, 0.6) z-value cutoff, respectively. Futility analyses are performed as long as there are at least two open experimental arms.

have various biomarkers assessed and are randomized into different treatment arms regardless of their biomarker values. One can then attempt to tease out which treatments work for which biomarker-defined subgroups. It is possible in this type of design to use adaptive randomization among the treatments rather than fixed randomization. Since different treatments may work better in different biomarker subgroups, the adaptive randomization should be done separately within each biomarker subgroup. Two trials that took this approach, I-SPY2 and BATTLE, are discussed in this section.

7.5.1 I-SPY2 Trial

In the phase II I-SPY2 trial (Barker et al. 2009), women with locally advanced breast cancer are randomized to various novel neoadjuvant chemotherapies or a standard neoadjuvant. The outcome is pathological complete response (pCR) rate, determined at the time of surgery (after the chemotherapy). An adaptive randomization is used to assign treatments based on a Bayesian analysis of the pCR rates, with the adaptive randomization taking place within various biomarker groups. The novel agents can be dropped from further testing in a biomarker subgroup if they have a low probability of being better than standard therapy in that subgroup or graduated from that biomarker subgroup if they have a high probability of being better than standard therapy in that subgroup (Barker et al. 2009).

As of this time, the results of the I-SPY2 are not available nor are the details of the design publicly available (e.g., sample sizes and targeted pCR rate differences between the novel and standard treatment arms). However, the simulation results presented here in Sections 7.3 and 7.4 suggest that, compared to the adaptive randomization being used in I-SPY2, equal randomization with interim monitoring would result in smaller required total sample sizes, but with a smaller overall pCR rate for the patients treated on the trial.

7.5.2 BATTLE Trial

In the phase II BATTLE trial (Kim et al. 2011), chemorefractory non–small cell lung cancer patients were randomized among four treatments: erlotinib, vandetanib, erlotinib + bexarotene, and sorafenib. Patients had biomarkers analyzed on their tumors and were grouped into five biomarker groups. The primary outcome of the trial was the 8-week disease control rate (DCR), defined by the proportion of patients with a complete or partial response, or with stable disease at 8 weeks. For simplicity of explication, we will refer to such a patient as being a responder. Unlike the previous trial designs discussed in this chapter, BATTLE was not designed to compare treatment arms to a control arm. Instead, each arm was to be compared to an historical DCR of 30%. Because the previous simulation results do not apply to this situation, we will have an extended discussion here of the implications for the randomization used for this trial.

TABLE 7.6

Results for the BATTLE Trial: Numbers of Patients with Disease Control at 8 Weeks/Number of Evaluable Patients (%)

	Treatment Group				
Biomarker Group	**Erlotinib**	**Vandetanib**	**Erlotinib + Bexarotene**	**Sorafenib**	**Total**
EGFR	6/17 (35%)	11/27 (41%)	11/20 (55%)	9/23 (39%)	27/87 (43%)
KRAS/BRAF	1/7 (14%)	0/3 (0%)	1/3 (33%)	11/14 (79%)	13/27 (48%)
VEGF/VEGFR-2	10/25 (40%)	6/16 (38%)	0/3 (0%)	25/39 (64%)	41/83 (49%)
RXR/Cyclin D1	0/1 (0%)	0/0.	1/1 (100%)	1/4 (25%)	2/6 (33%)
None	3/8 (38%)	0/6 (0%)	5/9 (56%)	11/18 (61%)	19/41 (46%)
Total	20/58 (34%)	17/52 (33%)	18/36 (50%)	57/98 (58%)	112/244 (46%)

Note: Data in this table were taken from Table 2 of Kim et al. (2011).

In BATTLE, equal randomization was used for the first 97 patients (except that patients who had prior erlotinib treatment were not randomized to erlotinib or erlotinib + bexarotene), and then adaptive randomization was used within each of five biomarker groups for the next 158 patients. An early stopping rule was applied to treatment–biomarker subgroups that were showing insufficient activity (Zhou et al. 2008). The design specified a type 1 error of 20% for the null hypothesis that the DCR was 30%.

The results of the BATTLE trial are displayed in Table 7.6 for the evaluable patients. The overall DCR was 46%, corresponding to 112 responders and 132 nonresponders among the 244 patients. We can approximate what would have happened if an equal randomization had been used throughout the trial by assuming that the observed response rates in Table 7.6 were the true probabilities of having a response. (We assume throughout that the true DCR is 33% for patients in the RXR/cyclin D1 marker group treated with vandetanib because there are no data for this combination.) We estimate that with equal randomization the overall DCR would have been 38%, corresponding to 93 responders and 151 nonresponders if 244 patients had been evaluated.

Although these results appear very good for adaptive randomization, the question arises as to whether the adaptive randomization is placing more patients on certain treatment arms than is necessary to answer the questions the trial is asking. The BATTLE trial used a Bayesian analysis, but we can apply a frequentist analysis and design to address this issue (Rubin et al. 2011; Simon 2013). The trial is stated to have 80% power (Kim et al. 2011) and simulations performed by the BATTLE investigators suggested that the trial has 80% power against an alternative hypothesis of a 60% DCR (Zhou et al. 2008). Targeting a 30% versus 60% DCR's would require (at most) eight patients for a particular biomarker–treatment group combination with a two-stage design: Initially treat three patients for a particular combination and if there is at least one response, treat a total of eight patients for that combination.

Considering a treatment to be effective for a combination if there are at least four responses out of the eight patients yields a type 1 error of 18% and a power of 80%. The maximum sample size for this design is 160 (= 20 × 8), but some combinations will stop after three patients and no responses. Assuming the four combinations that treated patients with no responses would have stopped after three patients (and, conservatively, no other combinations would have stopped) yields a sample size of 140. The expected DCR if this equal-randomization design had been used is 43%, corresponding to 60 responders and 80 nonresponders. This can be compared to the adaptive design used that had a DCR of 46%, with 112 responders and 132 nonresponders. Viewed in this manner, it would appear that equal randomization would have been better than adaptive randomization for this trial.

A different type of comparison with equal randomization may also be informative: Instead of accruing 140 patients, we can consider accruing up to 244 patients, keeping the trial open to treatment–biomarker groups that have passed the design criteria; that is, have at least one response in the first three patients and at least four responses in the first eight patients. This method of comparison has been used in the multiarm setting without biomarkers (Lee et al. 2012). We do not think it is a good method of comparison in the setting of no biomarkers because there will be no reason to accrue more patients in a trial than necessary to answer the clinical question being asked. However, in the present setting of biomarker-defined subgroups, one could argue that it is reasonable to keep treating on trial patients who are in a more prevalent subgroup while waiting for patients in a less prevalent subgroup to accrue. (If another trial was available for these patients, it would be preferable to offer them that option.)

To perform the equal-randomization (up to) 244 patient comparison, we again assume the observed response rates in Table 7.6 are the true response rates. We simulated 100,000 trial datasets, each with sample sizes 87, 27, 83, 6, and 41 in the five biomarker subgroups. We used equal randomization within each biomarker group among the treatment groups that have not been closed for inefficacy (after three and eight patients have been evaluated) for the biomarker subgroup. We find that the expected response rate is 48%, with on average 113 responders and 122 nonresponders (average total sample size = 235). These results compare favorably to the outcome-adaptive design used, which had a DCR of 46%, with 112 responders and 132 nonresponders.

7.6 Issues with Adaptive Randomization

A fundamental concern with adaptive randomization, which was noted early (Byar et al. 1976), is the potential for bias if there are any time trends in the prognostic mix of the patients accruing to the trial. In fact, time trends associated with the outcome due to any cause can lead to bias with straightforward implementations of adaptive randomization. There are approaches to eliminating this potential bias, for example, by performing a block randomization and a block-stratified analysis, but these approaches make the adaptive randomization much more inefficient (Korn and Freidlin 2011a). Although a change in the underlying patient population may be unlikely during a quickly accruing small trial, care is still required since the type of patients who choose to go on the trial may quickly change, especially if patients and their clinicians can see how well (or not well) the new treatment is doing based on the current randomization ratio if the trial is not blinded. This, along with the possibility that knowledge that the randomization ratio is favoring the control treatment arm may drastically diminish accrual, suggests the advisability of placebo-controlled designs whenever possible when using adaptive randomization.

Another issue in using adaptive randomization in a definitive trial is that the endpoint will usually be long term, such as overall survival. This can make adaptive randomization, which requires sufficient accruing outcome information to adapt, difficult to implement. It is possible to use whatever survival information is available adapt the randomization imbalance (Cheung et al. 2006), but this randomization will not adapt as quickly as when the outcome is available sooner. This can also be an issue with early clinical trials that, for example, use outcomes that are not immediate. For example, in the I-SPY 2 trial, the outcome (pCR) was determined at surgery that occurred 6 months after randomization. To perform the adaptive randomization more efficiently, the investigators used accruing information about the association of pCR and baseline and longitudinal markers (including multiple MRI scans) to allow the use of the baseline/longitudinal data to substitute for not-yet-available pCR data to update the randomization ratios (Barker et al. 2009).

7.7 Discussion

We are sometimes told by (nonstatistician) investigators that adaptive randomization will lead to smaller and quicker trials. As our results show, and as proponents of adaptive randomization acknowledge (Berry and Eick 1995, Lee et al. 2012), this is not true. We believe that the major source of confusion is that there may not be a realization that interim monitoring for efficacy and futility, which is a standard part of randomized clinical trial methodology, is not special to adaptive randomization. Interim monitoring leads to quicker and shorter trials, whether or not the randomization is adaptive. In fact, as compared to 1:1 randomization with appropriate interim monitoring, adaptive randomization leads to larger and longer trials.

This leaves the question as to the benefits and costs of adaptive randomization to the patients on a trial that uses it (Lee et al. 2010). When the experimental treatment is more effective than the control treatment, adaptive randomization will lead on average to an overall better outcome for the patients on the trial than 1:1 randomization (although the benefit may be slight). However, since adaptive randomization leads to a larger trial, in absolute numbers there will be not only more patients with good outcomes, but there will also be more patients with bad outcomes than if 1:1 randomization were used. If the experimental treatment is no more effective than the control treatment, the larger trial due to the adaptive randomization means that more patients will be exposed to the toxicities of the ineffective experimental treatment than if 1:1 randomization were used. Therefore, it is arguable that adaptive randomization offers net benefit to the patients on the trial.

In summary, given its complexity, its modest potential benefits to patients on the trial, and its requirement of larger trials to answer the clinical questions, we do not recommend outcome-adaptive randomization.

References

Barker, A.D., C.C. Sigman, G.J. Kelloff et al. 2009. I-SPY 2: An adaptive breast cancer trial design in the setting of neoadjuvant chemotherapy. *Clinical Pharmacology and Therapeutics* 86:97–100.

Berry, D.A. 2006. Bayesian clinical trials. *Nature Reviews Drug Discovery* 5:27–36.

Berry, D.A. 2011. Adaptive clinical trials: The promise and the caution. *Journal of Clinical Oncology* 29:606–609.

Berry, D.A. and S.G. Eick. 1995. Adaptive assignment versus balanced randomization in clinical trials: A decision analysis. *Statistics in Medicine* 14:231–246.

Biswas, S., D.D. Liu, J.J. Lee et al. 2009. Bayesian clinical trials at the University of Texas M.D. Anderson Cancer Center. *Clinical Trials* 6:205–216.

Brittain, E. and J.J. Schlesselman. 1982. Optimal allocation for the comparison of proportions. *Biometrics* 38:1003–1009.

Byar, D.P., R.M. Simon, W.T. Friedewald et al. 1976. Randomized clinical trials—Perspectives on some recent ideas. *The New England Journal of Medicine* 295:74–80.

Cheung, Y.K., L.Y.T. Inoue, J.Y. Wathen, and P.F. Thall. 2006. Continuous Bayesian adaptive randomization based on event times with covariates. *Statistics in Medicine* 25:55–70.

Cornfield, J., M. Halperin, and S.W. Greenhouse. 1969. An adaptive procedure for sequential clinical trials. *Journal of the American Statistical Association* 64:759–770.

Faderl, S., F. Ravandi, X. Huang et al. 2008. A randomized study of clofarabine versus clofarabine plus low-dose cytarabine as front-line therapy for patients aged 60 years and older with acute myeloid leukemia and high-risk myelodysplastic syndrome. *Blood* 112:1638–1645.

Freidlin, B. and E.L. Korn. 2009. Monitoring for lack of benefit: A critical component of a randomized clinical trial. *Journal of Clinical Oncology* 27:629–633.

Freidlin, B. and E.L. Korn. 2013. Adaptive randomization versus interim monitoring. *Journal of Clinical Oncology* 31:969–970.

Freidlin, B., E.L. Korn, and R. Gray. 2010a. A general inefficacy interim monitoring rule for randomized clinical trials. *Clinical Trials* 7:197–208.

Freidlin, B., E.L. Korn, R. Gray, and A. Martin. 2008. Multi-arm clinical trials of new agents: Some design considerations. *Clinical Cancer Research* 14:4368–4371.

Freidlin, B., L.M. McShane, and E.L. Korn. 2010b. Randomized clinical trials with biomarkers: Design issues. *Journal of the National Cancer Institute* 102:152–160.

Giles, F.J., H.M. Kantarjian, J.E. Cortes et al. 2003. Adaptive randomized study of idarubicin and cytarabine versus troxacitabine and cytarabine versus troxacitabine and idarubicin in untreated patients 50 years or older with adverse karyotype acute myeloid leukemia. *Journal of Clinical Oncology* 21:1722–1727.

Kim, E.S., R.S. Herbst, I.I. Wistuba et al. 2011. The BATTLE trial: Personalizing therapy for lung cancer. *Cancer Discovery* 1:44–53.

Korn, E.L. and B. Freidlin. 2011a. Outcome-adaptive randomization: Is it useful? *Journal of Clinical Oncology* 29:771–776.

Korn, E.L. and B. Freidlin. 2011b. Reply to Yuan Y. et al. *Journal of Clinical Oncology* 29: e393.

Lee, J.J., N. Chen, and G. Yin. 2012. Worth adapting? Revisiting the usefulness of outcome-adaptive randomization. *Clinical Cancer Research* 18:4498–4507.

Lee, J.J., X. Gu, and S. Liu. 2010. Bayesian adaptive randomization designs for targeted agent development. *Clinical Trials* 7:584–596.

Rubin, E.H., K.M. Anderson, and C.K. Gause. 2011. The BATTLE trial: A bold step toward improving the efficiency of biomarker-based drug development. *Cancer Discovery* 1:17–20.

Rubinstein, L.V., E.L. Korn, B. Freidlin et al. 2005. Design issues of randomized phase II trials and a proposal for phase II screening trials. *Journal of Clinical Oncology* 23:7199–7206.

Simon, R.M. 2013. *Genomic Clinical Trials and Predictive Medicine*. Cambridge, U.K.: Cambridge University Press, pp 31–33.

Thall, P.F. and J.K. Wathen. 2007. Practical Bayesian adaptive randomisation in clinical trials. *European Journal of Cancer* 43:859–866.

Thompson, W.R. 1933. On the likelihood that one unknown probability exceeds another in view of the evidence of the two samples. *Biometrika* 25:285–294.

Trippa, L, E.Q. Lee, P.Y. Wen et al. 2012. Bayesian adaptive randomized trial design for patients with recurrent Glioblastoma. *Journal of Clinical Oncology* 30:3258–3263.

Trippa, L, E.Q. Lee, P.Y. Wen et al. 2013. Reply to Freidlin B. et al. *Journal of Clinical Oncology* 31:970–971.

Zelen, M. 1969. Play the winner rule and the controlled clinical trial. *Journal of the American Statistical Association* 64:131–146.

Zhou, X., S. Liu, E.S. Kim, R.S. Herbst, and J.J. Lee. 2008. Bayesian adaptive design for targeted therapy development in lung cancer—A step toward personalized medicine. *Clinical Trials* 5:181–193.

8

Challenges of Using Predictive Biomarkers in Clinical Trials

Sumithra Mandrekar and Daniel Sargent

CONTENTS

8.1 Introduction

The Biomarkers Definitions Working Group defined a biomarker to be "a characteristic that is objectively measured and evaluated as an indicator of normal biological processes, pathogenic processes, or pharmacologic responses to a therapeutic intervention" [1]. The term biomarker in oncology refers to a broad range of markers and includes a range of measures derived from tumor tissues, whole blood, plasma, serum, bone marrow, or urine. From the perspective of clinical utility, biomarkers can be classified into three categories: prognostic biomarkers, predictive biomarkers, and surrogate endpoints, with the recognition that some biomarkers may fall into more than one category. Prognostic and predictive biomarkers focus on individual patient risk-classification and treatment selection, respectively, whereas biomarkers used as surrogate endpoints aid in the evaluation of the efficacy of a new treatment. It is critical to realize that the ultimate intended usage of a biomarker determines its definition and the required validation methods. A prognostic biomarker predicts the natural history of the disease process in a given individual, and thus aids in the decision of whether a patient needs an intensive and possibly toxic treatment as opposed to no treatment or standard therapy [2]. A predictive biomarker predicts whether an individual patient will respond to a particular therapy or not, and hence its clinical utility is in allowing for individualized therapy. A surrogate endpoint biomarker replaces the primary clinical outcome (i.e., endpoint) and informs the efficacy of a new treatment with greater cost-effectiveness than the primary clinical outcome (such as overall survival) at the population level [3]. We focus our discussion in this chapter on predictive biomarkers.

Predictive biomarker validation, both in an initial (i.e., phase II) and in a definitive (i.e., phase III) setting, is complex and requires the same level of evidence (for definitive validation) as is needed to adopt a new therapeutic intervention [4,5]. This implies that a predictive marker validation is prospective in nature, and the obvious strategy is to conduct an appropriately designed prospective randomized controlled trial (RCT). In the setting of phase II trials, RCTs also provide the opportunity to simultaneously assess multiple promising therapies (and multiple possible markers) for a given disease. Freidlin et al. [6] proposed guidelines for the design of randomized phase II trials with biomarkers that can inform the design of the subsequent phase III trial. Specifically, the results from the biomarker-driven phase II trial (if the treatment is found promising in the phase II setting) can lead to three possible phase III trial decisions: enrichment/targeted design, biomarker stratified (marker by treatment interaction) design, or an unselected design [6]. The crucial component of RCTs is, of course, randomization, which is essential for the following reasons:

1. RCT assures that the patients who are treated with the agent for whom the marker is purported to be predictive are comparable to those who are not.
2. Changes in patient population based on biological subsetting and/or evolution in imaging technologies can make comparisons against historical controls inaccurate.
3. RCTs are essential for making the distinction between a prognostic and predictive marker [7].
4. RCTs provide the opportunity to assess multiple promising therapies (and multiple possible markers) for a given disease simultaneously in a phase II setting.

In the absence of an RCT, it is impossible to isolate any causal effect of the marker on therapeutic efficacy from the multitude of other factors that may influence the decision to treat or not to treat a patient. For instance, a cohort of nonrandomized patients was used to evaluate the predictive utility of tumor microsatellite instability for the efficacy of 5-fluorouracil (5-FU)-based chemotherapy in colon cancer. In this cohort, the median age of the treated patients was 13 years younger than those of the nontreated patients, thus rendering any meaningful statements about the predictive value of the marker for the relevant endpoints of disease-free and overall survival impossibly confounded [8]. In some instances, where a prospective RCT is not possible in the phase III setting due to ethical and logistical considerations (large trial and/or long time to complete), a well-conducted prospectively specified retrospective validation can also aid in bringing forward effective treatments to marker defined patient subgroups in a timely manner [5]. In the phase II setting, a controversial yet pertinent question is whether it is necessary to randomize throughout the entire duration of a trial in a phase II setting. This might be relevant in the case, for example, where preliminary evidence for a new experimental agent is promising in a biomarker-defined cohort, but not sufficiently compelling to pursue a nonrandomized trial. In such cases, one might consider an alternative phase II design approach that starts as an RCT, but allows for a switch to direct assignment (i.e., all patients receive the experimental agent) after a prespecified interim analysis [9,10]. Regardless, the use of an RCT either in the prospective or retrospective setting is critical for initial as well as definitive predictive marker validation.

Another important component of biomarker validation relates to biomarker assay issues, including the choice of using a central facility versus local laboratories for patient selection [4,11]. This choice depends on three factors: (1) the reliability and reproducibility of the assay, (2) the complexity of the assay, and (3) potential for a repeat assessment of the marker status (when feasible and ethically appropriate) if the results from the first assessment are questionable. For the purposes of this chapter, we will assume that the issues surrounding technical feasibility, assay performance metrics, and the logistics of specimen collection are resolved and that initial results demonstrate promise with regard to the predictive ability of the marker(s).

Demonstrating clinical validity of predictive biomarkers poses unique challenges to the design, conduct, and analysis of clinical trials. In the remainder of this chapter, we review the design strategies for initial and definitive marker validation, along with a discussion of the relative merits and limitations of each design. We will use examples of real clinical trials, where available, to illustrate the design concepts.

8.2 Initial Validation: Phase II Setting

Phase II clinical trials are designed primarily to identify promising experimental regimens that are then tested further in definitive phase III trials. Trial designs in the phase II setting for initial marker validation can be classified under enrichment, all-comers, adaptive (specifically, outcome-based adaptive randomization), and direct assignment option categories as elaborated in Table 8.1 [12]. Examples of phase II trials utilizing one of these design strategies are outlined as follows:

- N0923 (Clinicaltrials.gov identifier (CT.gov id): NCT01017601) is an example of a phase II trial following an enrichment design strategy. This is a randomized double-blinded phase II study of a replication-competent picornavirus versus matching placebo, after standard

TABLE 8.1

Overview of Phase II Biomarker-Driven Designs

Design	Useful When
Enrichment designs screen all patients for the marker, but only randomize those with certain molecular features. These evaluate treatment in the marker-defined subgroup only.	• There is compelling preliminary evidence that treatment benefit, if any, is restricted to a subgroup of patients • The cut point for marker status determination is well established • Analytical validity has been well established • There is rapid turnaround time for the assay
All-comers designs screen all patients for the marker and randomize patients with a valid marker result with analysis plans to test the treatment by marker interaction effect.	• The new treatment has the potential to benefit both marker subgroups • If marker status used for stratification, then the cut point for marker status determination needs to be well established • The marker prevalence is high
Outcome-based adaptive randomization designs are a class of designs that adapt the design parameters during the course of the trial based on accumulated data.	• Prespecified biomarker-defined subgroups and/or multiple treatment options • Analytical validity well established • Rapid turnaround time for the assay
Direct assignment option designs have the option for direct assignment (i.e., stop randomization and assign all patients to the experimental arm) based on prespecified interim analysis (IA).	• The prevalence of the marker in question is moderate (between 20% and 50%), and the preliminary evidence is not compelling for an enrichment design • Recognizes the need for randomization but also acknowledges the possibility of promising but inconclusive results after preplanned IA • Allows randomization to the control to be stopped based on the interim analysis results • Leads to accrual savings and treating proportionally more patients with active versus control treatment, while maintaining desirable statistical properties

platinum-containing cytroreductive induction chemotherapy in patients with extensive stage small cell lung cancer with a neuro-endocrine histology as per presence of ≥1 neuroendocrine marker (synaptophysin, chromogranin, and CD56) [12].

- I-SPY 2 (investigation of serial studies to predict therapeutic response with imaging and molecular analysis 2; CT.gov id: NCT01042379) and BATTLE (biomarker-integrated approaches of targeted therapy of lung cancer elimination trial) are examples of trials in the phase II setting that utilized an outcome-based adaptive randomization strategy [13–15].

The key considerations when deciding between designs in a phase II setting include the marker prevalence, strength of the preliminary evidence, the assay reliability and validity, and turnaround times for marker assessment (see Table 8.2) [16]. The following discussion (and Table 8.2) is only intended as a generic guideline to help determine the choice of a design based on all of the criteria listed earlier.

Enrichment designs are clearly appropriate when there is compelling preliminary evidence to suggest benefit of a treatment only in a marker-defined subgroup(s) and/or when the marker prevalence is low (<10%–20%). Under these situations, it is not feasible to use an all-comers strategy as the treatment effect in the overall population will be diluted, thus requiring a prohibitively large sample size. For enrichment designs, it is also essential to have an established assay with good performance and short turnaround times for marker assessment. A direct assignment option design with a single early interim analysis or two interim analyses with option for direct at both analysis (Figure 8.1) are other potential options in this setting [10]. This is an enrichment strategy, but where the randomization to the control could be stopped based on the interim analysis results. Potential advantages of the direct assignment enrichment design strategy, compared to the enrichment design, include accrual savings and treating proportionally more patients with active versus control treatment, while maintaining desirable statistical properties. A direct assignment option design can be used in combination with an all-comers or an enrichment design strategy, depending on whether all patients (regardless of the marker status or all marker subgroups) or only a biomarker defined subgroup are included.

An all-comers design is appropriate when (1) the preliminary evidence is unclear and the marker prevalence is high (≥50%) and/or (2) the assay performance is not well established (i.e., no established cut point for marker status definition) and/or (3) the turnaround time for marker assessment is long (more than a week for example in second- or third-line treatment settings). In most instances, however, an all-comers design should incorporate a prospectively specified subgroup analyses of the treatment effect within biomarker-defined subgroups. This is critical to ensure that the effect of the drug is tested both on the overall and prospectively defined subsets of patients so as to not incorrectly conclude that the drug is not effective, when it may be effective for a smaller subset of the population [5]. If the preliminary evidence for a new experimental agent is promising in only the biomarker-positive subgroup, but is not sufficiently compelling or clear in the biomarker-negative cohort, then a direct assignment option design could be considered for each of the positive and the negative biomarker cohorts.

The outcome-based adaptive randomization designs have the greatest potential when assessing multiple treatments and marker subsets where many questions are addressed and are usually not recommended in the context of two-armed trials, fixed sample size, and no biomarkers [17–19]. They do require established assays and reasonable turnaround times for

TABLE 8.2

Criteria for Choice of Biomarker-Driven Design in a Phase II Setting

	Design			
Criteria	**Enrichment**	**All-Comers**	**Direct Assignment Option**	**Outcome-Based Adaptive Randomization**
Preliminary evidence				
1. Strongly suggest benefit in marker defined subgroups	Optimal	Not recommended	Appropriate (with an early single IA, or two IA with option for direct at both IA)	Appropriate (assess multiple treatments/biomarker subgroups)
2. Uncertain about benefit in overall population versus marker defined subgroups	Not recommended	Appropriate	Appropriate (direct assignment option within the biomarker positive and negative cohorts)	Appropriate (learn and adapt as the trial proceeds)
Assay reproducibility and validity				
1. Excellent (high concordance between local and central testing; commercially available kits, etc.)	Required	Appropriate	Required	Required
2. Questionable	Not recommended	Appropriate	Not applicable	Not applicable
Turnaround times				
1. Rapid (2–3 days; without causing delay in the start of therapy)	Optimal	Optimal	Optimal	Optimal
2. Slow to modest (1 week or more)	Not recommended	Appropriate (retrospective marker subgroup assessment)	Appropriate in some cases	Appropriate in some cases
Marker prevalence				
1. Low (<20%)	Optimal	Not recommended	Appropriate (with an early single IA, or two IA with option for direct at both IA)	Appropriate
2. Moderate (20%–50%)	Appropriate	Appropriate (stratified by marker status)	Appropriate, with 2 IA with direct assignment option only at the second IA	Appropriate
3. High (>50%)	Appropriate	Appropriate	Appropriate	Appropriate

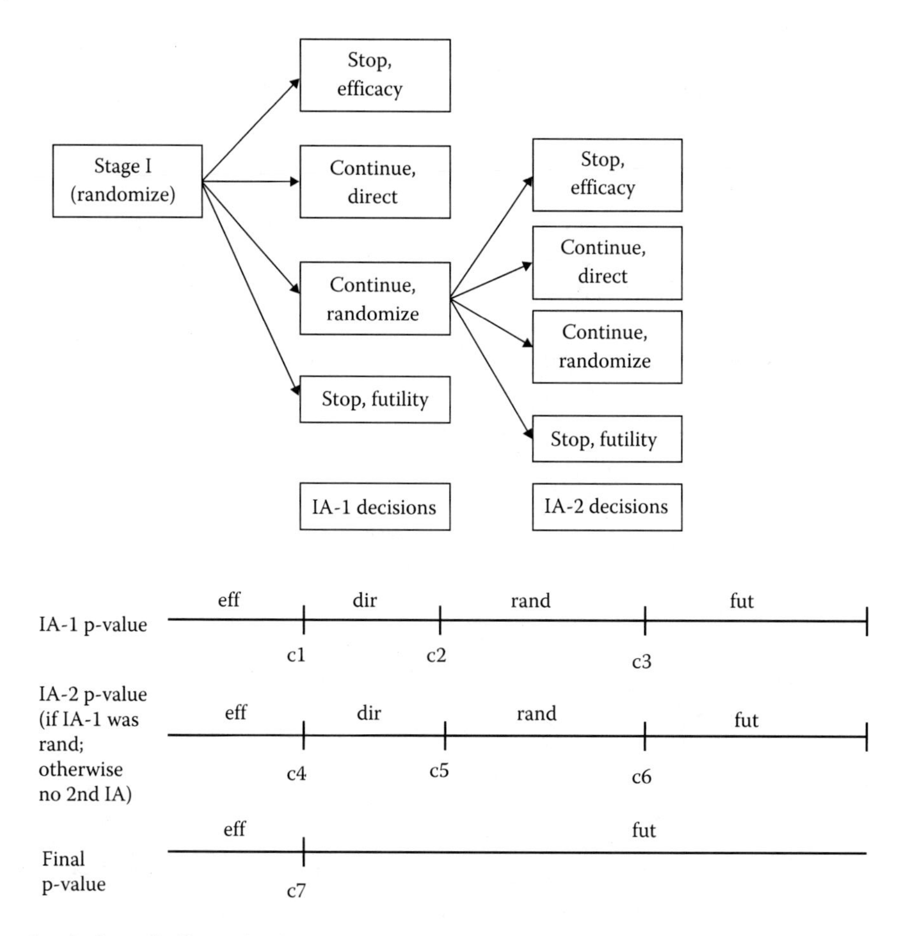

Fut, futility; eff, efficacy; dir, direct; rand, randomize

c1, c2, c3, c4 (=c2), c5 (=c7), c6, c7: O'Brien-Fleming stopping boundaries

FIGURE 8.1
Direct assignment option design with two planned interim analyses. (Reprinted with permission from Mandrekar, S.J. et al., *Contemp. Clin. Trials* 36, 597, 2013.)

marker assessment, but can be applied to any marker prevalence scenario (low, moderate, and high). Of course, a major consideration is the real-time access to outcome data for the adaptation to be informative in contrast to the direct assignment option design, which incorporates a simple adaptation but requires the same infrastructure as conventional designs. These designs can be regarded as a hybrid of enrichment and all-comers designs when they include an option to stop accrual to a biomarker-defined subgroup based on interim analysis or just as an all-comers design when such an option is not allowed.

In cases where the prevalence of the marker in question is moderate (between 20% and 50%), and the preliminary evidence is not compelling, two possible strategies are as follows:

- Strategy 1:
  - First, perform a single-arm enrichment trial (pilot) with a clear antitumor endpoint (such as tumor response) as proof of concept that the treatment likely has a major effect within the marker subgroup.
  - Second, based on data from the pilot trial, perform an all-comers phase II (randomized) trial, using either
    - An adaptive design where the relationship between markers to treatment success is assessed in an ongoing manner.
    - A trial stratified by marker status, with the primary hypothesis defined within the marker subgroup hypothesized to derive the most benefit. Accrue sufficient patients to the other subgroup(s) to demonstrate lack of benefit.
- Strategy 2: Instead of a two-step process, perform a direct assignment option design with two interim analyses, where the option for direct assignment is only possible at the second IA, which is a modification to the design proposed in Figure 8.1 [10].

In summary, incorporating biomarkers in the design of phase II studies of molecularly targeted agents informs the phase III trial design strategy, thus assuring optimal use of limited phase III financial and patient resources.

8.3 Definitive Validation: Phase III Setting

We begin with a discussion of retrospective versus prospective trial designs in the phase III setting. The terms retrospective and prospective can be confusing since they are used to describe both the nature of data collection (using existing versus collecting new data) and the planning of analysis (prior to versus after seeing the data). RCTs collect specimen and assay prospectively for newly accruing patients. However, these trials are resource-intensive in terms of both time and money. Further, we frequently do not fully understand the biology at the time of trial design, so may not prospectively plan to test for a particular biomarker within a trial. Thus, a study using archived specimens is sometimes used as an alternative. These studies are *retrospective* with respect to data collection. Often they use a convenience sample of specimens, which happen to be available and are assayed for the marker, with no prospective plan for subject eligibility, power calculation, marker cut-point specification, or analysis. Such *retrospectively planned* studies are very likely to result in biased conclusions. Simon et al. [20] emphasize the need to prospectively specify a protocol before the marker study is performed, labeling such designs as *prospective–retrospective*. They propose the following guidelines under which a prospective–retrospective design may be appropriate:

1. Adequate amounts of archived tissue are available from enough patients from a prospective randomized trial for analyses to have adequate statistical power.
2. Patients included in the evaluation are representative of the patients in the trial.
3. The test is analytically validated for use with archived tissue.
4. The plan for biomarker evaluation is completely prespecified before the performance of biomarker assays on archived tissue.
5. Results from archived specimens are validated using specimens from one or more similar, but separate, studies.

An example of a marker that was successfully validated retrospectively is KRAS as predictive of efficacy of panitumumab and cetuximab in advanced colon cancer [21].

Several designs have been proposed and utilized in the field of cancer biomarkers for the prospective validation of predictive markers [2,4,5,12]. Briefly, these designs can be classified as follows:

- Enrichment designs
- All-comers designs, which are further classified as
  - Hybrid designs
  - Marker by treatment interaction designs
  - Sequential testing strategy designs
- Adaptive analysis designs

Enrichment designs: As described in Table 8.1 for phase II trials, this design is based on the paradigm (when there is compelling preliminary evidence) that not all patients will benefit from the study treatment under consideration, but rather that the benefit will be restricted to a subgroup of patients who express (or not express) a specific molecular feature [22]. Prior to the launching of a trial with an enrichment design strategy, the assay reproducibility, accuracy, and turnaround times for marker assessment must be well established. An enrichment design strategy of enrolling only human epidermal growth factor receptor 2 (HER2)-positive patients (based on a local assessment of HER2 status) demonstrated that trastuzumab (i.e., herceptin) combined with paclitaxel after doxorubicin and cyclophosphamide significantly improved disease-free survival among women with surgically removed HER2-positive breast cancer [23]. Subsequent analyses raised questions regarding the assay reproducibility based on local versus central testing for HER2 status [24,25]. Since only patients deemed HER2 positive based on the local assessment were enrolled, and tissue from patients deemed HER2 negative were not collected, the question of whether trastuzumab therapy benefits a potentially larger group than the approximately 20% of patients defined as HER2 positive in these two trials is the subject of an ongoing trial [26].

All-comers design: hybrid designs: In this design strategy, only a certain subgroup of patients based on their marker status are randomized between treatments, whereas patients in the other marker defined subgroups are assigned the standard of care treatment(s) [5]. This design is an appropriate choice when there is compelling evidence demonstrating the efficacy of a certain treatment(s) for a marker-defined subgroup, thereby making it unethical to randomize patients with that particular marker status to other treatment options. However, unlike the enrichment design strategy, all patients regardless of the marker status are enrolled and followed. This provides the possibility for future testing for other potential prognostic markers.

Examples of marker validation trials that have utilized the hybrid design strategy [27–29] are (1) the phase III randomized study of oxaliplatin, leucovorin calcium, and fluorouracil with versus without bevacizumab in patients with resected stage II colon cancer and at high risk for recurrence based on molecular markers (Eastern Cooperative Oncology Group—ECOG 5202); (2) the TAILORx (Trial Assigning Individualized Options for Treatment [Rx]) trial designed to evaluate the Oncotype Dx (Genomic Health, Redwood City, CA), a 21-gene recurrence score (RS) in tamoxifen-treated breast cancer patients; and (3) the MINDACT (Microarray in Node-Negative Disease May Avoid Chemotherapy) trial for node negative breast cancer patients designed to evaluate MammaPrint (Agendia, Amsterdam, the Netherlands), the 70-gene expression profile discovered at the Netherlands Cancer Institute.

All-comers design: marker by treatment interaction design [30]: In this design, all patients meeting the eligibility criteria are entered into the trial. The ability to provide adequate tissue may be an eligibility criterion, but not the specific biomarker result [4,5]. The marker by treatment interaction design uses the marker status as a stratification factor and randomizes patients to the same treatments within each marker-based subgroup. While this is similar to conducting two independent RCTs under one large RCT umbrella, it differs from a single large RCT in two essential characteristics: (1) only patients with a valid marker result are randomized, and (2) there is a prospective sample size specification for each marker-based subgroup. The sample size planning for treatment-by-marker interaction design is based on the prespecified analysis plan. A separate evaluation of the treatment effect can be tested in the two marker-defined subgroups or a test of interaction can be carried out first. Different sequential analysis plans can also be implemented. For example, when the primary test of interaction is not significant at a prespecified significance level, then the treatment arms can be compared in the overall population (ignoring the biomarker status). If the interaction is significant, then the experimental treatment can be compared to the control arm within the strata determined by the marker status.

All-comers design: sequential testing strategy designs [31–33]: Sequential testing designs are similar in principle to an RCT design. These designs have a single primary hypothesis, which is either tested in the overall population first and then in a prospectively planned subset if the overall test is not significant (needs adjustment of the overall type I error rate), or in the marker-defined subgroup first and then tested in the entire population if the subgroup analysis is significant (does not require overall type I error rate adjustment). The first is recommended in cases where the experimental treatment is hypothesized to be broadly effective, and the subset analysis is ancillary. The latter (also known as the closed testing procedure) is recommended when there is strong preliminary data to support that the treatment effect is strongest in the marker-defined subgroup, and that the marker has sufficient prevalence that the power for testing the treatment effect in the subgroup is adequate. The sequential testing strategies are largely driven by three statistical parameters: (1) α, the type I error or probability of a false positive result; (2) β, the type II error or probability of a false negative result; and (3) δ, the targeted difference or targeted effect size. The sequential testing strategy designs differ in the choice of the values for these statistical parameters, which is dictated by the inference framework of the design. Both these sequential testing approaches appropriately control for the type I error rates associated with multiple testing. A modification to the first approach discussed earlier (testing in the overall population first and then in a planned subset if the overall test is not significant), taking into account potential correlation arising from testing the overall treatment effect and the treatment effect within the marker defined subgroup, has also been proposed [33]. The closed testing procedure was utilized to account for KRAS mutation status in the phase III trial testing cetuximab in addition to FOLFOX as adjuvant therapy in stage III colon cancer (N0147) [34].

Another class of designs that follow a similar sequential testing strategy is the adaptive threshold and the adaptive signature designs [35–38]. The former is used in situations where a marker is known at the start of the trial, but a cut point for defining marker positive and marker negative groups is not known. The latter is used when the marker and the threshold are both unknown at the start of the trial, and the design allows for the *discovery and validation* process of the marker within the realm of the single phase III trial, using either a cross-validation approach or the split-sample approach [36,37]. The adaptive threshold design can be implemented in one of two ways: (1) the new treatment is compared to the control in all patients at a prespecified significance level, and if not significant, a second-stage analysis involving finding an *optimal* cut point for the predictive marker is performed using the remaining alpha (similar to the first approach discussed under the sequential testing strategy designs section above); or (2) under the assumption that the treatment is effective only for a marker-driven subset, no overall treatment to control comparisons are made; instead, the analysis focuses on the identification of optimal cut points. Both these approaches were concluded to be superior (in terms of the power and number of events required to detect an effect at a prespecified overall type I error rate) to the classic nonadaptive design approaches in the simulation studies [35]. However, two issues need further consideration with such designs: (1) the added cost of a somewhat larger sample size and/or redundant power dictated by the strategy of partitioning the overall type I error rate; and (2) use of data from the same trial to both define and validate a marker cut point. The adaptive signature design uses approach #1 , where the new treatment is compared to the control in all patients at a prespecified significance level. If this overall comparison is significant, then it is taken that the treatment is broadly effective. If, however, the overall comparison is not significant, a second-stage analysis is undertaken for the development and use of a biomarker signature, using a split-sample or a cross-validated approach [36,37].

Adaptive designs: Clinical trials utilizing adaptive design strategies in the phase II setting, particularly the outcome-based adaptive randomization, were described earlier in this chapter. The adaptive accrual design outlines a strategy to adaptively modify accrual to two predefined marker defined subgroups based on an interim futility analysis [39]. Specifically, the trial follows the following scheme: (1) begin with accrual to both marker-defined subgroups; (2) at the interim analysis, if the treatment effect in one of the subgroups fails to satisfy a futility boundary, terminate accrual to that subgroup; and continue accrual to the other subgroup until the planned total sample size is reached, including accruing subjects that had planned to be included from the terminated subgroup. This design has demonstrated greater power than a nonadaptive trial in simulation settings; however, this strategy might lead to a substantial increase in the accrual duration depending on the prevalence of the marker for the subgroup that continues to full accrual. In addition, the futility boundary is somewhat conservative and less than optimal as it is set to be in the region where the observed efficacy is greater for the control arm than the experimental regimen. Another design to adaptively modify accrual was proposed by Liu et al. [40]. In this design, only the marker-positive group patients are accrued in the first stage. If the interim analysis shows promising results for the marker-positive cohort, then the second stage would continue accrual to the marker-positive cohort, but also include marker-negative patients. If the first stage shows no benefit in the marker-positive cohort, then the trial is closed permanently.

8.4 Summary

The choice of biomarker design depends on the study objectives, strength of preliminary evidence, assay performance, marker prevalence, and assay turnaround times. Simon and Maitournam [22] and Hoering et al. [41] showed that an enrichment design can dramatically reduce the number of patients required relative to an all-comers design, but that this result depends on assay performance and marker prevalence. Designs in which trials proceed based on the marker status (e.g., adaptive designs or the marker-by-treatment design that stratifies on marker status) require rapid turnaround times for assays.

A well-designed prospective biomarker-driven RCT that is analytically and clinically valid is a key step in translating basic science to clinically useful markers that improve clinical practice. To fully realize the clinical utility, it is imperative that there be (1) a strong biological basis for the target of therapy; (2) a clearly defined subgroup that will benefit from therapy and a practical method that can identify them from the general patient population; and (3) further studies demonstrating that the biomarker results truly influence clinical decisions and are cost-effective.

References

1. Biomarkers Definitions Working Group. Biomarkers and surrogate endpoints: Preferred definitions and conceptual framework. *Clin Pharmacol Ther* 69:89–95, 2001.
2. Mandrekar SJ, Sargent DJ. Clinical trial designs for biomarker evaluation. *Personal Med Oncol* 1(1), 2012.
3. Buyse M, Sargent DJ, Grothey A et al. Biomarkers and surrogate end points—The challenge of statistical validation. *Nat Rev Clin Oncol* 7:309–317, 2010.
4. Mandrekar SJ, Sargent DJ. Genomic advances and their impact on clinical trial design. *Genome Med* 1(7):69, 2009.
5. Mandrekar SJ, Sargent DJ. Clinical trial designs for predictive biomarker validation: Theoretical considerations and practical challenges. *J Clin Oncol* 27(24):4027–4034, 2009.
6. Freidlin B, McShane LM, Polley MY, Korn EL. Randomized phase II trial designs with biomarkers. *J Clin Oncol* 30(26):3304–3309, 2012.
7. Mandrekar SJ, Sargent DJ. All-comers versus enrichment design strategy in phase II trials. *J Thorac Oncol* 6(4):658–660, 2011.
8. Elsaleh H, Joseph D, Grieu F et al. Association of tumour site and sex with survival benefit from adjuvant chemotherapy in colorectal cancer. *Lancet* 355:1745–1750, 2000.
9. An MW, Mandrekar SJ, Sargent DJ. A 2-stage phase II design with direct assignment option in stage II for initial marker validation. *Clin Cancer Res* 18(16): 4225–4233, 2012.

10. Mandrekar SJ, An MW, Sargent DJ. A phase II trial design with direct assignment option for initial marker validation. *J Clin Oncol* 30:(suppl 30; abstr 34), 2012.
11. Moore HM, Kelly AB, Jewell SD et al. Biospecimen reporting for improved study quality (BRISQ). *Cancer (Cancer Cytopathol)* 119:92–101, 2011.
12. Mandrekar SJ, Sargent DJ. Design of clinical trials for biomarker research in oncology. *Clin Investig (Lond)* 1(12):1629–1636, 2011.
13. Barker AD, Sigman CC, Kelloff GJ, Hylton NM, Berry DA, Esserman LJ. I-SPY 2: An adaptive breast cancer trial design in the setting of neoadjuvant chemotherapy. *Clin Pharmacol Ther* 86(1):97–100, 2009.
14. Zhou X, Liu S, Kim ES. Bayesian adaptive design for targeted therapy development in lung cancer—A step towards personalized medicine. *Clin Trials* 5: 181–193, 2008.
15. Kim ES, Herbst RS, Wistuba II, Lee JJ, Blumenschein GR Jr, Tsao A et al. The BATTLE trial: Personalizing therapy for lung cancer. *Cancer Discov* 1(1):44–53, 2011.
16. Mandrekar SJ, An MW, Sargent DJ. A review of phase II trial designs for initial marker validation. *Contemp Clin Trials* 36(2):597–604, May 8, 2013.
17. Korn EL, Freidlin B. Outcome—Adaptive randomization: Is it useful? *J Clin Oncol* 29(6):771–776, 2011.
18. Korn E, Freidlin B. Outcome-adaptive randomization in early clinical trials. In *Design and Analysis of Clinical Trials for Predictive Medicine* (eds. Matsui S, Buyse M, Simon R). Chapman & Hall/CRC Press, 2015.
19. Berry DA. Adaptive clinical trials: The promise and the caution. *J Clin Oncol* 29(6):606–609, 2011.
20. Simon RM, Paik S, Hayes DF. Use of archived specimens in evaluation of prognostic and predictive biomarkers. *JNCI* 101(21):1446–1452, 2009.
21. Van Cutsem E, Köhne CH, Hitre E et al. Cetuximab and chemotherapy as initial treatment for metastatic colorectal cancer. *N Engl J Med* 360(14):1408–1417, 2009.
22. Simon R, Maitournam A. Evaluating the efficiency of targeted designs for randomized clinical trials. *Clin Cancer Res* 10(20):6759–6763, 2004.
23. Romond EH, Perez EA, Bryant J et al. Trastuzumab plus adjuvant chemotherapy for operable HER2-positive breast cancer. *N Engl J Med* 353(16):1673–1684, 2005.
24. Perez EA, Suman VJ, Davidson NE et al. HER2 testing by local, central, and reference laboratories in specimens from the North Central Cancer Treatment Group N9831 intergroup adjuvant trial. *J Clin Oncol* 24(19):3032–3038, 2006.
25. Paik S, Kim C, Wolmark N. HER2 status and benefit from adjuvant trastuzumab in breast cancer. *N Engl J Med* 358(13):1409–1411, 2008.
26. Hayes DF. Steady progress against HER2-positive breast cancer (editorial). *N Engl J Med* 365:14, 2011.
27. Sparano JA, Paik S. Development of the 21-gene assay and its application in clinical practice and clinical trials. *J Clin Oncol* 26(5):721–728, 2008.
28. Cardoso F, Van't Veer L, Rutgers E et al. Clinical application of the 70-gene profile: The MINDACT trial. *J Clin Oncol* 26(5):729–735, 2008.
29. Bogaerts J, Cardoso F, Buyse M et al. TRANSBIG consortium. Gene signature evaluation as a prognostic tool: Challenges in the design of the MINDACT trial. *Nat Clin Pract Oncol* 3(10):540–551, 2006.

30. Sargent DJ, Conley BA, Allegra C et al. Clinical trial designs for predictive marker validation in cancer treatment trials. *J Clin Oncol* 23(9):2020–2027, 2005.
31. Simon R, Wang SJ. Use of genomic signatures in therapeutics development. *Pharmacoenomics J* 6:1667–1673, 2006.
32. Bauer P. Multiple testing in clinical trials. *Stat Med* 10:871–890, 1991.
33. Song Y, Chi GYH. A method for testing a prespecified subgroup in clinical trials. *Stat Med* 26:3535–3349, 2007.
34. Alberts SR, Sargent DJ, Nair S, Mahoney MR et al. Effect of oxaliplatin, fluorouracil, and leucovorin with or without cetuximab on survival among patients with resected stage III colon cancer: A randomized trial. *JAMA* 307(13): 1383–1393, 2012.
35. Jiang W, Freidlin B, Simon R. Biomarker-adaptive threshold design: A procedure for evaluating treatment with possible biomarker-defined subset effect. *J Natl Cancer Inst* 99(13):1036–1043, 2007.
36. Freidlin B, Simon R. Adaptive signature design: An adaptive clinical trial design for generating and prospectively testing a gene expression signature for sensitive patients. *Clin Cancer Res* 11(21):7872–7878, 2005.
37. Freidlin B, Jiang W, Simon R. The cross-validated adaptive signature design. *Clin Cancer Res* 16(2):691–698, 2010.
38. Freidlin B, Simon R. Adaptive clinical trial designs with biomarker development and validation. In *Design and Analysis of Clinical Trials for Predictive Medicine* (eds. Matsui S, Buyse M, Simon R). Chapman & Hall/CRC Press, 2015.
39. Wang SJ, O'Neill RT, Hung HMJ. Approaches to evaluation of treatment effect in randomized clinical trials with genomic subset. *Pharm Stat* 6:227–244, 2007.
40. Liu A, Liu C, Li Q, Yu KF, Yuan VW. A threshold sample-enrichment approach in a clinical trial with heterogeneous subpopulations. *Clin Trials* 7(5):537–545, 2010.
41. Hoering A, LeBlanc M, Crowley JJ. Randomized phase III clinical trial designs for targeted agents. *Clin Cancer Res* 14(14):4358–4367, 2008.

Section III

Phase III Randomized Clinical Trials Using Biomarkers

9

Comparison of Randomized Clinical Trial Designs for Targeted Agents

Antje Hoering, Mike LeBlanc, and John Crowley

CONTENTS

9.1 Introduction

The treatment paradigm in oncology has shifted drastically over the last decade or so. Most cancers are now treated using so-called targeted or cytostatic therapies alone or in combination with more traditional cytotoxic agents. Targeted agents in this context refer to therapies that target specific pathways, molecules, or receptors that are essential in the tumor biology of a specific cancer. Conventional chemotherapies or cytotoxic agents, on the other hand, utilize various mechanisms important in mitosis to kill dividing cells, such as tumor cells.

Examples for targeted agents include antiantigenic agents that inhibit the formation of new blood vessels, proapoptotic agents that initiate tumor cell death or epidermal growth factor inhibitors that inhibit tumor cell division.

A biomarker is typically associated with a targeted therapy. Such a biomarker is hypothesized to be a predictive indicator of efficacy associated with a specific targeted agent (Sargent et al. 2005) and can be used to indicate which patients should be treated with a particular targeted agent. There are also prognostic markers that are prognostic for a specific disease independent of the actual treatment. It is not always known whether a marker is predictive or prognostic and some markers may be both.

9.2 Phase III Trial Designs for Targeted Agents

A variety of designs for assessing targeted treatments using biomarkers have been proposed. Figure 9.1 illustrates three such phase III trial designs for predictive markers. For illustration purposes, we restrict our discussion to two treatments T1 and T2, where T1 could be the standard of care and T2 the new therapy of interest. These do not have to be limited to single agents but can include entire treatment strategies, as is common for many cancers. We also assume that the marker distinguishes between two groups: marker-positive patients (M+) and marker-negative patients (M−). It is conjectured that the new therapy to be studied, T2, benefits M+ patients. For this illustration, we also assume that for continuous markers a cut-point has been determined to distinguish these two groups.

In the *randomize-all* or *all-comers* design, the marker status of the patient is assessed and all patients are randomized to one of two treatments. The treatment assignment for patients can also be stratified by observed marker status. If stratification is deemed not necessary, assessing the marker status of the patient can occur after randomization, which may speed up the start of treatment. If we hypothesize that the treatment is mostly efficacious in marker-positive patients, but it is unclear whether the therapy is beneficial (possibly to a lesser extent) for marker-negative patients as well, a variation

- *Randomize-all design*: randomize all patients, measure marker

Register → Assess Marker → Randomize → T2 (M+ M−) / T1 (M+ M−)

- *Targeted design*: randomize marker positive patients only

Register → Assess Marker → Randomize M+ → T2 M+ / T1 M+; (M− T1)

- *Strategy design*: randomize to marker based versus not marker-based

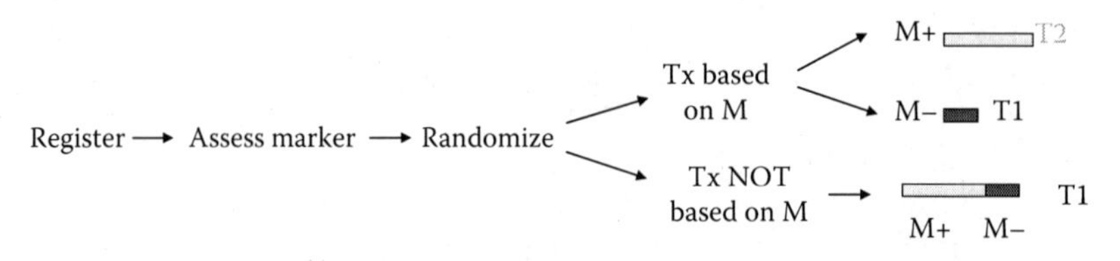

M+: marker positive pts., M−: marker negative pts., T1: Treatment 1, T2 : Treatment 2

FIGURE 9.1
Possible clinical trial designs for targeted therapy: randomize-all design, targeted design, and strategy design.

of this design is to test for overall benefit, regardless of marker status, and to explore the M− and M+ subsets. One possibility is to use this design and power it for the subgroup of marker-positive patients. This will then allow us to determine, with appropriate power, whether or not the treatment is effective overall and in the subgroup of M+ patients. Such a trial is sometimes referred to as a hybrid trial. A similar procedure in the context of hazard ratios was recently discussed by Jiang et al. (2007). SWOG has adopted this trial design for a Non–Small Cell Lung Cancer (NSCLC) trial (S0819) (Redman et al. 2012). In this trial, patients with advanced NSCLC are randomized to carboplatin and paclitaxel plus or minus cetuximab. Two hypotheses are being tested. The overall hypothesis tests whether cetuximab increases the efficacy of concurrent chemotherapy (carboplatin and paclitaxel) in patients with advanced NSCLC. The targeted hypothesis tests whether EGFR FISH+ patients benefit to a larger degree. More specifically, the hazard ratio to be tested in the EGFR FISH+ group was chosen to be larger than the hazard ratio to be tested in the entire study population.

A variation is the biomarker-stratified design, which tests the treatment effect in the biomarker-positive and biomarker-negative group instead of the biomarker-positive and the overall group, or even has quite different hypotheses in the strata. An example for such a design is the Marker Validation for Erlotinib in Lung Cancer (MARVEL) trial (Wakelee et al. 2008). The sample size in this case depends heavily on the sample size of the biomarker-defined subgroups and the treatment effect in each of those subgroups.

Simon and Manitournam (2004) evaluated the efficiency of a *targeted* trial design. In this design, patients are first assessed for their marker value and only marker-positive patients are enrolled in the trial and randomized to the two treatment options. This design is also referred to as an *enrichment* design or a *marker-positive* design. They evaluated the effectiveness of the *targeted* design versus the *randomize-all* design with respect to the number of patients required for screening and the number of patients needed for randomization. A *targeted* design proves to be a good design if the underlying pathways and biology are well enough understood, so that it is clear that the therapy under investigation only works for a specific subset of patients, namely marker-positive patients. Such a *targeted* design generally requires a smaller number of patients to be randomized than the *randomize-all* design to determine the efficaciousness of a new treatment in M+ patients; however, no insight is gained on the efficaciousness of the new treatment in M− patients, and a large number of patients still needs to be assessed for their marker status. There are similar designs in which only M+ patients are randomized to treatment, whereas M− patients are assigned to standard of care. Such a design is powered to detect differences in outcome in the M+ subgroup, similar to the *targeted* design. This design provides the additional value of offering treatment to all marker groups, but just as the targeted design, it cannot assess treatment efficacy for the marker-negative patients. Since the power and sample size considerations are the same as those for of the *targeted* design, we focus further discussion on the *targeted* design. Some recent examples were discussed by Mandrekar and Sargent (2009).

Freidlin and Simon (2005, Freidlin, Chapter 18) also proposed an adaptive two-stage trial design specifically for developing and accessing markers using gene expression profiling. We do not evaluate this trial design here as we focus our discussion on one-stage designs.

Hayes et al. (1998) suggested a trial design for predictive markers, where patients are randomized between marker-based treatment (M+ patients getting new therapy, M− patients getting standard of care) and every patient, independent of their marker status, getting standard of care. Such a trial is designed to test whether marker-based treatment strategy is superior to standard therapy. We refer to this trial design as the *strategy* design. Sargent and Allegra (2002) suggested an *augmented strategy* design, extending this strategy design to the case where patients are randomized between marker-based treatment (as in the strategy design) and treatment independent of marker, where in the latter arm a second randomization to new versus standard therapy is added. We evaluate the *strategy* design rather than the *augmented strategy* design since the former is more frequently used. As an example, the *strategy* design was recently used in an NSCLC trial to test individualized cisplatin-based chemotherapy dependent on the patients ERCC1 mRNA (Cobo et al. 2007).

These various trial designs test different hypotheses. The *randomize-all* design addresses the question whether the treatment is beneficial for all patients, with the possibility of testing whether or not the new treatment is beneficial in the subset of marker-positive patients. We also investigate testing both the *targeted* and the *overall* hypothesis in the *randomize-all* design with appropriate adjustment for multiple comparisons. The *targeted* design tests whether or not the treatment is beneficial for marker-positive patients. The *strategy* design addresses the question of whether the marker-based treatment strategy is better than everyone receiving standard of care (T1) regardless of marker status. The *strategy* design does not directly address the question of whether treatment T2 is more efficacious than treatment T1; however, it is frequently used in that context and thus we felt it important to assess its properties.

9.3 Possible Underlying Marker Scenarios and Simulation Studies

We evaluated the effectiveness of the *randomize-all*, the *targeted*, and the *strategy* phase III trial designs under the most common scenarios (Hoering et al. 2008, 2012). These scenarios include the presence of a prognostic marker, several possible scenarios for the presence of a predictive marker, and no valid marker. We assume that the underlying distribution of the biomarker is continuous in nature. We further assume that a cut-point is used to distinguish patients with marker values above (below) such a threshold, who are then referred to as marker-positive (negative) patients. We recently investigated the performance of several test statistics for the different trial designs discussed in this section as a function of the marker distribution and the marker cut-off (Hoering et al. 2008, 2012). The performance was evaluated as a function of the cut-point, the number of patients screened, and the number of patients randomized to obtain a certain power and significance for the various test statistics. We studied these designs under some simple marker and effect assumptions.

In practice, the underlying marker distribution and the response probability as a function of the marker value are often continuous. Assume that the log-transformed marker value X is normally distributed, $X \sim N(\mu,\sigma^2)$, and its density function is denoted by $f(X)$. Other distributional assumptions may be used instead. If multiple markers are of interest, a combined distribution of a linear combination of the markers can be used. We assume that two treatments T1 and T2 are being investigated and that the treatment assignment has been determined using one of the various trial designs discussed earlier. The treatment assignment is indexed by $j=1, 2$, and we focus our analysis on binary outcomes. However, this approach can be easily extended to a survival outcome. The expected outcome for the subgroup M+ patients, $M+=\{X:X>c\}$, can be written, assuming a logit link, as

$$g_j(c,\mathrm{M}+)=\int\limits_{x>c}\frac{e^{a_{0j}+a_{1j}x}}{1+e^{a_{0j}+a_{1j}x}}f(x)\,dx/v_{\mathrm{M}+}(c),$$

where c is the cut-point that distinguishes M+ from M− subjects and where the fraction of marker-positive patients is given by $v_{\mathrm{M}+}(c)=\int_{x>c}f(x)\,dx$ and the marker-negative fraction by $v_{\mathrm{M}-}(c)=1-v_{\mathrm{M}+}(c)$. Analogous calculations for the M− patients give the summary measures, $g_j(c,\mathrm{M}-)$ for those groups. We study design properties indexed by the cut-point c. Therefore, important parameters in the design assessments are $(g_j(c,\mathrm{M}+), g_j(c, \mathrm{M}-), v_{\mathrm{M}+}(c))$, which constitute the outcome and the fractions of patients in the M+ group.

Figure 9.2 presents several scenarios based on this simple marker treatment model. Scenario 1 is where the marker under investigation is a false marker, that is, it has no effect on the outcome. Scenarios 2 through 4 are different scenarios for a predictive marker. In scenario 2, the new treatment (T2) does not help M− patients more than the standard treatment (T1), but has additional benefit for marker-positive patients, increasing with the marker value. In scenario 3, the two treatment curves are diverging with increasing marker value. The marker does not have any effect on treatment 1, but the effect of treatment 2 is increasing with increasing marker value.

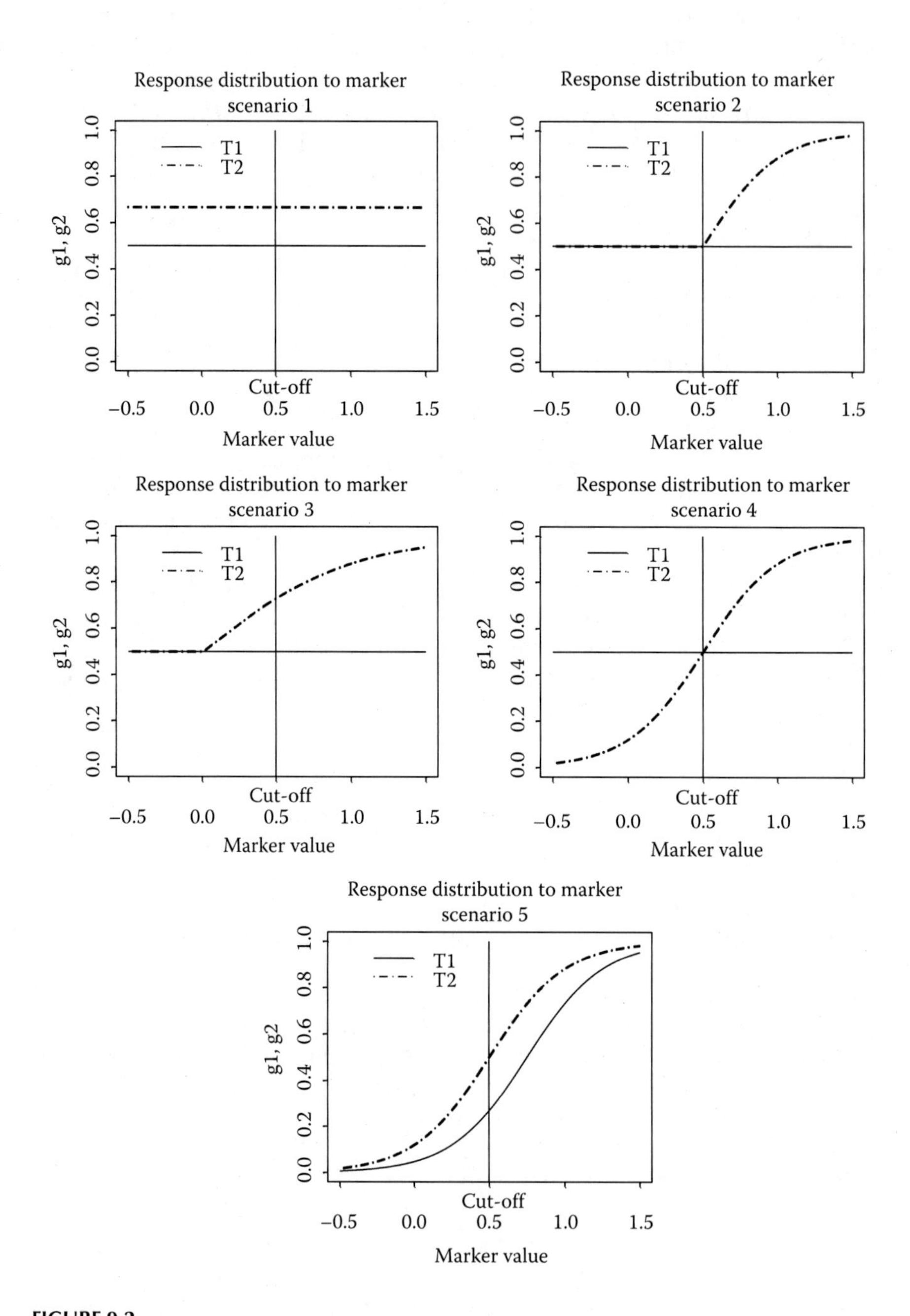

FIGURE 9.2
Scenarios for response distribution of marker. The response probability is plotted versus the log-transformed marker value X.

In scenario 4, the new therapy benefits M+ patients, but has a negative impact on M− patients. Finally, for a prognostic marker, where T2 is overall better than T1, both are increasing with increasing marker value (scenario 5). All these graphs are on a logit scale.

We investigated the overall performance of the different designs in the various scenarios discussed earlier (Hoering et al. 2008, 2012). We simulated the underlying log-marker distribution from a normal distribution $X \sim N(\mu,\sigma^2)$. We then evaluated the response probability to the marker using the distribution functions discussed earlier for the various scenarios. The actual parameters used to evaluate the response probabilities for the five different scenarios can be found in Hoering et al. (2008). We performed 5000 simulations to calculate $g_j(c,\text{M}-)$ and $g_j(c,\text{M}+)$. These derived quantities were then used to evaluate power or sample size for the different scenarios assuming an underlying binomial distribution. For the power calculations, we used a one-sided significance level α of 0.05. We investigated the overall performance of the different designs in the various scenarios discussed earlier (Hoering et al. 2008, 2012).

9.4 Results

Figure 9.3 shows the power of the three designs as a function of the sample size of patients randomized for each of the five scenarios discussed earlier. In scenario 1, which is the scenario with no valid marker, the *randomize-all* and the *targeted* design achieve the same power for all sample sizes, as response to treatment is independent of the marker status. The lowest power is achieved with the *strategy design* as this design assigns subsets of patients in both of the randomized arms to the identical treatment and is thus inefficient if there is no true underlying marker. For scenario 2, in which the new treatment T2 only helps patients with the marker, the *targeted* design outperforms both the *randomize-all* and the *strategy* design, as this is the scenario of a true marker for which this trial has been designed. The *randomize-all* design and the *strategy* design achieve the same power. This is due to the fact that in the experimental arm the same fraction of marker-positive patients are treated with the effective treatment T2 and the same fraction of marker-negative patients are treated with T1 (in the *strategy* design) or T2 (in the *randomize-all* design), and the effect of both treatments is the same for marker-negative patients. Scenario 3 is the scenario in which M− patients benefit less than M+ patients. In that scenario, the *targeted* design performs the best, followed by the *randomize-all* design, and then the *strategy* design. In this case, the efficacy is the largest in the M+ patients and thus best picked up by the *targeted* design. However, the new therapy also helps M− patients. This fact is missed by the *targeted* design since no information is obtained on M− patients. In the

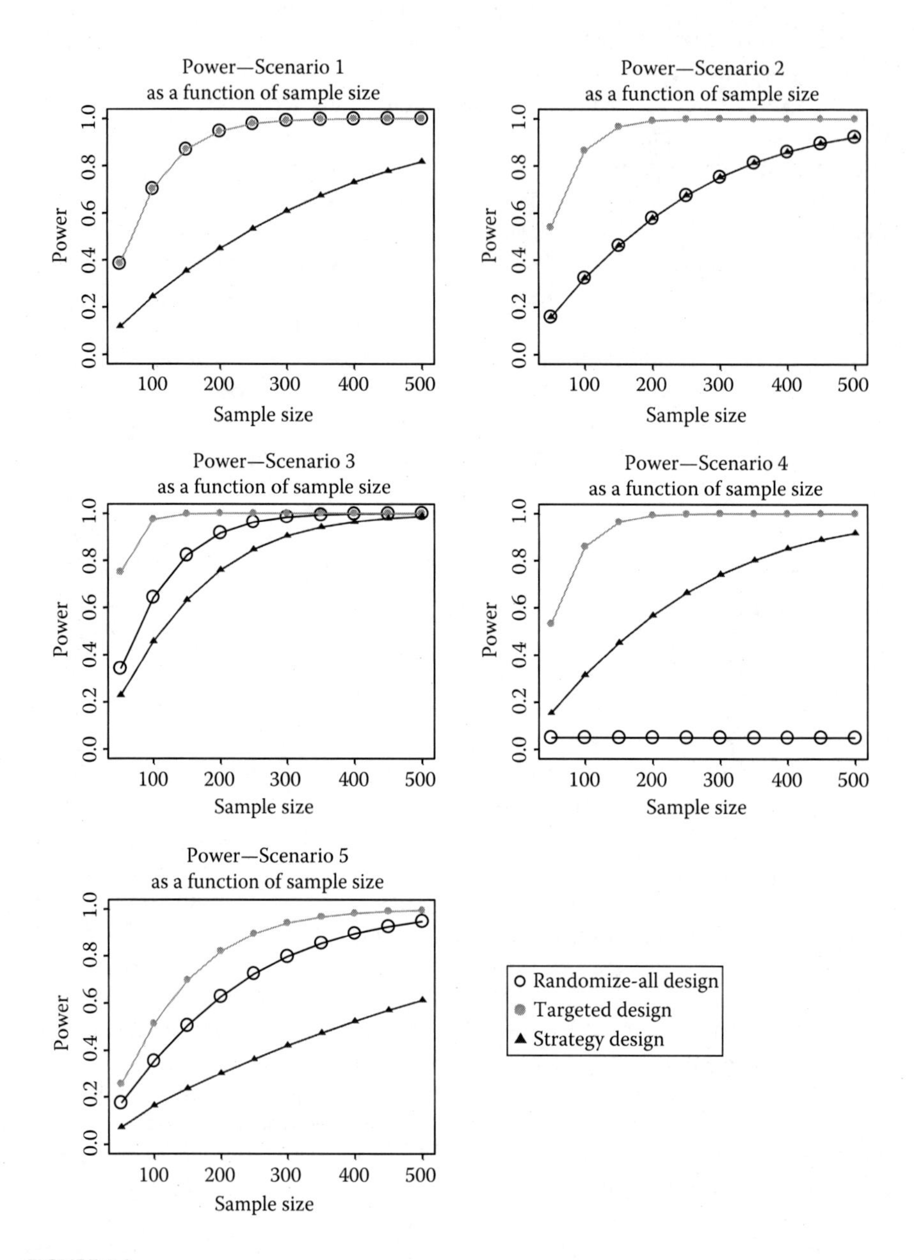

FIGURE 9.3
Power of the randomize-all, targeted, and strategy designs as a function of sample size (number or randomized patients) for the different scenarios.

strategy design, the M− patients in the experimental arm are treated with the less effective treatment T1 and the power of that design is thus lower than that of the other two designs. In scenario 4, where the new therapy is beneficial for M+ patients, but is actually harmful for M− patients, the *targeted* design outperforms the others. The *randomize-all* design does the worst as the two effects in this example cancel each other out. Lastly, in scenario 5, the example for a purely prognostic marker, the *targeted* design performs the best, followed by the *randomize-all* design and lastly the *strategy* design.

For a new marker or a new assay that has not been thoroughly tested yet, the cut-point corresponding to the strongest therapeutic effect is often not known precisely. Using an underlying continuous marker model makes it possible to investigate this effect on power and sample size for the various scenarios. We thus performed simulation studies in which we vary the cut-point c, which distinguishes M+ from M− patients. Shifting the cut-point results in some patients being incorrectly (or inappropriately) classified as M+, when treatment T2 is not more effective for these patients and vice versa. We investigated the effect on sample size for the targeted versus the randomize-all design. Figure 9.4 displays the impact of misclassification of the marker. In our examples, the correct cut-point is at 0.5 (50% of patients are M+). Moving the cut-point does not affect power in the *randomize-all* design as all patients are being randomized independent of their marker status and the underlying marker distribution is not affected by moving the cut-point. Moving the cut-point has an effect on whether a subject is

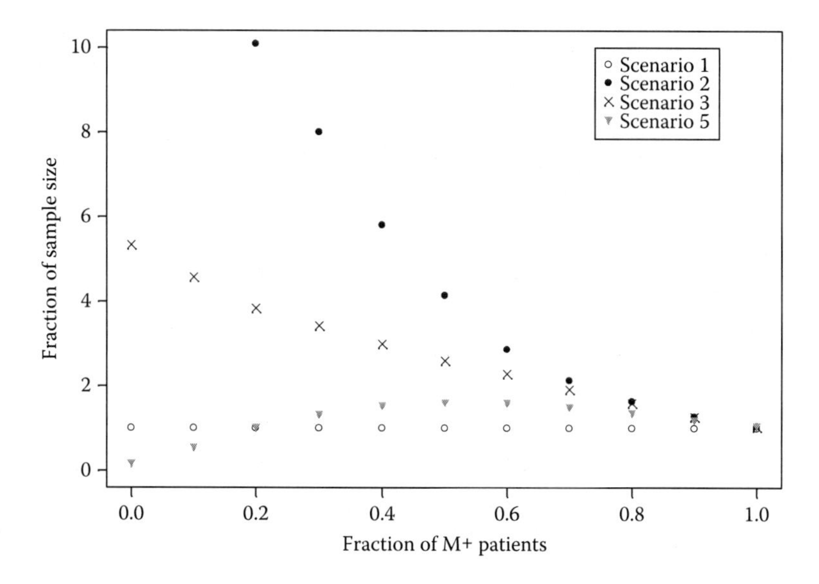

FIGURE 9.4
Sample size needed for the randomize-all versus the targeted design as a function of shifting the cut-point. Scenario 4 is outside the range of the graph.

classified as being marker positive or being marker negative and thus has a large effect on sample size for the *targeted* and the *strategy* design. If the cut-point is moved all the way to the left, everyone is classified as marker positive and the randomize-all and the targeted designs are identical. On the other hand, if the cut-point is moved toward the right, only patients with the most extreme marker values are considered marker positive. For the scenarios with an underlying predictive marker (scenarios 3–5), those are the patients benefitting the most from the new therapy, thus the targeted design performs the best, but also misses the fact that many more patients with less extreme marker values would have benefitted from this new therapy. In summary, we found that overall the improvements in power for the *targeted* design are impressive for most scenarios. Only in the case in which there is a constant odds ratio between treatment arms is there a decrease in power for the *targeted* design and then only for the most extreme marker group. The worst case for the *randomize-all* design is the hypothetical total interaction model of scenario 4, where the overall treatment effect is null. This is also the only case in which the *strategy* design performs slightly better than the *randomize-all* design (not shown in Figure 9.4).

We also evaluated the effect of maker prevalence in the patient population on power and sample size for the different designs and scenarios. In our simulations, we achieve this by shifting the marker distribution, but leaving the cut-point at $X = 0.5$. Shifting the marker distribution increases or decreases the fraction of M+ and M− patients. Figure 9.5 shows the effect of prevalence

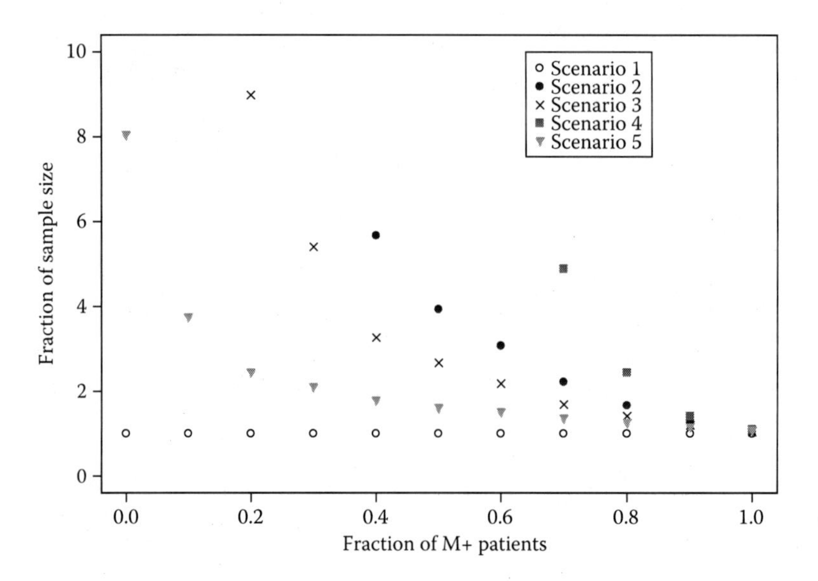

FIGURE 9.5
Sample size needed for the randomize-all versus the targeted design as a function of marker prevalence.

in terms of sample size needed for randomize-all versus targeted design. If the mass of the distribution is moved all the way to the right, everyone is marker positive and the randomize-all and the targeted design are the same. As the mass of the distribution is moved toward the left, marker prevalence is getting smaller and the targeted design performs much better than the randomize-all design. The *targeted* design performs the best in all scenarios with an underlying true predictive marker (scenarios 2–4). In those scenarios, the treatment benefit for M+ patients is diluted in the *randomize-all* and the *strategy* design and many more patients are needed to test the respective hypothesis. However, the *targeted* design misses the benefit of the T2 for marker-negative patients in scenario 3. In the case of a prognostic marker (scenario 5) with a constant odds ratio between treatment arms, the *targeted* design has smaller power than the *randomize-all* design but only for the extreme marker values when the cut-point is shifted such that most patients are marker negative. The *randomize-all* design performs as well or in most cases better than the *strategy* design except for the hypothetical total interaction model of scenario 4, where the overall treatment effect is null (not shown in Figure 9.5).

We also studied the feasibility and performance of testing both the overall and the targeted hypothesis in the *randomize-all* design with appropriate adjustment for multiple comparisons. We split the significance level α and test the overall hypothesis at $\alpha=0.04$ and the targeted hypothesis at $\alpha=0.01$. Other splits of the significance level can be considered, but the outcome would qualitatively stay the same. In general, there is little change in power for the overall hypothesis for $\alpha=0.04$ versus $\alpha=0.05$ (Hoering et al. 2008, 2012). The change in power for the targeted hypothesis for $\alpha=0.01$ versus $\alpha=0.05$ is slightly larger since there is a larger difference in alpha. The main question however is whether it is feasible to test both the targeted and the overall hypothesis in the scenarios with a predictive marker using this trial design. In the scenarios with a predictive marker (scenarios 2–4), with exception of the scenario of total interaction (scenario 4), the power for the two hypotheses (with Bonferroni-adjusted alpha levels) is comparable and only a modest increase of sample size (compared to the *randomize-all* design with just the overall hypothesis and $\alpha=0.05$) is needed to test both hypotheses. We note that in the context of a given real study, one can simulate from the large sample joint normal distribution of the two test statistics to less conservatively control for the overall type 1 error. For instance, if the overall hypothesis is fixed at $\alpha=0.04$, then by using this calculation one could increase alpha for subgroup test to greater than .01, yet still have overall $\alpha=0.05$ (Song and Chi 2007, Wang et al. 2007, Spiessens and Debois 2010).

Finally, we investigated the effect of the marker prevalence on the ratio of the number of patients randomized in the *randomize-all* design and the number of patients screened in the *targeted* design (Hoering et al. 2008, 2012). The number of patients required to be screened in the *targeted* design is given by the ratio of the number of patients randomized in the *targeted* design divided

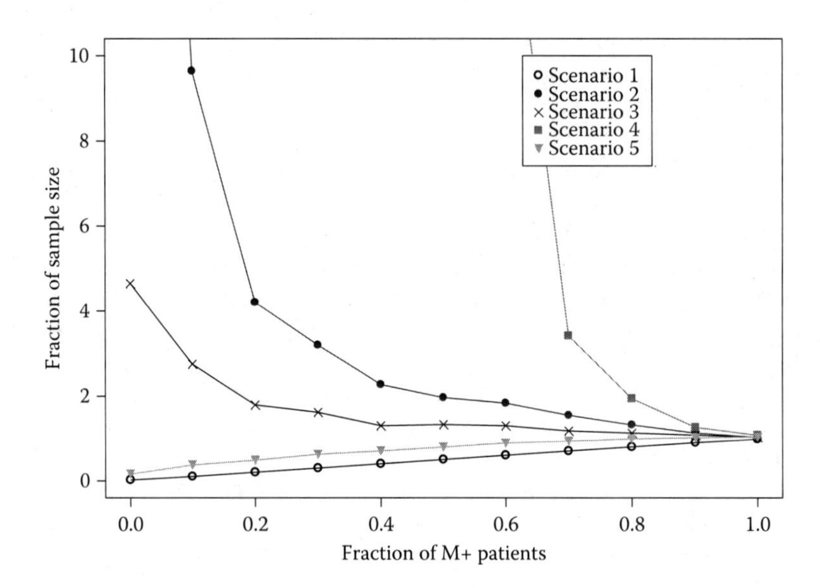

FIGURE 9.6
Ratio of the number or patients randomized in the randomize-all design and the number of patients screened in the targeted design.

by the fraction of M+ patients. If the fraction of M+ patients is equal to 1, the *targeted* and the *randomize-all* design are equivalent. For a small fraction of M+ patients, the mass of the marker distribution is centered at very low marker values. Scenarios 1 and 5 are similar. In the case of no marker (scenario 1) and a constant difference in treatment efficacy independent of the marker value, this ratio increases linearly with the fraction of M+ patients. In scenario 5, this ratio increases too, but is not linear as the difference in response is not constant. Scenarios 2–4, the scenarios with an underlying predictive marker, are also similar. The ratio of the number of patients randomized in the *randomize-all* design and the number of patients screened in the *targeted* design gets larger with smaller M+ prevalence. If the marker prevalence is small in those scenarios, we have to screen more patients in the targeted design. However, we have to randomize even more patients in the randomize-all design than screen in the targeted design, as the treatment effect gets diluted (Figure 9.6).

9.5 Example

The approach of testing both the overall and the targeted hypothesis in the *randomize-all* design was recently used in the SWOG trial S0819, a randomized, phase III study comparing carboplatin/paclitaxel or carboplatin/paclitaxel/bevacizumab with or without concurrent cetuximab in patients with advanced NSCLC (Redman et al. 2012). This study was designed to have two primary objectives. The primary objective for the entire study population is to compare overall survival (OS) in advanced NSCLC patients treated with chemotherapy plus bevacizumab (if appropriate) versus chemotherapy and bevacizumab (if appropriate) and cetuximab. The addition of cetuximab will be judged to be superior if the true increase in median OS is 20% (overall hypothesis). The second primary objective is to compare progression-free survival (PFS) by institutional review in EGFR FISH-positive patients with advanced NSCLC treated with chemotherapy plus bevacizumab (if appropriate) versus chemotherapy and bevacizumab (if appropriate) and cetuximab. The addition of cetuximab will be judged to be superior in this subset of patients if the true increase in median PFS is 33% (targeted hypothesis). The overall sample size for this study is 1546 patients, which includes approximately 618 EGFR FISH+ patients. The overall one-sided significance level, α, was chosen to be 0.025. The overall hypothesis was tested at $\alpha = 0.015$ and the targeted hypothesis at $\alpha = 0.020$; the split of α was determined using simulation studies. The power for the overall hypothesis is 86% and the power for the targeted hypothesis is 92%. These calculations are based on 4-year accrual and 1-year follow-up. The estimate for OS and PFS in the EGFR FISH+ subgroup and the entire patient population for the control arm were determined by estimating the proportion of patients deemed to be in the bevacizumab-appropriate versus the bevacizumab-inappropriate. A targeted design testing the targeted hypothesis only with the same statistical properties as used in S0819 (except for using a one-sided $\alpha = 0.025$) would take 582 patients. The strategy design testing the marker-based treatment (only EGFR FISH+ patients receiving the addition of cetuximab) versus treatment not based on marker (none of the patients receiving cetuximab independent of marker status) results in testing a hazard ratio of 1.14 and would require approximately 2580 patients. These calculations are based on using the aforementioned parameters and statistical assumption for the overall hypothesis and a one-sided $\alpha = 0.025$. This design and the many considerations that went into it were recently discussed by Redman et al. (2012). Determining the best interim monitoring plan for this study was another challenge. Decisions whether efficacy and/or futility should be monitored in the overall group or only in the EGFR FISH+ group and how to best spend alpha between the different tests had to be made.

9.6 Discussion

We evaluated three different trial designs commonly considered for situations when an underlying predictive marker is hypothesized. We consider the *randomize-all* design, the t*argeted* design, and the *strategy* design. We also evaluate testing both the overall and the targeted hypothesis in the *randomize-all* design. Even if a promising marker is found in the laboratory, it is not clear that this marker is an actual predictive marker for the treatment of patients or that the new treatment under investigation only helps marker-positive patients. We investigated five realistic scenarios, considering several different types of predictive markers, a prognostic marker, and no marker. Since many biological markers are continuous in nature, we assume an underlying continuous marker distribution rather than a discrete distribution as has been used in the current literature. This is more realistic for most markers and thus allows for a more precise design and analysis of clinical trial data. It also allows us to determine the effect of range of cut-points on the performance of the various designs. For a newly developed marker or assay, the cut-point has often not been determined precisely. This formulation also allows us to take into account marker prevalence in the patient population by shifting the underlying marker distribution. Finally, while the results are stated for a single continuous marker, the same strategy holds for a linear combination potentially based on two or more biological markers. For instance, the continuous marker could be a linear combination of gene expression measurements.

The large impact on power we have observed due to differences in treatment efficacy as a function of marker values and fraction of selected marker-positive patients highlights the need for a thorough investigation of properties prior to committing to a specific design and initiating a phase III study with targeted agents. Freidlin et al. (2012) discuss ways to guide the choice of design based on phase II data. If the actual underlying scenario (marker response distribution) is known, it is easy to decide on the most appropriate trial design using our results. In reality, however, the true underlying marker response distribution is often unknown and we have to consider several possibilities.

The SWOG trial S1007 provides a recent example when using a continuous marker is essential (Barlow 2012). S1007 is a phase III randomized clinical trial of standard adjuvant endocrine therapy ± chemotherapy in patients with 1–3 positive nodes, hormone receptor-positive, and HER2-negative breast cancer with recurrence score (RS) of 25 or less. Women who have been diagnosed with node-positive (1–3 positive nodes), HER2-negative, endocrine-responsive breast cancer who meet the eligibility criteria will undergo testing by the 21-gene RS assay (OncotypeDX®). Enough patients will initially be tested to obtain a total of 4000 eligible women with RS of 25 or less accepting to be randomized. The primary question is to test whether chemotherapy benefit (if it exists) depends on the RS. Thus, the underlying hypothesis is that there is an interaction of chemotherapy and RS. This trial tests scenario 4 (interaction) versus scenario 5 (prognostic marker). The interaction is tested in a Cox regression model of disease-free survival. If the interaction of chemotherapy and the linear RS term is statistically significant (two-sided α)

and there is a point of equivalence between the two randomized treatments for some RS value in the range 0–25, then additional steps are undertaken. Based on simulation studies, power to find a significant interaction with an equivalence point is 81%. Assuming there is a significant predictive effect of RS on chemotherapy benefit, a clinical cut-point for recommending chemotherapy will be estimated. This estimated cut-point is the upper bound of the 95% confidence interval on the point of equivalence. If there is no statistical interaction between linear RS and chemotherapy, then chemotherapy will be tested in a Cox model adjusting for RS, but without an interaction term. This test will be conducted at a one-sided $\alpha = 0.025$ since chemotherapy would be expected to improve outcomes.

We suggest some general guidelines to help with the decision on which trial design is most appropriate. In general, the *targeted* design performs the best in all scenarios with an underlying true predictive marker in terms of the required number of randomized patients, that is, sample size. There is only one exception, which is in the case of a prognostic marker with constant odds ratio between treatment arms (scenario 5) when the *targeted* design has less power than the *randomize-all* design, but only for the extreme marker values when the cut-point is shifted such that most patients are marker negative. In addition, more patients still need to be assessed for their marker status compared to the *randomize-all* and the *strategy* designs. If the new treatment may also help marker-negative patients, there is the question whether the targeted design is appropriate. The *strategy* design tends to be inefficient to compare the efficacy difference of two treatments as patients in different randomized arms are treated with the same therapy. The *randomize-all* design performs as well or in most cases better than the *strategy* design except for the hypothetical total interaction model on scenario 4, where the overall treatment effect is null. We thus recommend using the *randomize-all* design over the *strategy* design except for cases where the actual strategy hypothesis is of greater interest than the efficacy hypothesis or if almost all patients in the marker-based treatment arm receive the experimental treatment T2. An example for when the *strategy* design may be appropriate is in the setting of personalized therapy, where patients are evaluated on a variety of biomarkers and treatment is chosen form a large portfolio of agents. In that case, a randomization between patients being treated by that treatment strategy versus standard of care may be the most appropriate design as it answers the strategy hypothesis.

We recommend using the *targeted* design if it is known with little uncertainty that the new treatment does not help all patients to some degree, if the marker prevalence (indicating patients helped by the new therapy) is small, and if the cut-point of marker-positive and marker-negative patients is relatively well established. If the cut-point is not well established yet, the power of the study can be severely compromised. Likewise, if only the most extreme marker values are classified as marker positive, but if the treatment is more broadly effective, then some patients who are classified as marker negative will not get randomized even though they would have benefitted from the new treatment.

Scenario 3 is a very likely scenario. In this scenario, the treatment works better for M+ subjects but also benefits M− subjects, for instance, to a lesser extent. Even if one pathway of action is well understood for M+ patients, there is always the possibility that the new agent works via a different pathway for the M− patient. This has recently been observed in the case of Her-2 overexpression in breast cancer, there is still the possibility that the new therapy under investigation works through other pathways not yet investigated (Shepherd et al. 2005, Menendez et al. 2006). If there is the possibility that the new treatment helps marker-negative patients, that the cut-point determining marker status has not yet been well established, and if the marker prevalence is large enough to make the study effective, we recommend using the *randomize-all* design with the power adjusted for multiple comparison such that both the overall and the targeted hypothesis can be tested. Our results show that if there is an underlying predictive marker and if the cut-point determining marker status is not too far off the correct cut-point, the targeted hypothesis and the overall hypotheses (with split alpha level) achieve similar power as the overall hypothesis tested at $\alpha = 0.05$ and thus both hypotheses can be tested with only a modest increase in sample size compared to testing the overall hypothesis alone in the *randomize-all* design. In addition, we found that even in the case of extreme (large or small) marker prevalence, both the targeted and the overall hypotheses (with split alpha level) achieve comparable power as the overall hypothesis tested at $\alpha = 0.05$ and again both hypotheses can be tested with only a modest increase in sample size compared to testing the overall hypothesis only in the *randomize-all* design.

References

Barlow W. 2012. Design of a clinical trial for testing the ability of a continuous marker to predict therapy benefit. In Crowley J, Hoering A (eds.). *Handbook of Statistics in Clinical Oncology*, 3rd ed. Boca Raton, FL: Chapman & Hall/CRC.

Cobo M, Isla D, Massuti B et al. 2007. Customizing cisplatin based on quantitative excision repair cross-complementing 1 mRNA expression: A phase III trial in non-small-cell lung cancer. *J Clin Oncol* 25(19): 2747–2754.

Freidlin B et al. 2012. Randomized phase II trial designs with biomarkers. *J Clin Oncol* 30(26): 3304–3309.

Freidlin B and Simon R. 2005. Adaptive signature design: An adaptive clinical trial design for generating and prospectively testing a gene expression signature for sensitive patients. *Clin Cancer Res* 11(21): 7872–7878.

Hayes DF, Trock B, and Harris AL. 1998. Assessing the clinical impact of prognostic factors: When is "statistically significant" clinically useful? *Breast Cancer Res Treat* 52(1–3): 305–319.

Hoering A, LeBlanc M, and Crowley J. 2008. Randomized phase III clinical trial designs for targeted agents. *Clin Cancer Res* 14: 4358–4367.

Hoering A, LeBlanc M, and Crowley J. 2012. Seamless phase I/II trial design for assessing toxicity and efficacy for targeted agents. In Crowley J, Hoering A (eds.), *Handbook of Statistics in Clinical Oncology*, 3rd ed. Boca Raton, FL: Chapman & Hall/CRC.

Jiang W, Freidlin B, and Simon R. 2007. Biomarker-adaptive threshold design: A procedure for evaluating treatment with possible biomarker-defined subset effect. *J Natl Cancer Inst* 99(13): 1036–1043.

Mandrekar SJ and Sargent DJ. 2009. Clinical trial designs for predictive biomarker validation: Theoretical considerations and practical challenges. *J Clin Oncol* 27(24): 4027–4034.

Menendez JA, Mehmi I and Lupu R. 2006. Trastuzumab in combination with heregulin-activated Her-2 (erbB-2) triggers a receptor-enhanced chemosensitivity effect in the absence of Her-2 overexpression. *J Clin Oncol* 24(23): 3735–3746.

Redman M, Crowley J, Herbst R et al. 2012. Design of a phase III clinical trial with prospective biomarker validation: SWOG S0819. *Clin Cancer Res* 18(15): 4004–4012.

Sargent D and Allegra C. 2002. Issues in clinical trial design for tumor marker studies. *Semin Oncol* 29(3): 222–230.

Sargent DJ, Conley BA, Allegra C et al. 2005. Clinical trial designs for predictive marker validation in cancer treatment trials. *J Clin Oncol* 9: 2020–2027.

Shepherd FA, Rodrigues Pereira J, Ciuleanu T et al. 2005. Erlotinib in previously treated non-small-cell lung cancer. *N Engl J Med* 353(2): 123–132.

Simon R and Maitournam A. 2004. Evaluating the efficiency of targeted designs for randomized clinical trials. *Clin Cancer Res* 10(20): 6759–6763.

Song Y and Chi GYH. 2007. A method for testing a prespecified subgroup in clinical trials. *Stat Med* 26: 3535–3549.

Spiessens B and Debois M. 2010. Adjusted significance levels for subgroup analyses in clinical trials. *Contemp Clin Trials* 31: 647–656.

Wakelee H, Kernstine K, Vokes E. et al. 2008. Cooperative group research efforts in lung cancer 2008: Focus on advanced-stage non-small-cell lung cancer. *Clin Lung Cancer* 9(6): 346–351.

Wang S. et al. 2007. Approaches to evaluation of treatment effect in randomized clinical trials with genomic subset. *Pharm Stat* 6: 227–244.

10

*Phase III All-Comers Clinical Trials with a Predictive Biomarker**

Shigeyuki Matsui, Yuki Choai, and Takahiro Nonaka

CONTENTS

10.1 Introduction

This chapter considers phase III clinical trials to confirm treatment efficacy based on a single predictive biomarker or signature that is analytically validated and completely specified. When evidence from biological or early trial data suggests that the biomarker is so reliable and the use of the treatment for biomarker-*negative* patients predicted by the biomarker not to benefit from the treatment is considered unethical at the initiation of a phase III trial, an enrichment or targeted design that randomizes only a subgroup of biomarker-*positive* patients (predicted to benefit from the treatment) can be an efficient trial design (e.g., Simon and Maitournam, 2005; see also Chapters 8 and 9). However, it is more common that, at the initiation of phase III trials, there is no compelling evidence regarding the capability of the biomarker in

* The views expressed herein are the result of independent work and do not necessarily represent the views of the Pharmaceuticals and Medical Devices Agency.

predicting treatment effects or there is uncertainty about a cut-point of an analytically validated predictive assay. In such situations, it is generally reasonable to include all patients as eligible for randomization as done in traditional clinical trials, but to plan for *prospective* subgroup analysis based on the biomarker (Pusztai and Hess, 2004; Sargent et al., 2005; Simon and Wang, 2006; Simon, 2008; Wang et al., 2007; Mandrekar and Sargent, 2009; Freidlin et al., 2010, 2013; Buyse et al., 2011; Freidlin and Korn, 2014; Matsui et al., 2014).

In this chapter, we focus on such all-comers or randomize-all designs and discuss the three approaches of statistical analysis plans: fixed-sequence, fallback, and treatment-by-biomarker interaction approaches (Figure 10.1). An important feature of these approaches is that they can demonstrate treatment efficacy for either the overall patient population or a biomarker-based subgroup of patients based on the observed clinical trial data. We provide a comparison of these approaches in terms of the probability of asserting treatment efficacy for the right patient population (i.e., either the overall population or the biomarker-based subgroup) (Matsui et al., 2014). Discussion also includes sample size calculations and criteria for clinical validation of predictive biomarkers.

10.2 Approaches to Statistical Analysis Plan

We consider a phase III randomized trial to compare a new treatment and its control on the basis of survival outcomes. We suppose that at the time the trial is initiated, a candidate predictive biomarker will be available. In many cases, biomarker values are dichotomous or cut-points are used to classify the biomarker results as either *positive* or *negative*, denoted by M+ and M−, respectively. Typically, M+ represents the subgroup of patients that is expected to be responsive to the treatment, while M− represents the remainder. Let p_+ denote the prevalence of M+ in the patient population. Randomization can be either stratified or unstratified on the basis of the predictive biomarker. We suppose a stratified trial because of possible prognostic effects of the biomarker. It also ensures observation of the biomarker status for all randomly assigned patients (Freidlin et al., 2010).

For a particular patient population, we assume proportional hazards between treatment arms and use the asymptotic distribution of a log-rank test statistic S to compare survival outcomes between the two arms under equal treatment assignment and follow-up, $S \sim N(\theta, 4/E)$ (Tsiatis, 1981). Here, θ is the logarithm of the ratio of the hazard function under the new treatment relative to that under the control treatment, and E is the total number of events observed. For a clinical trial with a given number of events, we express a standardized test statistic for testing treatment efficacy in the M+ subgroup of patients as $Z_+ = \hat{\theta}_+/\sqrt{V_+}$, where $\hat{\theta}_+$ is an estimate of θ_+

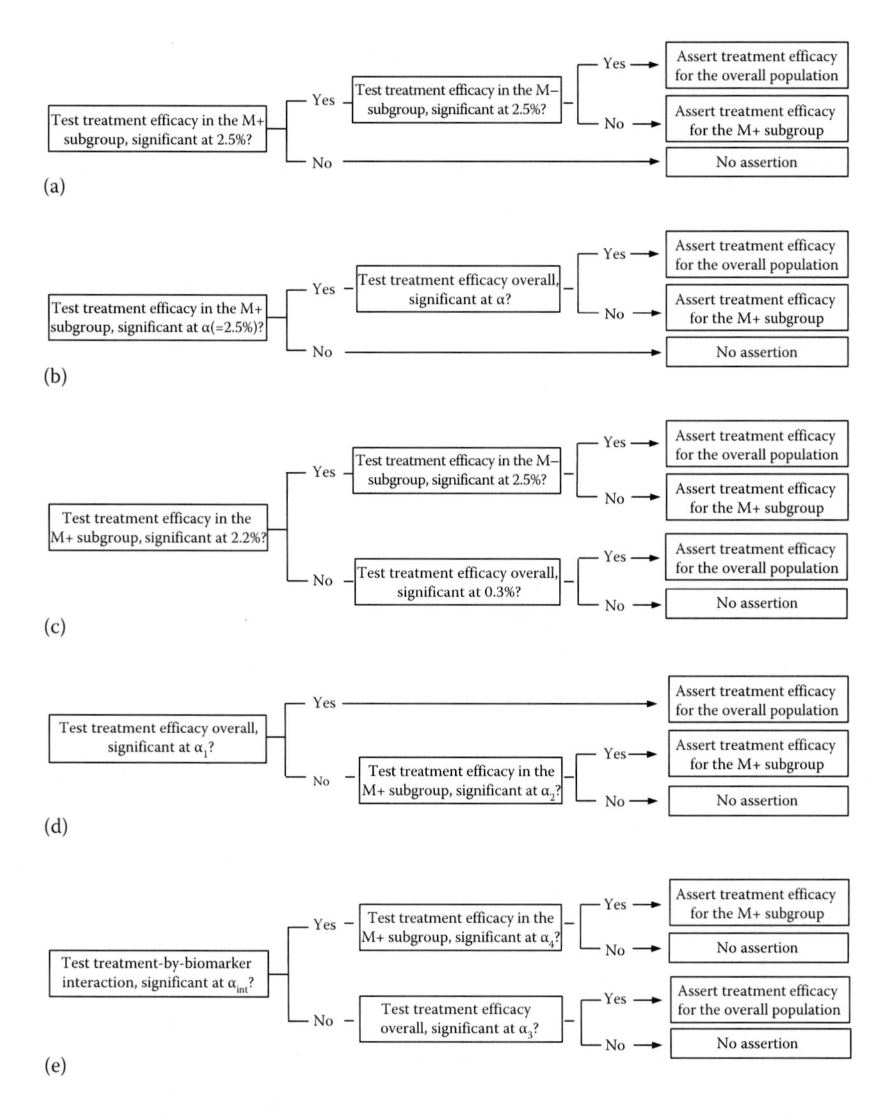

FIGURE 10.1
Approaches of statistical analysis plan for all-comers phase III trials with a predictive biomarker. All alpha levels are one sided. (a) Fixed-sequence-1 approach; (b) fixed-sequence-2 approach; (c) MaST approach; (d) fallback approach; and (e) treatment-by-biomarker interaction approach.

and $V_+ = 4/E_+$ in this subgroup. Similarly, for the M− patients, we consider a similar standardized statistic, $Z_- = \hat{\theta}_- / \sqrt{V_-}$, where $\hat{\theta}_-$ is an estimate of θ_- and $V_- = 4/E_-$ in this subgroup. We also express a standardized test statistic for testing overall treatment efficacy as $Z_{\text{overall}} = \hat{\theta}_{\text{overall}} / \sqrt{V_{\text{overall}}}$, where $\hat{\theta}_{\text{overall}}$ is an estimate of θ_{overall} and $V_{\text{overall}} = 4/E_{\text{overall}} = 4/(E_+ + E_-)$. By using an approximation, $\hat{\theta}_{\text{overall}} \approx \{(1/V_+)\hat{\theta}_+ + (1/V_-)\hat{\theta}_-\}/(1/V_+ + 1/V_-)$, we have the following stratified statistic for testing overall treatment effects:

$$Z_{\text{overall}} = \frac{\sqrt{V_{\text{overall}}}}{V_+}\hat{\theta}_+ + \frac{\sqrt{V_{\text{overall}}}}{V_-}\hat{\theta}_-.$$

We assume that the aforementioned standardized statistics follow asymptotically normal distributions with variance 1, where the means of Z_+, Z_-, Z_{overall} are $\theta_+/\sqrt{V_+}$, $\theta_-/\sqrt{V_-}$, and $\sqrt{V_{\text{overall}}}(\theta_+/V_+ + \theta_-/V_-)$, respectively.

In what follows, we outline the three approaches to the statistical analysis plan: fixed-sequence, fallback, and treatment-by-biomarker interaction approaches. Each approach can demonstrate treatment efficacy for either the overall patient population or the M+ subgroup of patients with a control of the study-wise type I error rate α (Figure 10.1). In the following presentations, all alpha levels are one sided.

10.2.1 Fixed-Sequence Approaches

Where evidence from biological or early trial data suggests the predictive ability of the biomarker and one would not expect the treatment to be effective in the M− patients unless it is effective in the M+ patients, a fixed-sequence analysis that first tests treatment efficacy in the M+ subgroup is reasonable. As a *fixed-sequence-1* approach, the treatment effect is tested in the M+ patients using Z_+ at a significance level $\alpha = 0.025$. If this is significant, then the treatment effect is also tested in the M− patients using Z_- at the same significance level α (Figure 10.1a) (Simon, 2008). This sequential approach controls the study-wise type I error at α. As an example of this approach, in a randomized phase III trial of panitumumab with infusional fluorouracil, leucovorin, and oxaliplatin (FOLFOX) versus FOLFOX alone for untreated metastatic colorectal cancer (Douillard et al., 2010), the treatment arms were first compared on progression-free survival (PFS) for patients with wild-type *KRAS* tumors. Treatment comparison in patients with mutant *KRAS* tumors was conditional on a significant difference in the first test for the wild-type *KRAS* subgroup.

In another variation of the fixed sequence approaches, *fixed-sequence-2*, the second stage involves testing treatment efficacy for the overall population using Z_{overall} rather than for the subgroup of M− patients (Figure 10.1b) (Mandrekar and Sargent, 2009). An example of this approach is a phase III trial testing cetuximab in addition to FOLFOX as adjuvant therapy in stage III colon cancer (N0147). In the analysis plan, the efficacy of the regimen on disease-free survival is first tested in the patients with wild-type *KRAS* using a log-rank test at a significance level of 2.5%. If this subgroup test is statistically significant, then a test for the overall population is performed at a significance level of 2.5% (Mandrekar and Sargent, 2009).

In the fixed-sequence 1 and 2 approaches, when both first and second tests are significant, one may assert treatment efficacy for the overall patient population. When only the first test is significant, one may assert treatment efficacy only for future patients who are biomarker positive (Figure 10.1a,b).

As a more complex variation of statistical analysis plan, Freidlin et al. (2013, 2014) recently proposed an analysis plan called marker sequential test (MaST). In this approach, a fixed-sequence-1 approach using a reduced significance level, such as 0.022, is performed. If the test in the M+ subgroup is not significant, treatment efficacy in the overall population is tested using a significance level of 0.003 (=0.025 – 0.022) (see Figure 10.1c). The use of this overall test intends to improve the power for detecting homogenous treatment effects between biomarker-based subgroups. Recommended significance levels for the test in the M+ subgroup are 0.022 and 0.04 for the study-wise type I error rate of $\alpha = 0.025$ and 0.05, respectively (Freidlin et al., 2014). This is to control the probability that erroneously asserting treatment efficacy for the M– patients at the level α under the hypothesis that the treatment is effective for the M+ patients, but not for the M– patients, in addition to controlling the study-wise type error rate at the level α under the global null hypothesis of no treatment effects in both M+ and M– patients. Rather than using the Bonferroni approach, a more powerful analysis is to determine significance levels for $Z_{overall}$ and Z_+ for a given α, through taking their correlation into consideration, where the correlation $corr(Z_{overall}, Z_+)$ reduces to $\sqrt{p_+}$ approximately (Song and Chi, 2007; Wang et al., 2007; Spiessens and Debois, 2010).

10.2.2 Fallback Approach

When there is no convincing evidence on the predictive value of the biomarker and it is considered that the treatment has a potential to be broadly effective, it is reasonable to evaluate treatment efficacy in the overall population and prepare a biomarker-based subgroup analysis as a fallback option. Specifically, the treatment effect is first tested in the overall population using $Z_{overall}$ at a reduced significance level α_1 ($<\alpha$). If this is not significant, the treatment effect is tested in the M+ patients using Z_+ at a reduced significance level α_2 ($<\alpha$) (Figure 10.1d) (Simon and Wang, 2006). The significance level α_2 can be specified by taking into account the correlation between $Z_{overall}$ and Z_+ (Song and Chi, 2007; Wang et al., 2007; Spiessens and Debois, 2010). When the first test is significant, one may assert treatment efficacy for the overall population. Meanwhile, when only the second subgroup test is significant, one may assert treatment efficacy only for future M+ patients (Figure 10.1d).

Parallel testing for the overall population and the M+ subgroup can also be considered. For example, in the SATURN trial (Cappuzzo et al., 2010) to assess the use of erlotinib as maintenance therapy in patients with nonprogressive disease following first-line platinum-doublet chemotherapy, PFS after randomization was tested in all patients at a significance level of 1.5% and in the patients whose tumors had EGFR protein overexpression at a significance level of 1%. The parallel testing will have the same statistical properties with the sequential fallback test when the result of the overall test is prioritized (Freidlin et al., 2013).

10.2.3 Treatment-by-Biomarker Interaction Approach

Another approach when there is limited confidence in the predictive biomarker is to decide whether to compare treatments overall or within the biomarker-based subgroups on the basis of a preliminary test of interaction of treatment and biomarker (Sargent et al., 2005; Simon, 2008). For example, in the MARVEL trial (Wakelee et al., 2008) to compare erlotinib and pemetrexed as second-line treatment for non-small-cell lung cancer, the analysis was planned to be conducted separately in *EGFR*-positive and *EGFR*-negative patients, with the use of an interaction test on the difference in treatment effects between the two subgroups of patients. For the interaction test, we can use the following standardized statistic:

$$Z_{\text{int}} = \frac{\hat{\theta}_+ - \hat{\theta}_-}{\sqrt{V_+ + V_-}}.$$

It is reasonable to consider a one-sided test to detect larger treatment effects in the M+ patients (Simon, 2008). As an asymptotic approximation for Z_{int}, we assume a normal distribution with mean $(\theta_+ - \theta_-)/\sqrt{V_+ + V_-}$ and variance 1.

In order to control the study-wise type I error rate, Matsui et al. (2014) proposed the following approach: a preliminary one-sided test of interaction is performed as the first stage using a significance level of α_{Int}. If this test is not significant, the treatment effect is tested in the overall population using a reduce significance level α_3 ($<\alpha$). Otherwise, the treatment effect is tested in the M+ subgroup using a significance level α_4 ($<\alpha$). When the interaction is significant and the test in the M+ patients is significant, one may assert treatment efficacy only for the M+ patients. When the interaction is not significant and the overall test is significant, one may assert treatment efficacy for the overall population (Figure 10.1e).

The significance levels, α_{int}, α_3, and α_4, are chosen to control the study-wise type I error rate of asserting treatment efficacy at the level α under the global null hypothesis of no treatment efficacy for the M+ and M− patients (and thus no effects for the overall population). The study-wise type I error rate (and power) is evaluable based on the asymptotic distribution of Z_{int}, Z_{overall}, and Z_+. Here, the correlations between Z_{int} and Z_{overall} or Z_+ may reduce to $corr(Z_{\text{int}}, Z_{\text{overall}}) = 0$ or $corr(Z_{\text{int}}, Z_+) =$

$\sqrt{V_+/(V_+ + V_-)} = \sqrt{E_-/(E_+ + E_-)} = \sqrt{R/(1+R)}$, where $R = E_-/E_+$. When $E_+ = p_+E$ or $R = (1 - p_+)/p_+$ can be supposed, we have $corr(Z_{\text{int}}, Z_+) = \sqrt{1-p_+}$. This is reasonable for many cases, for example, when the number of events is slightly less than the number of patients under adequate follow-up for advanced diseases or when the event rates are comparable across the biomarker-based subgroups. In general situations, we search for the significance levels based on $corr(Z_{\text{int}}, Z_+) = \sqrt{R/(1+R)}$ rather than $corr(Z_{\text{int}}, Z_+) = \sqrt{1-p_+}$. We need an expected value for the event ratio R under the global null effects, which may depend on the respective (baseline) event rates (possibly, with some prognostic effects) and the censoring distributions across biomarker-based subgroups.

10.3 Comparison of the Approaches

10.3.1 Criteria: Probabilities of Asserting Treatment Efficacy

The statistical analysis plans described in Section 10.2 can make either of two kinds of assertions regarding treatment efficacy, one for the overall population and the other for the subgroup of M+ patients. Which of the two assertions is considered to be valid depends at least on the underlying treatment effects in the biomarker-based subgroups as discussed in Matsui et al., (2014). Let HR_+ and HR_- be the hazard ratios of the treatment relative to the control in the M+ and M− subgroups, respectively. If the treatment truly has homogeneous effects that are clinically meaningful in both M+ and M− subgroups, for example, $HR_+ = HR_- = 0.7$, the assertion of treatment efficacy for the overall population would be more valid than that for the M+ subgroup because the latter assertion would deprive the M− patients of the chance of receiving the effective treatment. On the other hand, if the treatment can exert a clinically important effect only in the M+ subgroup, for example, $HR_+ = 0.5$, and no effect in the M− subgroup, for example, $HR_- = 1.0$, indicating a qualitative interaction between treatment and biomarker, the assertion of treatment efficacy for the M+ subgroup would be more valid than that for the overall population because the latter assertion would yield overtreatment for the M− patients using the ineffective, even toxic treatment.

However, there can be other scenarios in which it is not clear which of the two assertions is valid. For example, the treatment can exert a clinically important effect for the M+ subgroup, for example, $HR_+ = 0.5$, but some moderate or small effects for the M− subgroup, for example, $HR_- = 0.8$, indicating a quantitative interaction between treatment and biomarker. Such a profile of treatment effect could be explained by the treatment having multiple mechanisms of action, the misclassification of responsive patients into the M− subgroup (low sensitivity of the biomarker), and so on. Which of the two assertions is considered to be valid will be determined on a case-by-case basis incorporating many factors, including the prevalence of M+, possible adverse effects, treatment costs, prognosis of the disease, availability of other treatment choices, and so on. In such situations, the probability of asserting treatment efficacy for either the overall population or the M+ subgroup could be another meaningful criterion. From the point of view of treatment developers (e.g., pharmaceutical companies), this probability would be always important because it can be interpreted as the *probability of success* in treatment development.

Let $P_{overall}$, $P_{subgroup}$, and $P_{success}$ denote the probability of asserting treatment efficacy for the overall population and for the M+ subgroup, and that of success, respectively. Apparently, $P_{overall} + P_{subgroup} = P_{success}$ for the statistical analysis plans in Section 10.2, indicating that there is a trade-off between $P_{overall}$ and $P_{subgroup}$ for a given value of the total probability $P_{success}$.

10.3.2 Numerical Evaluations

We assessed the probabilities $P_{overall}$, $P_{subgroup}$, and $P_{success}$ for the statistical analysis plans based on the asymptotic distributions of $Z_{overall}$, Z_+, and Z_{int} given in Section 10.2. For a total number of events $E = E_+ + E_-$, we supposed that $E_+ = p_+E$ and $E_- = (1 - p_+)E$ (or $R = (1 - p_+)/p_+$) under both null and non-null treatment effects (see Section 10.2.3). The asymptotic distributions are adequate approximations for a wide range of the underlying survival time distributions. Adequacy of using the approximations under limited sample sizes was checked by simulations with exponential survival times (Matsui et al., 2014).

We considered the prevalence of M+ in the patient population to be $p_+ = 0.2$, 0.4, or 0.6. With respect to the underlying treatment effects within biomarker-based subgroup, we considered the following scenarios: $(HR_+, HR_-) = (1.0, 1.0)$, (0.7, 0.7), (0.5, 1.0), or (0.5, 0.8), that is, null effects, constant effects, qualitative interaction, and quantitative interaction, as described in Section 10.3.1. The study-wise type I error rate ($P_{success}$ under the global null effects) was specified as $\alpha = 0.025$. In the MaST approach, following the recommendation by Freidlin et al. (2014), we used the significance level of 0.022 for the M+ subgroup, but that for the test in the overall population was determined, such that $P_{success} = 0.025$ under the global null, through taking account of the correlation between $Z_{overall}$ and Z_+, to avoid a conservative analysis and have a fair comparison with the other approaches (while the inflation of the type I error that erroneously asserting treatment effects for the M− patients when the treatment is effective for the M+ patients, but not for the M− patients, was minimal; see Figure 10.3). In the treatment-by-biomarker interaction approach, the significance level for the one-sided interaction test, α_{int}, was specified as 0.1, a small level such that the interaction test could serve as evidence in clinical validation of the predictive biomarker. For the significance levels in the fallback approach, α_1 and α_2, and the treatment-by-biomarker

TABLE 10.1

Significance Levels of the Fallback and Treatment-by-Biomarker Interaction Approaches That Satisfy $P_{overall}=0.015$ and $P_{subgroup}=0.01$ under the Global Null Effects

	Fallback Approach		Treatment-by-Biomarker Interaction Approach	
p_+	α_1	α_2	α_3	α_4
0.2	0.0150	0.0116	0.0167	0.0101
0.4	0.0150	0.0133	0.0167	0.0116
0.6	0.0150	0.0157	0.0167	0.0154

Notes: The significance level of the interaction test was specified as $\alpha_{int}=0.1$. We supposed $E_+=p_+E$ for calculating significance levels α_3 and α_4 in the treatment-by-biomarker interaction approach.

interaction approaches, α_3, and α_4, we specified them so that $P_{overall}$ and $P_{subgroup}$ ($=\alpha - P_{overall}$) under the global null hypothesis were identical for these approaches for a fair comparison. We considered setting an intermediate or balanced level $P_{overall}=0.015$ ($P_{subgroup}=0.01$) under the global null. See Table 10.1 for resultant significance levels. For more unbalanced levels, such as $P_{overall}=0.005$ or 0.02 ($P_{subgroup}=0.02$ or 0.005), under the global null, similar conclusions would be obtained (see the Supplemental Data of Matsui et al., 2014). We also evaluated the traditional approach without use of the biomarker as a reference, for which $P_{overall}=P_{success}$ and $P_{subgroup}=0$, because there is no option for asserting treatment efficacy for the M+ subgroup. Note that the values of $P_{success}$ for the fixed-sequence-1 and fixed-sequence-2 approaches are always identical to the probability that the test for the M+ subgroup (the first test in the fixed-sequence approaches) is statistically significant.

We first ascertained the control of type I error rates. Under the global null effects $(HR_+, HR_-)=(1.0, 1.0)$, the probabilities $P_{overall}$, $P_{subgroup}$, and $P_{success}$ calculated based on the asymptotic distributions were constant for any values of E. Table 10.2 provides these values as well as those obtained by simulations with exponential survival times when $E=200$. Agreement of these two indicates adequacy of using the asymptotic approximations under the global null effects.

With regard to the results under nonnull treatment effects, Figures 10.2 through 10.4 show $P_{overall}$, $P_{subgroup}$, and $P_{success}$ calculated based on the asymptotic distributions for various values of E under constant effects, qualitative interaction, and quantitative interaction, respectively.

For the scenarios with constant treatment effects, $(HR_+, HR_-)=(0.7, 0.7)$, where $P_{overall}$ would be a relevant criterion, the traditional approach provided the greatest values of $P_{overall}$, as was expected (Figure 10.2). The fallback and treatment-by-biomarker interaction approaches provided slightly reduced values of $P_{overall}$ than those of the traditional approach. On the other hand, the fixed-sequence-1 and fixed-sequence-2 provided much smaller

TABLE 10.2

$P_{overall}$, $P_{subgroup}$, $P_{success}$ under the Global Null $(HR_+, HR_-) = (1.0, 1.0)$ for $p_+ = 0.4$

	Probability	Traditional	Fixed-Sequence-1	Fixed-Sequence-2	MaST	Fallback	Treatment-by-Biomarker Interaction
Asymptotic approximations	$P_{overall}$	0.025	0.001	0.007	0.004	0.015	0.015
	$P_{subgroup}$	0.000	0.024	0.018	0.021	0.010	0.010
	$P_{success}$	0.025	0.025	0.025	0.025	0.025	0.025
Simulations[a]	$P_{overall}$	0.026	0.000	0.007	0.004	0.016	0.016
	$P_{subgroup}$	0.000	0.025	0.018	0.022	0.010	0.010
	$P_{success}$	0.026	0.025	0.025	0.025	0.026	0.026

[a] Exponential survival times were generated in the M+ and M− patients with the baseline event rates, $\lambda_+ = \lambda_- = 1.0$, and treatment effects (HR_+, HR_-) for a total number of patients of 200. Survival times were uncensored so that $E_+ = p_+ E$ holds. Use of other values of the baseline hazards λ_+ and λ_- (possibly $\lambda_+ \neq \lambda_-$) may not change the results with the use of the stratified statistic $Z_{overall}$ for the overall test. 10,000 simulations were conducted for each configuration.

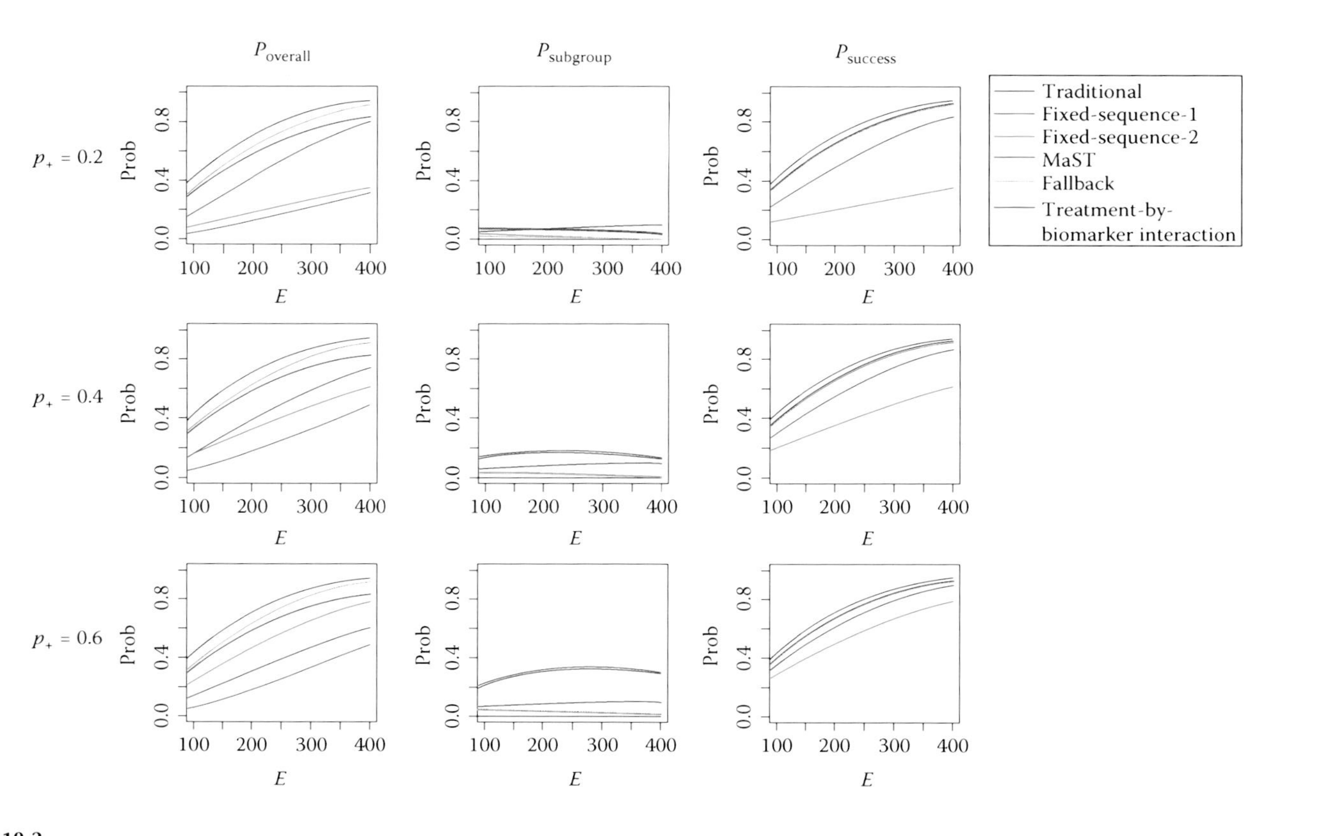

FIGURE 10.2

$P_{overall}$, $P_{subgroup}$, and $P_{success}$, for various numbers of events, E, under constant effects $(HR_+, HR_-) = (0.7, 0.7)$. The $P_{success}$ curve for the fixed-sequence-1 is always coincident with that for the fixed-sequence-2. The $P_{subgroup}$ curves for the fixed-sequence-1 and MaST were nearly identical.

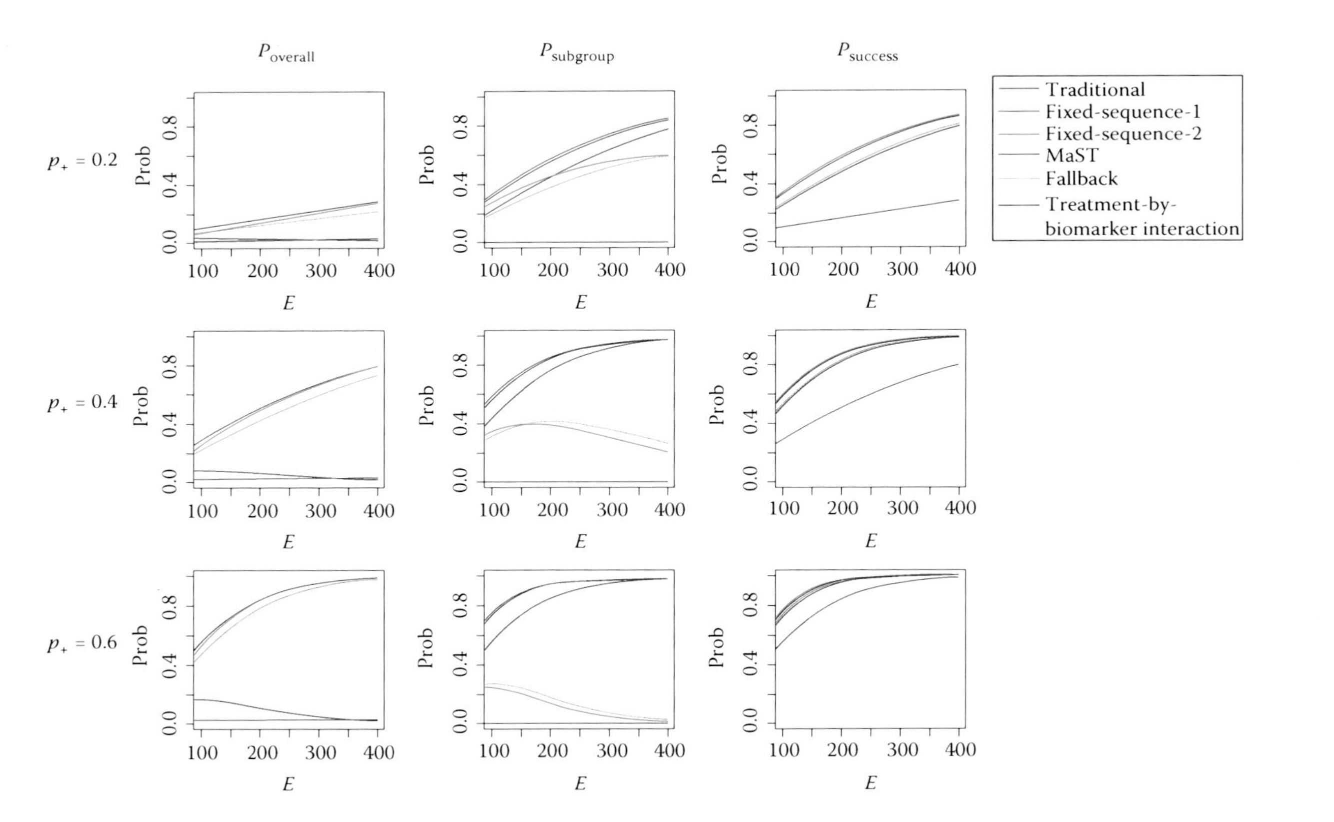

FIGURE 10.3
$P_{overall}$, $P_{subgroup}$, and $P_{success}$, for various numbers of events, E, under a qualitative interaction (HR_+, HR_-) = (0.5, 1.0). The $P_{success}$ curve for the fixed-sequence-1 is always coincident with that for the fixed-sequence-2.

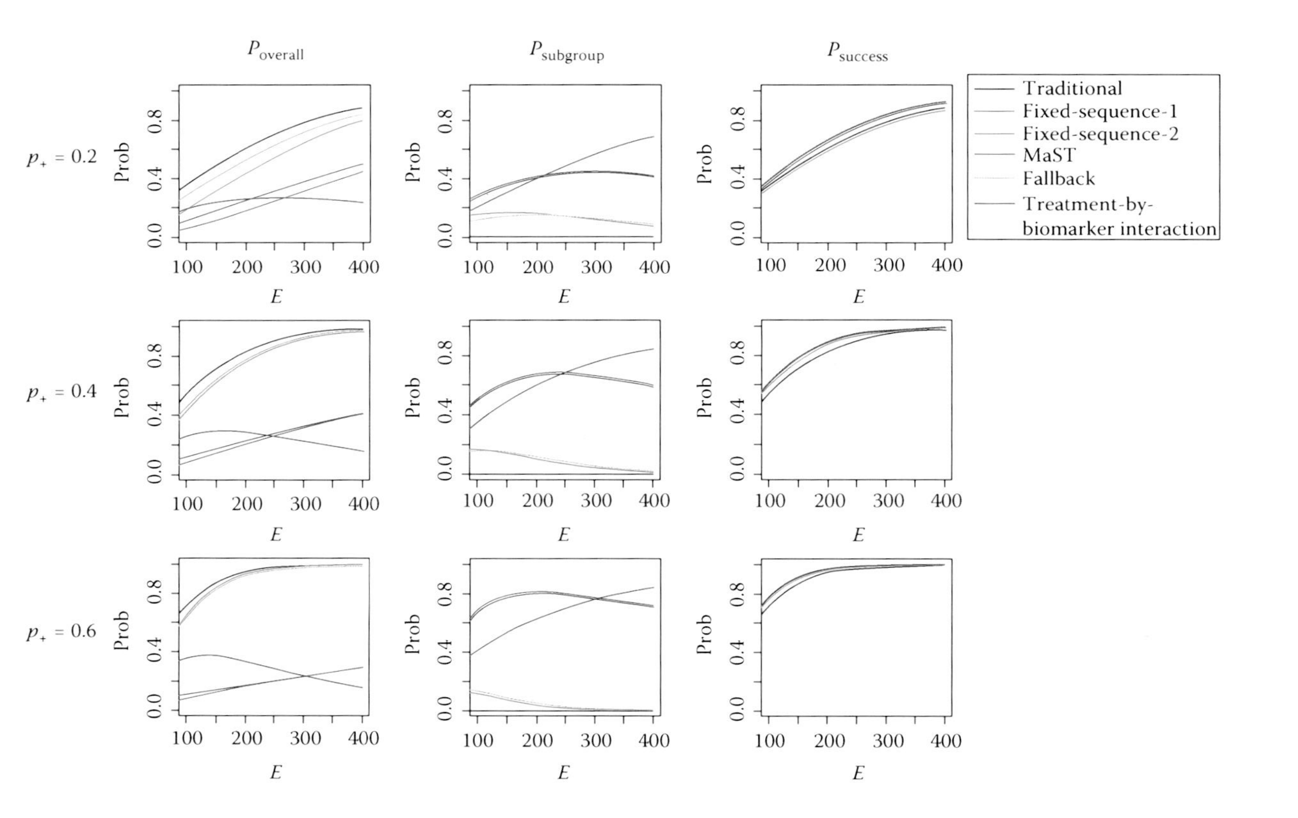

FIGURE 10.4
$P_{overall}$, $P_{subgroup}$, and $P_{success}$, for various numbers of events, E, under a quantitative interaction $(HR_+, HR_-) = (0.5, 0.8)$. The $P_{success}$ curve for the fixed-sequence-1 is always coincident with that for the fixed-sequence-2.

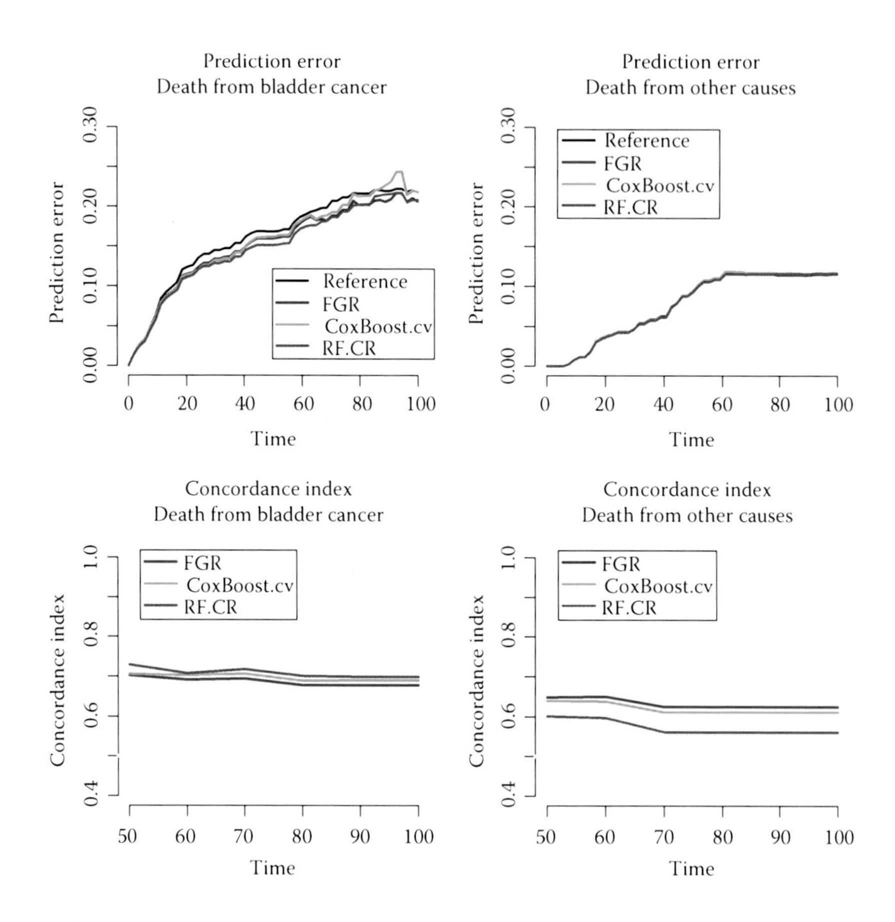

FIGURE 15.2
Estimated Brier scores (upper panels) and time-truncated concordance index (lower panels) for risk prediction models from Fine–Gray regression with clinical covariates only (FGR), componentwise boosting (CoxBoost.cv), and random forests (RF.CR) for predicting progression and cancer-related death (left panels) and death from other causes (right panels). All estimates are obtained by averaging 100 bootstrap subsample cross-validation runs. In each run, training data are drawn without replacement and include 90% of all patients.

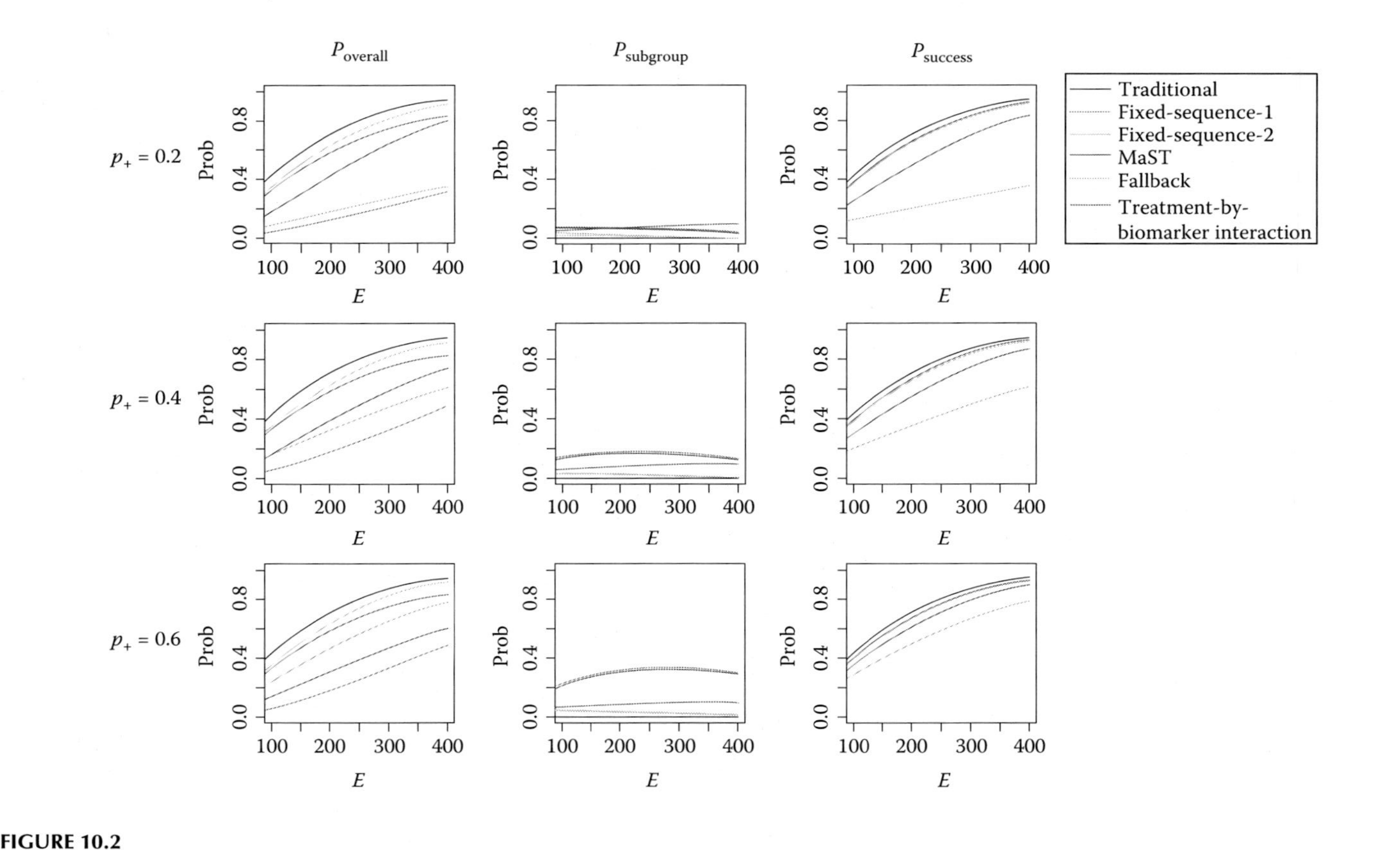

FIGURE 10.2
(See color insert.) $P_{overall}$, $P_{subgroup}$, and $P_{success}$, for various numbers of events, E, under constant effects $(HR_+, HR_-) = (0.7, 0.7)$. The $P_{success}$ curve for the fixed-sequence-1 is always coincident with that for the fixed-sequence-2. The $P_{subgroup}$ curves for the fixed-sequence-1 and MaST were nearly identical.

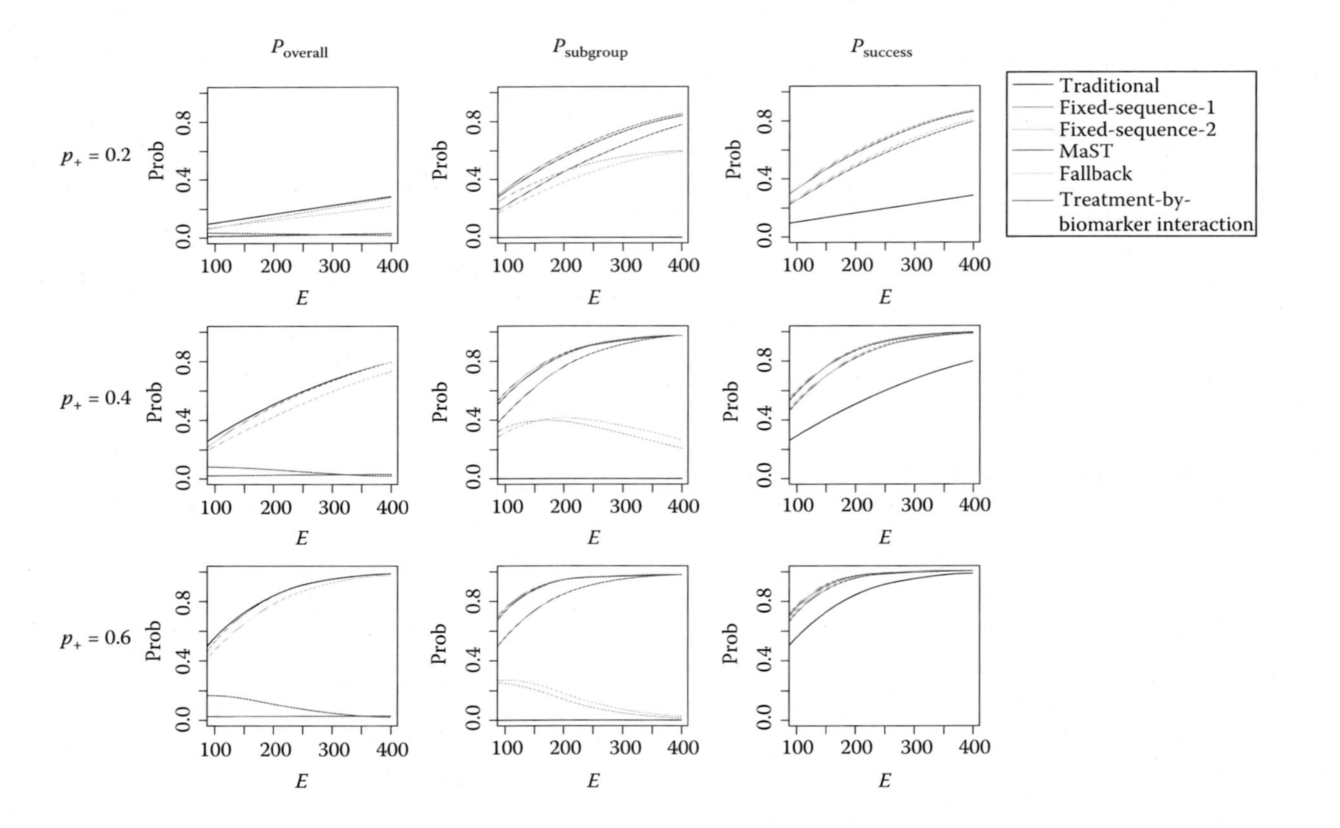

FIGURE 10.3
(See color insert.) $P_{overall}$, $P_{subgroup}$, and $P_{success}$, for various numbers of events, E, under a qualitative interaction $(HR_+, HR_-) = (0.5, 1.0)$. The $P_{success}$ curve for the fixed-sequence-1 is always coincident with that for the fixed-sequence-2.

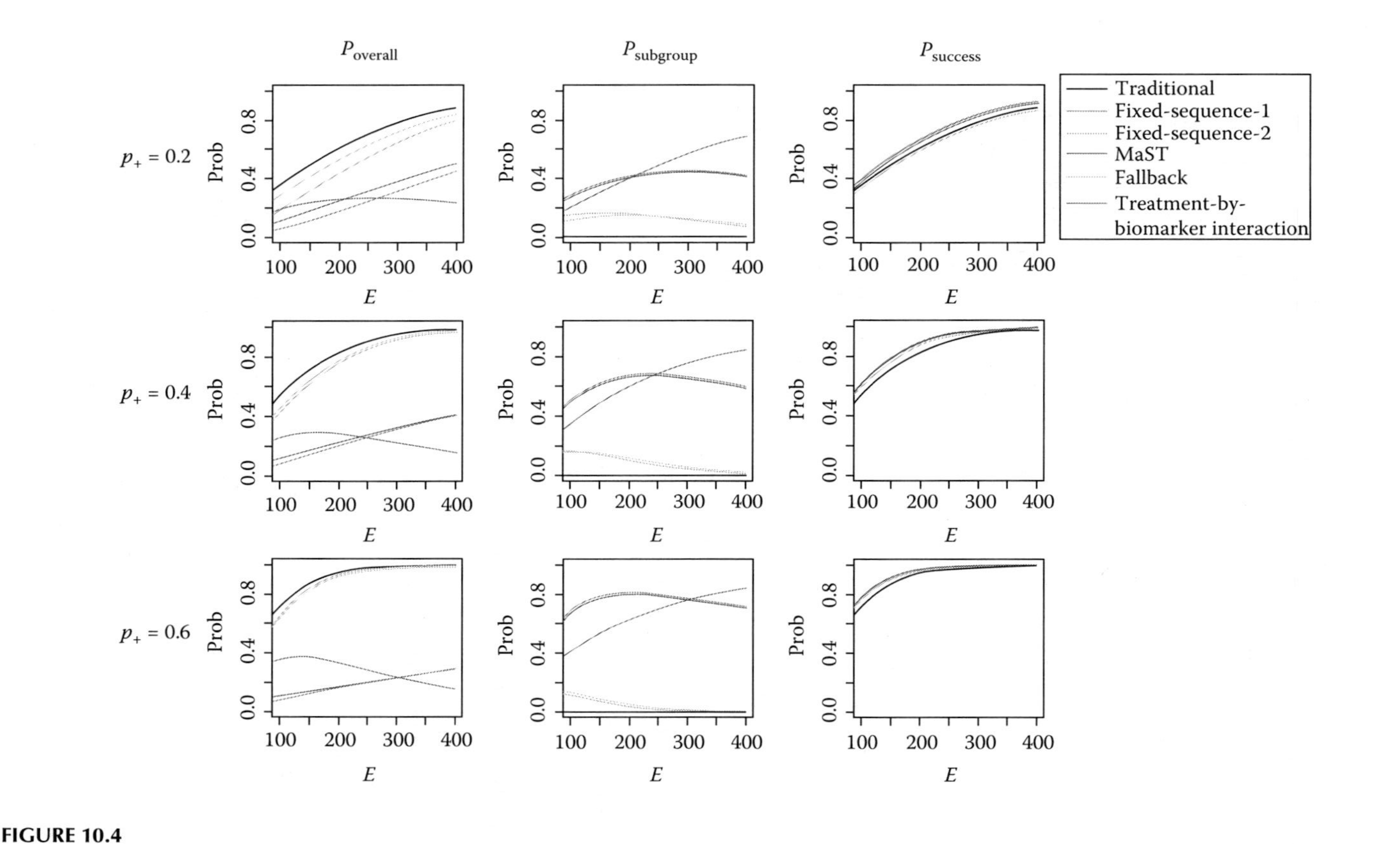

FIGURE 10.4
(See color insert.) $P_{overall}$, $P_{subgroup}$, and $P_{success}$, for various numbers of events, E, under a quantitative interaction (HR_+, HR_-) = (0.5, 0.8). The $P_{success}$ curve for the fixed-sequence-1 is always coincident with that for the fixed-sequence-2.

values of $P_{overall}$. The MaST approach also provided smaller values of $P_{overall}$, but showed some improvement over the fixed-sequence-1 approach. Similar trends were observed for $P_{success}$.

For the scenarios with a qualitative interaction, $(HR_+, HR_-) = (0.5, 1.0)$, where $P_{subgroup}$ would be relevant, the fixed-sequence-1 and MaST approaches performed best, followed by the treatment-by-biomarker interaction approach with some reduction in $P_{subgroup}$ (Figure 10.3). The fixed-sequence-2 and fallback approaches provided much smaller values of $P_{subgroup}$. Besides, as E became large, $P_{subgroup}$ of these approaches could decrease with an increment of $P_{overall}$. In contrast, the fixed-sequence-1, MaST, and treatment-by-biomarker interaction approaches suppressed the increment of $P_{overall}$, the probability of overassertion (overtreatment) in this scenario. With respect to $P_{success}$, the fallback and the treatment-by-interaction interaction approaches provided slightly reduced values of $P_{success}$, compared with the fixed-sequence-1, fixed-sequence-2, and MaST approaches. The traditional approach provided much smaller $P_{success}$ values, reflecting $P_{subgroup} = 0$.

Lastly, for the scenarios with a quantitative interaction, $(HR_+, HR_-) = (0.5, 0.8)$, the characteristics of the respective approaches became clearer (Figure 10.4). The fallback and fixed-sequence-2 approaches tended to provide larger $P_{overall}$, like the traditional approach, while the fixed-sequence-1, MaST, and treatment-by-biomarker interaction approaches tended to provide larger $P_{subgroup}$ values. For the fallback, fixed-sequence-1, fixed-sequence-2, and MaST approaches, $P_{subgroup}$ can decrease (with an increment in $P_{overall}$) as E increases. On the contrary, for the treatment-by-biomarker interaction approach, $P_{overall}$ can decrease (with an increment in $P_{subgroup}$) as E increases. With respect to $P_{success}$, all the biomarker-based approaches provided comparable $P_{success}$ values. The traditional approach provided slightly smaller values of $P_{success}$.

10.3.3 Discussion

The numerical evaluations indicated that the approaches of statistical analysis plans have their advantages and disadvantages depending on the underlying profile of treatment effects across biomarker-based subgroups (Matsui et al., 2014).

Generally, the fixed-sequence-1 approach would be suitable for cases where there are large treatment effects in the M+ patients (Figures 10.3 and 10.4), but could suffer from a serious lack of power for nearly homogeneous treatment effects with relatively moderate effect sizes in the overall population (Figure 10.2). Interestingly, the fixed-sequence-2 approach has quite different properties. This approach had similar characteristics with those of the fallback approach under qualitative and quantitative interactions (Figures 10.3 and 10.4), but suffered from a serious lack of power under constant treatment effects, like the fixed-sequence-1 approach (Figure 10.2).

As is expected, the MaST approach showed some improvement in $P_{overall}$ over the fixed-sequence-1 approach under constant treatment effects

(Figure 10.2), while providing comparable $P_{subgroup}$ values under the qualitative interaction (Figure 10.3). This approach uses a stringent significance level for the overall test to control a type I error under the hypothesis that the treatment is effective for the M+ subgroup, but not for the M− subgroup, as an extension of the fixed-sequence-1 approach (Freidlin et al., 2014). The need of a strict control of this type of error rate, in addition to the strict control of type I error rate under the global null, could be arguable, especially when there is limited confidence in the predictive biomarker to assume that the treatment will not be effective in the M− subgroup unless it is effective in the M+ subgroup. The performance under homogeneous treatment effects further improved by considering larger significance levels for the overall test (by specifying smaller significance levels in testing for the M+ subgroup than 0.022) (data not shown). This modification, which only controls the study-wise type I error rates under the global null, can be regarded as a hybrid of fix-sequence-1 and fallback approaches. This approach has the potential to be effective for both homogenous and heterogeneous treatment effects across biomarker-based subgroups.

The fallback approach would be suitable for cases with homogenous treatment effects in the overall population (Figure 10.2), but could suffer from a serious lack of power for qualitative interactions between treatment and biomarker (Figure 10.3). In other words, the chance of asserting treatment effects for the M+ patients (or the effect of introducing the fallback test) could be at most moderate. One major concern for the fallback approach (and the fixed-sequence-2 approach) is that, under qualitative interactions, the chance of asserting treatment effects for the overall population can be very large (Figure 10.3). This suggests the importance of a subgroup analysis based on the biomarker to assess the treatment effects in the M− and M+ subgroups even when the primary analysis ended with a significant result of the overall test. This is to protect against the overassertion (overtreatment). When incorporating possible assertions only for the M+ subgroup based on an additional subgroup analysis for the M− patients outside the formal analysis plan, higher $P_{subgroup}$ (and smaller $P_{overall}$) values are expected. As the fallback approach provided a high chance of asserting treatment efficacy for the overall population under quantitative interactions (Figure 10.4), it can work well when the treatment with moderate or even small effects is acceptable for the M− patients, as is the case where there are no effective treatments for such patients.

The treatment-by-biomarker interaction approach had an intermediate property between the fallback and fixed-sequence-1 approaches. This approach performed similar to the fallback approach under homogenous treatment effects (Figure 10.2) and also well with the fixed-sequence-1 approach under a qualitative interaction (Figure 10.3). In addition, it generally provided high $P_{success}$ values under all the scenarios. The good performance of this approach can be explained by the effectiveness of the preliminary interaction test in selecting the appropriate population for testing treatment effects based on the observed data. Like the fixed-sequence-1 approach (and the MaST approach), the treatment-by-biomarker interaction approach can be effective to detect large treatment effects in the M+ patients, as seen in Figures 10.3 and 10.4. This is because a larger interaction (one-sided) can be interpreted as a larger treatment effect in the M+ subgroup, and vice versa. In contrast to the fallback approach, the treatment-by-biomarker interaction approach can work well when the treatment with moderate effects is clinically unimportant for the M− patients, for example, as is the case where established standard treatments are already available for such patients. In practical application, it is important to note that the treatment-by-biomarker interaction approach can perform well even when there is limited confidence in the predictive biomarker unlike the fixed-sequence-1 approach.

Another important indication from our numerical assessment is that the traditional approach has two critical limitations when there is a moderate-to-large treatment-by-biomarker interaction, as is the case for many targeted treatments. One is a serious lack of power in terms of P_{success} because $P_{\text{subgroup}}=0$ (Figure 10.3). The other is its inability in discerning whether a significance result in the overall test is brought by large treatment effects only in the M+ patients (Figures 10.3 and 10.4) because of no incorporation of any biomarker in this approach. Hence, when a candidate biomarker is available for targeted treatments, it is generally advisable to plan for randomize-all phase III trials using biomarker-based analysis plans, such as the treatment-by-biomarker interaction, fixed-sequence-1, MaST, and fallback approaches, taking account of the aforementioned properties of the respective approaches.

10.4 Sample Size Calculation

Some methods for sample size calculation have been proposed for all-comers phase III trials with a predictive biomarker. In the fixed-sequence-1 approach, E_+ is determined to ensure the prespecified level of power, such as 90%, for the first test in the M+ patients. This coincides with the required number of events for randomized patients in the enrichment designs. In this calculation, E_- is not determined at the design stage. That is, the M− patients are enrolled concurrently until sufficient numbers of the M+ patients with E_+ are enrolled. As such, E_- can depend on the prevalence of M+, p_+, and the event rates λ_+ and λ_- in the M+ and M− control groups, respectively, at the time that there are E_+ events in the M+ subgroup. Specifically,

$$E_- = E_+\left(\frac{\lambda_-}{\lambda_+}\right)\left(\frac{1-p_+}{p_+}\right)$$

is held approximately (Simon, 2008, 2012). We expect a small (large) E_{-}, especially when p_{+} is large (small). A small E_{-} can lead to a lack of power for detecting clinically important treatment effects in the M− patients at the second stage. On the other hand, a large E_{-} can yield ethical and practical concerns about enrolling a large number of the M− patients who are unlikely to benefit from the treatment (Simon, 2008, 2012). Hence, sample size determination and/or planning of an interim futility analysis for the M− patients would be warranted.

For the fixed-sequence-2 and MaST designs, a similar approach can be applied, but the power of the test on treatment efficacy for the overall population would also be ensured. Here, in calculating the total power (i.e., $P_{success}$ in Section 10.3), we can assume independence between Z_{+} and Z_{-}, but not between Z_{+} and $Z_{overall}$ (see Sections 10.2.1 and 10.2.2).

As discussed in Section 10.5, another approach to sample size calculation in the fixed-sequence-1, and possibly MaST approaches, is that the M+ and M− subgroups are sized separately on the basis of specification of reference levels of effect size that are clinically meaningful for the biomarker-based subgroups.

For the fallback approach, sample size calculation will be based on the first test on treatment efficacy for the overall population, like in the traditional randomized trials, apart from the use of the significance level α_1 (<0.05) (Hoering et al., 2008; Simon, 2012; see also Chapter 9). Because of possible treatment effects that are clinically important in the M+ patients, it is advisable to perform sample size calculation for the second test for the M+ patients and plan for the option of delaying the second stage analysis until collection of the required number of events for the M+ patients when it is needed (Simon, 2012).

The treatment-by-biomarker interaction approach has been discussed in the literature as a design for clinical validation of the predictive biomarker itself, although it can suffer from a serious lack of power in detecting an interaction (Sargent et al., 2005; Simon, 2008; Mandrekar and Sargent, 2009). When positioning this type of analysis as one for assessing the medical utility of a new treatment with the aid of a biomarker, as is the case for the approach with a strict control of the study-wise type I error rate given in Section 10.2.3, it can become efficient as indicated by our numerical evaluations. One practical issue is that the choice of the significance levels depends on an unknown value of the event ratio R under the global null hypothesis. Optimality of chosen significance levels under nonnull treatment effects and methods for sample size calculation are a subject of future studies.

It is reasonable from the discussions in Section 10.3.1 that sample size calculations are based on the probabilities, $P_{overall}$, $P_{subgroup}$, and $P_{success}$. In Figures 10.2 through 10.4, we should note that the prevalence of M+, p_{+}, which pertains to the study patients enrolled in the trial, is not necessarily that of the general population in clinical practice. When sample size calculation is performed for testing treatment efficacy for the overall patients and the M+ subgroup (or for the M+ and M− subgroups) separately, the expected prevalence, p_+, in the trial may not be equivalent with the prevalence of the general population. As such, our results (Figures 10.2 through 10.4) can apply to a wide range of situations, possibly with modulated values of the prevalence for p_+, to evaluate which analysis plan is efficient for plausible values of the effect sizes (HR_+, HR_-) and to calculate required sample sizes for a selected analysis plan to assure desired levels for P_{overall}, P_{subgroup}, and P_{success} under some specified values of (HR_+, HR_-). An R-code is available upon request to the authors to depict figures such as Figures 10.2 through 10.4, possibly using different values of p_+, (HR_+, HR_-), and R, to help design actual clinical trials.

10.5 Clinical Validation of Predictive Biomarkers

Clinical validation of predictive biomarkers is important, particularly when asserting treatment efficacy for the M+ subgroup. Probably one of the most widely accepted ways to clinical validation is to conduct a test of interaction between treatment and biomarker. This is built into the treatment-by-biomarker interaction approach. Although a one-sided interaction test *per se* is intended to detect larger treatment effects in the M+ subgroup, not to detect a qualitative interaction of treatment and biomarker, a significant interaction may suggest a qualitative interaction (or no meaningful effects in the M− subgroup) because the power of the test under quantitative interactions is generally much lower than that under qualitative interactions.

Another criterion for clinical validation would be to demonstrate that the size of treatment effects for the M+ subgroup is greater than a clinically important effect size, ψ_1, but that for the M− subgroup is less than a minimum size of clinical importance, ψ_2, where ψ is an absolute log-hazard ratio between treatment arms and $\psi_1 \geq \psi_2$. The fixed-sequence-1, and possibly MaST, approaches can incorporate this criterion if the M+ and M− subgroups are sized separately on the basis of these thresholds as reference levels of effect size. In this case, again, a plan for interim futility analysis would be warranted for the M− subgroup because enrolling a large number of these patients who are unlikely to benefit from the treatment can yield ethical concerns (Simon, 2012).

Another possible criterion for clinical validation is to demonstrate treatment efficacy with the aid of the biomarker when a test for treatment efficacy in the overall population without use of the biomarker is not significant. The fallback approach seems to employ this criterion. However, this is a rather indirect or informal criterion compared with the aforementioned criteria, so one may argue the need for additional clinical validation based on the other criteria described earlier, outside the formal fallback analysis plan.

Interval estimation of the treatment difference (e.g., in terms of hazards ratio) within biomarker subgroup is generally useful for assessing the profile of treatment efficacy across subgroups under possible limitation in sample sizes of subgroups. This can help determine the recommended treatment for each subgroup if the confidence intervals are sufficiently narrow (Polley et al., 2013).

10.6 Concluding Remarks

In this chapter, we have discussed various statistical analysis plans and related design issues in all-comers phase III trials with a predictive biomarker. Our numerical evaluations in terms of the probability of asserting treatment efficacy for the right patient population would provide a benchmark for designing actual clinical trials. As one general recommendation, if there was some evidence that the treatment would work better in the M+ subgroup than the M− subgroup, then the fixed-sequence approaches would be favored, whereas if evidence was weak that there would be much difference in responsiveness between the two subgroups, then the fallback approach would be favored. If there was substantial uncertainty in the difference in treatment effects between the subgroups, the treatment-by-biomarker interaction approach (and possibly a modified MaST approach as a hybrid of fixed-sequence-1 and fallback approaches; see Section 10.3.3) could be a reasonable choice.

Interim monitoring is an important aspect in designing clinical trials. In biomarker-based all-comers designs, early stopping rules for superiority and inefficacy of the treatment can be considered for the overall population and biomarker-based subgroups (e.g., Freidlin et al., 2010). One difficulty is how to incorporate these rules in a biomarker-based analysis plan without compromising its integrity. For example, compared to a trial with only a single analysis (e.g., fallback analysis) without interim monitoring, an early stopping for one subgroup (e.g., the M+ subgroup in superiority) can need a modification of the procedure of subsequent analysis (e.g., at least, the decision on treatment efficacy has already been done for the M+ subgroup) and also change the outcome data used in it (e.g., accumulated data from the M+ patients until the interim monitoring combined with those from the rest M− patients collected until the end of the trial in testing treatment efficacy for the overall population). Any possible changes in evaluation and follow-up of patients in the other subgroups by knowing the early stopping for a particular subgroup can bias the evaluation of treatment effects after the early stopping. Even if such changes can be minimized, a pooling of the subgroup data that have already provided evidence for early stopping for this subgroup with the other subgroup data may cause a biased estimation for the pooled data. Some practical considerations are provided by Redman et al. (2012). Full-fledged statistical researches are needed for this area.

Unbiased estimation of treatment effects is particularly crucial in definitive phase III trials. Owing to the sequential nature of the biomarker-based analysis plans, however, estimation bias can arise at the second stage of the analysis (even in trials without interim monitoring) because of possible correlations between the tests, for example, $Z_{overall}$ and Z_+ in the fallback and MaST approaches and Z_{int} and Z_+ in the treatment-by-biomarker interaction approach. Recently, Choai and Matsui (2014) proposed a bias-corrected estimation in the fallback approach. Further researches on bias corrections are warranted in the fallback and other approaches.

In conclusion, many important statistical issues still remain in the field of biomarker-based clinical trials for personalized medicine. We hope this chapter helps guiding the design and analysis of actual clinical trials and also stimulates further methodological researches in this active field.

References

Buyse M, Michiels S, Sargent DJ et al. Integrating biomarkers in clinical trials. *Expert Rev Mol Diagn*. 2011; 11: 171–182.

Cappuzzo F, Ciuleanu T, Stelmakh L et al. Erlotinib as maintenance treatment in advanced non-small-cell lung cancer: A multicentre, randomised, placebo-controlled phase 3 study. *Lancet Oncol*. 2010; 11: 521–529.

Choai Y, Matsui S. Estimation of treatment effects in all-comers randomized clinical trials with a predictive marker. *Biometrics*. 2014; (In press).

Douillard JY, Siena S, Cassidy J et al. Randomized, phase III trial of panitumumab with infusional fluorouracil, leucovorin, and oxaliplatin (FOLFOX4) versus FOLFOX4 alone as first-line treatment in patients with previously untreated metastatic colorectal cancer: The PRIME study. *J Clin Oncol*. 2010; 28: 4697–4705.

Freidlin B, Korn EL. Biomarker enrichment strategies: Matching trial design to biomarker credentials. *Nat Rev Clin Oncol*. 2014; 11: 81–90.

Freidlin B, Korn EL, Gray R. Marker sequential test (MaST) design. *Clin Trials*. 2014; 11: 19–27.

Freidlin B, McShane LM, Korn EL. Randomized clinical trials with biomarkers: Design issues. *J Natl Cancer Inst*. 2010; 102: 152–160.

Freidlin B, Sun Z, Gray R, Korn EL. Phase III clinical trials that integrate treatment and biomarker evaluation. *J Clin Oncol*. 2013; 31: 3158–3161.

Hoering A, LeBlanc M, Crowley JJ. Randomized phase III clinical trial designs for targeted agents. *Clin Cancer Res*. 2008; 14: 4358–4367.

Mandrekar SJ, Sargent DJ. Clinical trial designs for predictive biomarker validation: Theoretical considerations and practical challenges. *J Clin Oncol*. 2009; 27: 4027–4034.

Matsui S, Choai Y, Nonaka T. Comparison of statistical analysis plans in randomize-all phase III trials with a predictive biomarker. *Clin Cancer Res*. 2014; 20: 2820–2830.

Polley MY, Freidlin B, Korn EL, Conley BA, Abrams JS, McShane LM. Statistical and practical considerations for clinical evaluation of predictive biomarkers. *J Natl Cancer Inst*. 2013; 105: 1677–1683.

Pusztai L, Hess KR. Clinical trial design for microarray predictive marker discovery and assessment. *Ann Oncol*. 2004; 15: 1731–1737.

Redman MW, Crowley JJ, Herbst RS, Hirsch FR, Gandara DR. Design of a phase III clinical trial with prospective biomarker validation: SWOG S0819. *Clin Cancer Res*. 2012; 18: 4004–4012.

Sargent DJ, Conley BA, Allegra C, Collette L. Clinical trial designs for predictive marker validation in cancer treatment trials. *J Clin Oncol*. 2005; 23: 2020–2027.

Simon R. The use of genomics in clinical trial design. *Clin Cancer Res*. 2008; 14: 5984–5993.

Simon R. Clinical trials for predictive medicine. *Stat Med*. 2012; 31: 3031–3040.

Simon R, Maitournam A. Evaluating the efficiency of targeted designs for randomized clinical trials. *Clin Cancer Res*. 2005; 10: 6759–6763.

Simon R, Wang SJ. Use of genomic signatures in therapeutics development in oncology and other diseases. *Pharmacogenomics J*. 2006; 6:166–173.

Song Y, Chi GY. A method for testing a prespecified subgroup in clinical trials. *Stat Med*. 2007; 26: 3535–3549.

Spiessens B, Debois M. Adjusted significance levels for subgroup analyses in clinical trials. *Contemp Clin Trials*. 2010; 31: 647–656.

Tsiatis AA. The asymptotic joint distribution of the efficient score test for the proportional hazards model calculated over time. *Biometrika*. 1981; 68: 311–315.

Wakelee H, Kernstine K, Vokes E et al. Cooperative group research efforts in lung cancer 2008: Focus on advanced-stage non-small-cell lung cancer. *Clin Lung Cancer*. 2008; 9: 346–351.

Wang SJ, O'Neill RT, Hung HM. Approaches to evaluation of treatment effect in randomized clinical trials with genomic subset. *Pharm Stat*. 2007; 6: 227–244.

11

Evaluation of Clinical Utility and Validation of Gene Signatures in Clinical Trials

Stefan Michiels and Federico Rotolo

CONTENTS

11.1 Introduction

With the advent of the targeted therapy era, molecular signatures are becoming increasingly important for anticipating the prognosis of individual patients (*prognostic* biomarkers) or for predicting how individual patients will respond to specific treatments (*predictive* biomarkers, more generally called *effect modifiers*).

Once a gene signature has been identified, its analytical validity performs satisfactory and its clinical validity has been shown to be robust in several independent patient cohorts, one can consider to design a clinical trial to establish the clinical utility. Clinical utility can be defined according to Evaluation of Genomic Applications in Practice and Prevention initiative as "evidence of improved measurable clinical outcomes, and its usefulness and added value to patient management decision-making compared with current management without genetic testing" (Teutsch et al. 2009). In practice, the gene signatures have to be incorporated in a clinical trial in order to evaluate their utility as prognostic factors or their predictive value as *treatment modifiers*, which is their ability to discriminate patients who will benefit from the treatment from others.

In Section 11.2, we will discuss trial designs integrating prognostic gene signatures such as the Mindact trial, which compares the MammaPrint™ gene signature to traditional clinical–pathological methods for assessing the risk of breast cancer recurrence. The operating characteristics of this design will be contrasted to a trial aiming at showing clinical utility for Oncotype Dx™.

Many of the current *targeted* drugs under development in oncology have a well-defined mechanism of action at the molecular level, allowing clinical researchers to measure the effect of these drugs on the gene expression level, as well as select patients likely to respond to these drugs based on gene expression. Neoadjuvant clinical trials, in which a treatment is administered before surgery, have become very attractive in the clinical development of targeted agents in oncology because biomarkers can be measured repeatedly in biopsies and the availability of a short-term endpoint at surgery, defined as pathological complete response rate (Fumagalli et al. 2012). The Food and Drug Administration has even outlined an accelerated approval strategy for new drugs in a guidance document (FDA 2014). Using data from multiple neoadjuvant clinical trials in breast cancer, we investigate the association between chemotherapy response and gene expression modules describing important biological processes and pathways, beyond established clinicopathological factors (Section 11.3).

In standard randomized clinical phase III trials of an experimental treatment versus standard treatment, it has become common to test multiple candidate predictive biomarkers on tumor samples for a possible interaction with treatment effect. A global permutation approach has been proposed to control the type I error when there is correlation among the biomarkers (Michiels et al. 2011b) without too much loss of power when there are 10 candidate biomarkers as compared to testing only a single biomarker. We illustrate in Section 11.4 how this global permutation test can be used as a green light before identifying a treatment-effect-modifying gene signature in a randomized clinical trial. However, the arrival of next-generation sequencing has led to the use of mutation panels of at least 100 cancer genes or more in retrospective analyses of clinical trials. Therefore, in Section 11.5, we extend the previously proposed permutation approach to a higher-dimensional setting of 100 candidate biomarkers and explore the added value of a ridge regression and a variable selection using Akaike's information criterion (AIC).

11.2 Evaluation of Prognostic Gene Signatures for Treatment Decisions in Randomized Trials

Results from randomized clinical trials are often difficult to translate into predictions for individual patients, but estimated absolute risk reductions from large trial results do still provide the best guidance (Rothwell 2005).

The absolute gain from the experimental arm as compared with the control arm depends on the event risk in the control arm and the relative risk reduction obtained by the treatment comparison. For example, if we assume a 33% relative risk reduction using a second-generation chemotherapy regimen in an estrogen receptor (ER)-positive breast cancer population that does not vary according to patients' characteristics or time (Early Breast Cancer Trialists' Collaborative et al. 2012), we can translate predictions of 10-year prognosis with the control arm treatment into predictions of average 10-year prognosis that would be obtained by the treatment arm (Stewart and Parmar 1993). For 10-year breast cancer–specific survival predictions of a patient treated with endocrine therapy alone (control) of 97%, 95%, 92%, and 88%, the absolute benefit when adding chemotherapy is estimated by 1%, 2%, 3%, 4%, and 5%. It is thus of importance to reliably predict the prognosis of patients to assist treatment counseling (Windeler 2000). In early breast cancer, while several clinical prediction models exist based on clinical and pathological characteristics—such as age, tumor size, nodal status, tumor grade, ER—there have been several attempts to develop prognostic gene signatures to improve prognostic information beyond that provided by the classic clinicopathological variables. At least six different genomic tests have been developed for this purpose in early breast cancer (Oncotype Dx, MammaPrint, Genomic Grade Index, PAM50, Breast Cancer Index, and EndoPredict) and several of these can currently be ordered by medical oncologists although they currently may have not yet reached the highest level of evidence (Azim et al. 2013). This can lead to an awkward situation where the treatment decision does not depend anymore on the clinician but on the genomic test ordered. Once a gene signature has shown sufficient analytical and clinical validity through consecutive validation studies, clinical trials can be set up to show possible clinical utility. Trial designs that aim at showing that, when patients are offered a prognostic gene signature, this will have a clinical impact are actually quite similar to available trial designs for diagnostic procedures (Bossuyt et al. 2000; deGraaff et al. 2004; Lu and Gatsonis 2013; Rodger et al. 2012).

The 70-gene MammaPrint signature is a microarray signature developed by the Netherlands Cancer Institute to predict among patients early diagnosed for breast cancer those who will present distant metastases within 5 years. Considering that patients with concordant low risk of relapse based on both a clinical prediction model and the gene signature could receive standard therapy (i.e., hormone therapy for ER-positive breast cancer) and that patients with concordant high risk of relapse could receive an aggressive treatment, it could be most efficient to conduct a randomized controlled trial in the discordant risk population. This type of discordant risk randomized trial design was implemented for the MammaPrint gene signature. The MINDACT (Microarray In Node negative Disease may Avoid ChemoTherapy) trial is a clinical trial from the European Organisation for Research and Treatment of Cancer, in which the primary objective was to evaluate the ability of MammaPrint signature to identify patients in whom

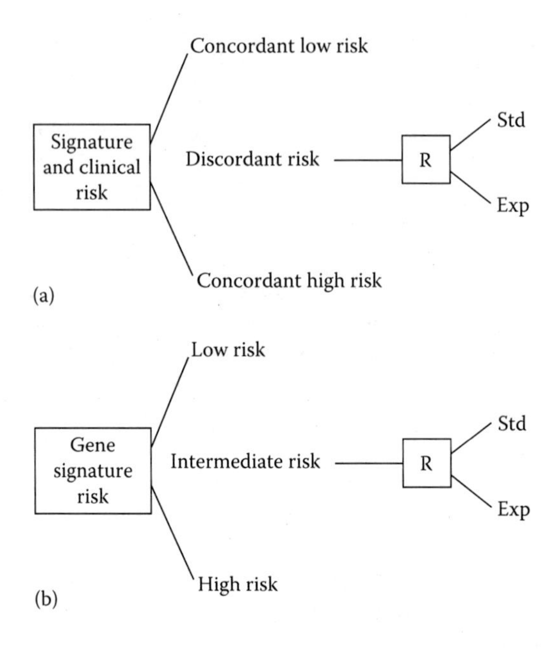

FIGURE 11.1
(a) Discordant risk design. (b) Intermediate signature risk randomized design. R, randomization; Std, standard; Exp, experimental.

chemotherapy can be avoided whatever their clinicopathological characteristics. To address this issue, the treatment (chemotherapy versus no chemotherapy) was randomized only in patients whose predicted categories of risk of relapse (high or low) were discordant according to the clinical prediction model and the signature (Figure 11.1a). Actually, randomizing the chemotherapy arm in patients with discordant clinical features and signature is strictly equivalent with randomizing the clinical strategy versus the gene signature strategy (Buyse and Michiels 2013). The trial's sample size was calculated for a primary test in the subset of patients who have a low gene signature risk and a high clinical prediction risk and did not receive chemotherapy by the randomization (Bogaerts et al. 2006). Among 1920 randomized patients out of 6600 recruited patients, the expected number of patients in this subgroup is only 672, corresponding to 80% power at a 2.5% significance level to reject the null hypothesis of 5-year distant metastasis-free survival of a 92% when the true distant metastasis-free survival is 95%. This primary test statistic is thus in a strict sense not taking the randomization into account. However, Hooper and colleagues recently showed that, if two tests disagree 32% of the time (gene signature and clinical prediction), and the experimental treatment reduces 10-year mortality in the overall population from 24% to 20%, then the absolute difference between the gene signature and the clinical prediction strategy is overall only 0.5% and a randomized trial of a size of

50,000 patients would be necessary to identify this mortality difference in a statistically satisfactory manner (Hooper et al. 2013).

The 21-gene Oncotype Dx signature is a continuous score combining expression of ER and human epidermal growth factor receptor 2, ER-regulated transcripts and proliferation-related genes to discriminate, among patients with ER-positive, node-negative cancers treated with endocrine therapy alone, those with low, intermediate, or high risk of recurrence at 10 years (Paik et al. 2004). In the TAILORx (Trial Assigning IndividuaLized Options for treatment [Rx]) trial, run under the auspices of the US NCI program for the assessment of clinical cancer tests, 10,000 women diagnosed with node negative breast cancer were recruited. Patients with low-risk Oncotype Dx signature score did not receive chemotherapy whereas patients with high risk did. In the subset of women with intermediate Oncotype Dx signature risk score, the chemotherapy arm was randomized. The primary objective of TAILORx trial was to evaluate in the intermediate signature risk group the noninferiority of the no chemotherapy arm as compared with the chemotherapy arm (Figure 11.1b). Noninferiority was defined using an unacceptable decrease in 5-year disease-free survival in the intermediate risk category from 90% (with chemotherapy) to 87% or less (no chemotherapy) at a one-sided type one error of 10% and 95% power, leading to a sample size of 4500 randomized patients. It can be argued that the relative effect of chemotherapy is rather well known in early breast cancer, and that for validating the prognostic effect of the gene signature in question a new prospective clinical trial is not always needed when retrospective cohort or cross-sectional studies have provided satisfactory level of evidence of a test. In both these trials, since the rate of distant relapse is quite low in early breast cancers, a very long follow-up is required to answer the clinical questions (Buyse and Michiels 2013).

These two examples illustrate that, in the context of a relative good prognosis population and a small absolute treatment benefit, developing a randomized controlled trial to demonstrate the clinical utility of a prognostic gene signature is challenging. In the next section, we will study whether the prognostic gene signature is susceptible to add a lot of supplementary information to the risk determined by a clinical prediction model.

11.3 Gene Signatures as Prognostic Biomarkers in Neoadjuvant Trials

The neoadjuvant setting provides a rather unique opportunity to study the effect of systemic treatments on breast cancer biology, thanks to repeated biopsies and to identify prognostic and predictive biomarkers (Fumagalli et al. 2012). Patients whose tumors show pathological complete response (pCR, binary endpoint) at surgery after neoadjuvant chemotherapy have better long-term survival outcome than patients whose tumors do not (Rastogi et al. 2008; vonMinckwitz et al. 2012). It is therefore of interest to identify biological factors associated with the presence or absence of pCR following preoperative chemotherapy. Clinicopathological characteristics such as clinical stage at diagnosis, ER status, histological grade, and age are known to be associated with pCR after anthracycline ± taxane-based neoadjuvant chemotherapy. Our aim was to quantify the net gain in predictive accuracy from gene signatures when added to these clinicopathological characteristics (Dunkler et al. 2007). We used the publicly available microarray data of 859 patients (189 pCRs) from 8 clinical studies with complete clinicopathological information and normalized the Affymetrix U133 microarrays as outlined in Ignatiadis et al. (2012). We computed 17 gene modules that approximate previously published gene signatures in early breast cancer and correspond to oncogenic pathways, the microenvironment, chromosomal instability, and tumor proliferation, including an approximate MammaPrint signature that we will denote as Gene70. Because the gene signatures are often derived on other microarray platforms from different laboratories and heterogeneous retrospective patient cohorts, we computed the gene module as a weighted average (Wirapati et al. 2008):

$$\text{Module score(s)} = \frac{\sum_{i=1}^{k} w_i x_i}{\sum_{i=1}^{k} |w_i|}$$

where k is the number of genes in module s, x_i is the expression of the gene in the module, and gene-specific weights w_i are equal to +1 or −1 depending on the direction of their association with the phenotype in the original publication. Only genes that can be mapped to Entrez Gene identifications (Maglott et al. 2007) are included and if multiple probes correspond to a single gene, the one with the maximum variance is picked. Additionally, in order to reduce the batch effects across the eight different studies, each module score was scaled within a study so that the 2.5% and 97.5% quantiles equaled −1 and +1, respectively. Based on the scaling of the 2.5% and 97.5% quantiles into the [−1, 1] range and our previous experience in microarray datasets in breast cancer (data not shown), we assumed that the 17 scaled gene modules would follow a normal distribution centered around 0 with standard deviation $\sigma = 0.50$. Thus, a one-unit increase in scaled module scores would correspond to a 2σ change. For the overall patient series, we assumed the pCR among patients with an average gene module value to be 24% (the overall pCR rate). With the sample size at hand, we calculated the statistical power to identify an association between a gene module and pCR beyond the clinicopathological characteristics in a logistic regression model as a function of the proportion of the variance of pCR explained by the remaining covariates (Hsieh et al. 1998). We assumed the clinicopathological model and dataset effect would explain 18% of the variation in pCR. For detecting an odds ratio of 2 in pCR for a one-unit change in a single gene module at significance level 0.05, the power would be approximately 97%.

We calculated odds ratios for pCR for a unit increase in a scaled module score after adjustment for study but also for treatment (anthracyclines versus anthracyclines + taxanes), age (≤50 versus >50), clinical tumor size (cT0, 1, 2 versus cT3, 4), clinical nodal status (negative versus positive), histological grade (1, 2 versus 3), ER status (negative versus positive), and HER2 status (negative versus positive): they are visualized in Figure 11.2. No strong departures from linearity were found using restricted cubic splines with three knots. To adjust for multiple module testing, the false discovery rate (FDR) was calculated (Benjamini and Hochberg 1995). A one-unit change in the Gene70 module corresponded to an adjusted odds ratio of 2.02 (95% CI 1.29–3.2) for patients who experience a pCR versus those who do not. Of note, at an FDR cut-off of 5%, high-expression modules of the two immune gene modules (Immune1, Immune2), of the proliferation modules (GGI, Gene70, PTEN), and of an E2F3 module were significantly associated with increased pCR probability in their respective multivariate models.

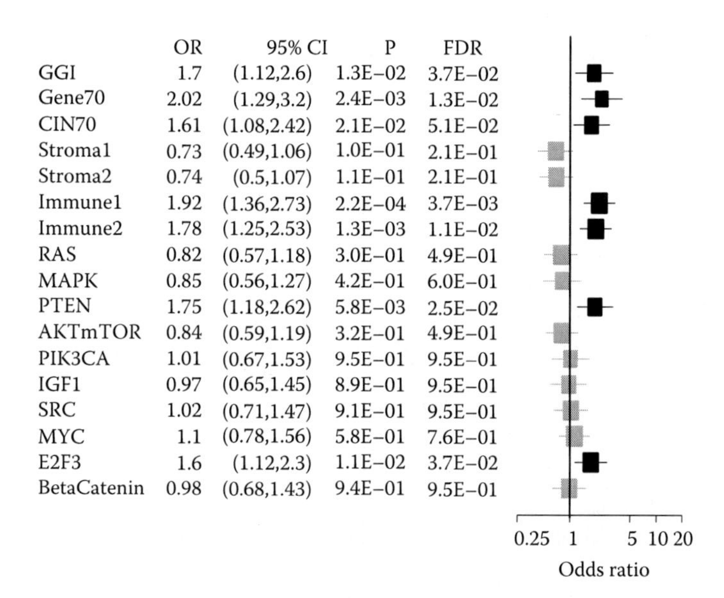

FIGURE 11.2
Forest plot of adjusted odds ratios of the selected 17 modules and pathological complete response rate. Each line corresponds to an odds ratio (OR) for pathological complete response for a unit increase in module score after adjustment for clinicopathological factors and study in a logistic regression model. The size of the square is inversely proportional to the standard error; horizontal bars represent the 95% confidence intervals of ORs. Modules with nominal significant effect ($p < 0.05$) are shown in black. FDR, false discovery rate.

We also estimated the ability to classify patients as having a pCR or no pCR through the area under the receiver operating characteristic curve (AUC) for the clinicopathological model with and without a module score. The AUC is a measure of discrimination ranging from 0.5 (no discriminative ability) to 1 (perfect discrimination). While the AUC of the clinicopathological model was given by 0.696, the highest increase when adding a gene module was obtained by adding Gene70, with an AUC equal to 0.708. A gene signature would be of interest if it provides additional and strong prognostic value, over and above that of all easily measured clinical and pathological characteristics of the patients. However, in many applications in oncology such as the neoadjuvant example in breast cancer presented here, the added prognostic value is moderate. However, a gene signature could also be of interest if it provides a more reproducible, cheaper, and more accurate measurement of an already existing tumor measurement that has proven clinical utility so that the clinical prediction rule could be updated (Michiels et al. 2011a).

Of note, none of the published gene signatures we reanalyzed in this section were actually developed for predicting the magnitude of a treatment effect, that is, they were fitted in the development patient series using only main effects. We will therefore focus in the next section on gene signatures that are quantitatively associated with a treatment benefit in randomized clinical trials through interaction tests.

11.4 Development of Gene Signatures as Treatment Modifiers in a Randomized Clinical Trial

In the context of an all-comers or randomize-all clinical trial, it is often the case that many candidate biomarkers (k) are tested as a possible treatment-effect modifier. It has been put forward that the only reliable statistical approach is to test for interaction between a subgroup and the treatment effect (Rothwell 2005), acknowledging the need for prespecification of subgroups. We assume a time-to-event outcome and that the test for interaction is for a multiplicative effect on a relative scale. It is not very uncommon that multiple candidate biomarkers are tested on tumor samples collected from phase III clinical trials to identify predictive biomarkers. Previously, we proposed a global permutation approach for controlling the family-wise type I error, accounting for dependence structures (Michiels et al. 2011b). Five different permutation procedures using single-biomarker statistics and composite statistic based on treatment-by-biomarker interactions in a Weibull accelerated failure time (AFT) model were proposed. Three tests are considered here. Two of these tests calculate for each permutation a Wald statistic for interaction in a biomarker-specific AFT model (containing a treatment effect, a main biomarker effect, and an interaction effect) and take either the maximum or the sum of all Wald statistics (max single Wald [MSW] or sum single Wald [SSW]). The idea behind the third test is to define a scaled linear combination of all k biomarkers, called composite biomarker score that combines the individual interaction signals. It is based on the parameters of the interaction effects of a full AFT model with $2k+1$ variables (a treatment effect, k main effects, and k interaction effects). An absolute difference in two concordance probabilities—called the composite difference (CD)—was proposed as statistic to permute (the concordance probability that a randomly chosen control patient will outlive a treated patient for a biomarker score positive patient minus the same concordance probability for a biomarker score negative patient) (Michiels et al. 2011b). For the permutation test to be valid, the data do not need to follow a Weibull or any distribution. The permutation rearranges the patients only within a treatment group.

A simulation study was performed illustrating type I error control under null scenarios and power under alternative scenarios when there are one or more true treatment-effect modifiers and different correlation patterns among 10 binary biomarkers. Under the simulated null scenarios, all five tests provided an appropriate control of the global type I error, but we observed slight conservatism for the CD when there was just one prognostic biomarker. Under the alternative scenarios, we found the MSW followed by the SSW to be optimal when there is one truly treatment-modifying biomarker, and the SSW or CD statistic to be optimal when there are two or three independent treatment-modifying biomarkers (Michiels et al. 2011b).

Based on the global permutation test, an analysis strategy for developing a signature from many candidate treatment-effect-modifying biomarkers in a phase III trial can be devised. In step 1, a global test for interaction (MSW, SSW, CD) is performed to control the type I error at a prespecified α level such as 5%. Only when the global interaction test is significant, a gene signature can be developed in step 2. For this purpose, the AFT Weibull model will be applied (or another AFT distributional model if this fits the data better). A resampling procedure such as cross-validation can be used to estimate treatment effects in biomarker-defined patient subsets (Matsui et al. 2012). The application of the AFT model to the full randomized clinical trial development data leads to an *indication* classifier to use for future patients (Simon 2012).

We applied this analysis strategy on tissue microarray data of two French breast cancer randomized trials of adjuvant anthracycline-based chemotherapy with long-term follow-up (Conforti et al. 2007). A total of 320 disease-free survival events occurred among the 798 patients with clinicopathological characteristics and the 11 candidate biomarkers (10 binary and 1 continuous biomarker). Kaplan–Meier estimated survival curves are provided in Figure 11.3a. The overall treatment effect of adjuvant chemotherapy versus no chemotherapy on disease-free survival was estimated by a hazard ratio of HR = 0.78 (95% CI [0.62–0.97]). If we had studied a single binary biomarker with 0.5 prevalence for which the number of events in the

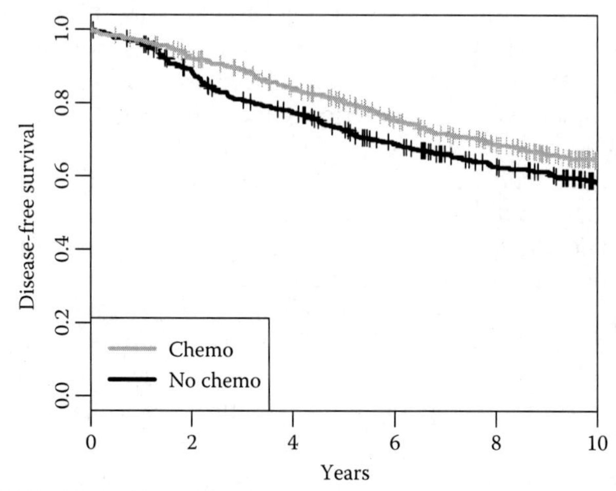

No. at risk						
No chemo	389	335	286	237	195	148
Chemo	409	368	321	266	223	161

(a)

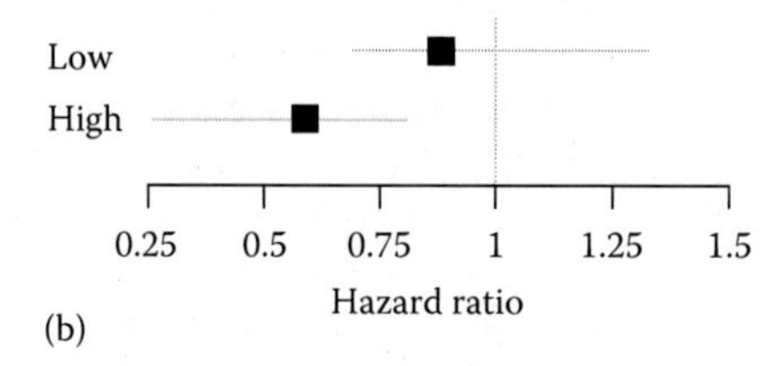

(b)

FIGURE 11.3
(a) Disease-free survival according to treatment in the two randomized trials of adjuvant chemotherapy (chemo) in breast cancer. (b) Cross-validated treatment effects according to the composite biomarker score, with a cut-off at 0.5 to define *high* and *low* composite biomarker scores. Confidence intervals are obtained by bootstrapping (2000 resamples, use of bootstrap percentiles).

four treatment-by-biomarker groups did not vary by more than a factor of 2 and had assumed exponential survival, then the observed number of 320 events would have provided approximately 86% power to detect a treatment-by-biomarker interaction when the ratio of the HR for the effect of chemotherapy on disease-free survival in the biomarker-positive group to the HR in the biomarker-negative group is equal to 2 (or 0.5) at a 5% significance level (Peterson and George 1993). In step 1, we applied the global interaction tests and obtained permutation p-values from the SSW, MSW, and CD test of $p=0.039$, $p=0.007$, and $p=0.010$, respectively, leading to a rejection of the global null hypothesis at a 5% significance level. In step 2, we used the AFT model and a 10-fold cross-validation scheme to estimate the treatment effects according to the composite biomarker score (cut-off at 0.5) so that the patients on which the treatment effects are estimated are not used to train the AFT model. As highlighted in Figure 11.3b, patients with high composite biomarker score benefited most from adjuvant chemotherapy (HR = 0.59, 95% CI [0.26–0.80]) as compared to patients with low composite biomarker scores (HR = 0.88, 95% CI [0.69–1.31]).

11.5 Extension of the Global Interaction Tests to a Higher-Dimensional Setting

In this section, we explore whether the overall type I error of the interaction tests can still be appropriately controlled when there is a higher number of candidate biomarkers that are tested on samples of a randomized clinical trial. In particular, we increase here the number of binary biomarkers k from 10 to 100 and investigate the performances of the global interaction tests SSW, MSW, and CD. Since the number of biomarkers and interaction effects to test becomes dangerously close to the number of events typically observed in a phase III trial in oncology, a reduction of the dimensionality of the problem might improve the performances of global tests. We considered two possible solutions: penalization and variable selection.

A huge literature exists on penalized regression for time-to-event data. Moving from regression models with L_2 (Verweij and VanHouwelingen 1994) to L_1 (Tibshirani 1997) penalties, also known as ridge and least absolute shrinkage and selection operator (LASSO) respectively, many extensions have been proposed (Zou and Hastie 2005; Zou 2006; Zhang and Lu 2007). Since our primary interest was control of global type I error and not the variable selection per se, we explored the added value of ridge regression when fitting an AFT model with $2k+1$ variables before calculating the CD test (denoted as L_2+CD). In this ridge Weibull AFT model, the L_2 penalties were chosen by minimizing AIC over a grid of values.

Another manner of simplifying the problem is to compute the global tests after a preselection of the most relevant biomarkers. Here, we consider a stepwise model selection based on the minimum AIC, starting from the Weibull AFT model containing only the main treatment effect. In the selection procedure we used, the main effects of the biomarkers and their interactions with the treatment could be iteratively added or dropped, under three constraints: the main effect for the treatment could not be removed; the main effect of a biomarker could be removed provided that its interaction with the treatment was not in; and the interaction between a biomarker and the treatment could be added provided that its main effect was in. Once the final model was chosen via this AIC stepwise procedure, we calculated the global tests using the parameter estimates of the retained interaction effects and their estimated variances (AIC+SSW, AIC+MSW, and AIC+CD).

We performed a simulation study to investigate, in the presence of 100 candidate biomarkers, the performance of the aforementioned global interaction tests and without and with penalization or preselection. As in Michiels et al. (2011b), we considered a metastatic setting with median survival of about 1 year. We first present the case of $n = 300$ patients, 150 per treatment arm, then we double the sample size to $n = 600$ patients, 300 per arm. We generated survival times via exponential random variables. Assuming 3-year uniform accrual and 2-year follow-up, uniform censoring times from 2 to 5 years were generated independently of event times.

A hundred binary biomarkers with prevalence of 1/2 were generated by truncation of normal multivariate random variables. Biomarkers were independent of each other in all but one scenario, in which correlation of the underlying normal random variables was specified for 10-biomarker blocks. Table 11.1 describes the five scenarios in which the tests have been compared. The first is the complete null scenario, with median survival time of 1 year, irrespective of the treatment arm and the biomarkers. In the second null scenario, there was a strong prognostic biomarker doubling the median survival times and also a relatively strong treatment effect with a 50% increase in median survival time, none of the biomarkers are interacting with treatment effect. In alternative scenario 3, there is no treatment effect for biomarker-negative patients, whereas the median survival time of treated biomarker-positive patients is doubled. The fourth scenario is similar to the previous one, except that the number of active biomarkers is five instead of only one, the improvement of each being smaller (50% increase of median survival time in the treated biomarker-positive patients). The last scenario is a variant

TABLE 11.1

Description of the Five Treatment by True Biomarker Scenarios Used in Simulation Study

	Median Survival Time (Years)				Average Censoring Probability			
	Control		Treatment		Control		Treatment	
Scenario	**B−**	**B+**	**B−**	**B+**	**$\rho = 1$**	**$\rho = 1.25$**	**$\rho = 1$**	**$\rho = 1.25$**
1. Complete null	1.0	1.0	1.0	1.0	0.10	0.06	0.11	0.06
2. One prognostic marker, strong effect size	0.6	1.2	0.9	1.8	0.09	0.05	0.18	0.13
3. One treatment modifier, strong effect size	0.8	0.8	0.8	1.6	0.06	0.03	0.15	0.10
4. Five treatment modifiers, medium effect size	0.8	0.8	0.8	1.2	0.06	0.03	0.35	0.32
5. Five treatment modifiers, medium effect size, correlation = 0.5 by 10	0.8	0.8	0.8	1.2	0.06	0.03	0.35	0.32

Note: B−, biomarker-negative; B+, biomarker-positive.

of the fourth one, with the addition of correlation within random blocks of 10 biomarkers: correlation 0.5 was used for the underlying normal random variables. The censoring proportions, provided in the last four columns of Table 11.1 according to treatment arm, ranged between 3% and 35%.

The global tests were evaluated in terms of the rejection probabilities and p-values. For each scenario, 250 trials were simulated. For each of them, the p-values of the global tests were computed by permuting independently 500 times the biomarker vectors of patients within each treatment arm, without moving any of them from an arm to the other. P-values are estimated by the proportion of the 500 permutations for which the test statistic is greater than for the data prior to permutation. Our approach is particularly sensitive to the presence of interaction effects, even though in fact it tests the broader hypothesis of neither main nor interaction effects. Permutation tests, indeed, are not able to test for interaction only (Potthoff et al. 2001). We provide the power estimates at a significance level $\alpha = 0.05$, that is, the proportion of the 250 datasets for which the null hypothesis is rejected at level α. Of note, if the rejection probability of a test is actually 0.05, then the exact 95% confidence interval for its empirical rejection probability over 250 repetitions is (0.024, 0.080). However, as the tests are computed via permutations, these power estimates can be biased (Potthoff et al. 2001). Therefore, unbiased estimates of the mean p-values are computed as the average across the 250 replications of the p-values. Table 11.2 shows the results of the simulation study for exponentially distributed survival times. The empirical rejection probabilities, estimates of the power at a significance level $\alpha = 0.05$, are provided in Table 11.2a, whereas the mean p-values are given in Table 11.2b.

Under the complete null scenario 1, the empirical power is always within the exact 95% confidence interval computed for an actual rejection probability of 0.05. In the presence of one prognostic biomarker (null scenario 2), some of the tests are more conservative notably with $n = 600$. In particular, the CD test has low rejection probabilities and neither penalization nor preselection (L_2+CD or AIC+CD) can alleviate this issue appreciably. The SSW test also has empirical power that is significantly different from 0.05 with $n = 600$, but its mean p-value is reassuring.

In the three alternative scenarios, the power of the global tests is generally quite low with $n = 300$ (3%–40%), whereas it is substantially higher if $n = 600$ (14%–80%). The MSW and the AIC+MSW tests perform the best in the presence of only one strongly predictive biomarker, but also the AIC+CD test has competitive power. The SSW and MSW tests are the best in the case of five predictive biomarkers (scenario 4), together with their preselection counterparts AIC+SSW and AIC+MSW. These latter are appreciably better in case of large data ($n = 600$). The CD test has generally poor power in alternative scenarios (7%–9% for $n = 300$; 14%–25% for $n = 600$) as compared to the other tests, with mean p-values that are often the highest. Even though penalization seems able to improve its performances for the larger sample size (3%–17% with $n = 300$; 28%–57% with $n = 600$), minimum AIC stepwise

TABLE 11.2

Results of the Simulation Study with $n = 300$ and $n = 600$

(Weibull shape = 1)			SSW	MSW	CD	L_2 + CD	AIC + SSW	AIC + MSW	AIC + CD
(a) *Rejection probabilities*									
Scenario	1	$n = 300$	0.06	0.03	0.05	0.06	0.06	0.05	0.04
		$n = 600$	0.05	0.05	0.07	0.07	0.04	0.03	0.07
	2	$n = 300$	0.05	0.05	0.01	0.00	0.03	0.05	0.01
		$n = 600$	0.02	0.05	0.01	0.01	0.04	0.02	0.02
	3	$n = 300$	0.12	**0.30**	0.07	0.05	0.09	*0.23*	*0.23*
		$n = 600$	0.28	*0.69*	0.14	0.28	0.38	**0.75**	*0.69*
	4	$n = 300$	**0.16**	*0.14*	0.09	0.03	*0.14*	**0.16**	0.13
		$n = 600$	0.44	0.42	0.18	0.29	**0.50**	*0.47*	0.36
	5	$n = 300$	**0.40**	*0.31*	0.07	0.17	0.11	0.16	0.24
		$n = 600$	**0.80**	*0.70*	0.25	0.57	0.48	0.48	0.51
(b) *Mean p-values*									
Scenario	1	$n = 300$	0.50	0.49	0.49	0.47	0.51	0.52	0.48
		$n = 600$	0.48	0.53	0.48	0.50	0.51	0.52	0.48
	2	$n = 300$	0.51	0.53	0.66	0.64	0.53	0.54	0.63
		$n = 600$	0.52	0.54	0.70	0.70	0.55	0.54	0.64
	3	$n = 300$	0.39	**0.28**	0.50	0.50	0.37	*0.31*	0.32
		$n = 600$	0.22	0.10	0.35	0.24	0.15	**0.07**	*0.08*
	4	$n = 300$	**0.32**	0.36	0.49	0.52	*0.35*	0.36	0.36
		$n = 600$	*0.15*	0.18	0.29	0.22	**0.13**	*0.15*	0.17
	5	$n = 300$	**0.17**	*0.24*	0.45	0.38	0.33	0.31	0.27
		$n = 600$	**0.05**	*0.06*	0.25	0.13	0.11	0.12	0.11

Notes: This table shows the rejection probabilities (a) and the unbiased estimate of mean p-value (b) for the five scenarios. For the alternative scenarios, the best performing test is shown in bold, and the second best is shown in italics.

SSW, sum single Wald statistic; MSW, maximum single Wald statistic, CD, composite difference statistic; L_2+CD, composite difference statistic in an L_2-penalized model (ridge); AIC+SSW, sum single Wald statistic after AIC model selection; AIC+MSW, maximum single Wald statistic after AIC model selection; AIC+CD, composite difference statistic after AIC model selection.

preselection increases substantially the power of the CD test for both samples sizes (13%–24% with $n = 300$; 36%–69% with $n = 600$).

AIC preselection is able to improve the power of the SSW and MSW tests provided that enough data are at hand ($n = 600$, scenarios 3 and 4). This result suggests that in the case of few observations and many candidate biomarkers ($n = 300$), stepwise selection does not select the right biomarkers, yielding to possibly wrong conclusions. Nevertheless, results in the last scenario suggest that a strong correlation pattern between active and inactive biomarkers can compromise the correctness of preselection. Globally, in the alternative scenarios, doubling the sample size ($n=600$) makes the mean p-values of all the tests about 2.6-fold smaller and their power is on average 3.4 times higher than for $n=300$.

11.6 Conclusion

In this chapter, we have illustrated the challenges in designing clinical trials to show clinical utility of prognostic gene signatures, which are related to the relatively small added prognostic information to clinicopathological models as seen in the neoadjuvant chemotherapy example. Clinical trial designs originally proposed for diagnostic tests can be adopted for trials with prognostic gene signatures. We propose to move away from prognostic gene signatures to genes signatures specifically developed on randomized controlled trial data as a treatment effect modifier. Our approach consists of applying first a global permutation test—by permuting a statistic in an AFT Weibull regression model—to control the overall type I error at a prespecified α level. If many candidate predictive biomarkers are expected to be truly associated with differential treatment efficacy, the SSW test with or without AIC preselection may be preferred for this step. If the global test is significant, a treatment-modifying gene signature can be developed on the trial data using a particular variable selection method in an AFT model and a cross-validation scheme to estimate treatment effects within biomarker score defined subgroups. More research is needed to develop approaches that combine the inference step—that is, the global test—and the variable selection step (Wang and Lagakos 2009). Last but not least, in clinical trials of gene signatures some of the strongest challenges are to control confounding that can arise through the handling of the specimens, batch effects within and between laboratories, measurement error, and tumor heterogeneity.

References

Azim, H.A., Jr., Michiels, S., Zagouri, F. et al. (2013) Utility of prognostic genomic tests in breast cancer practice: The IMPAKT 2012 working group consensus statement, *Ann Oncol*, **24**, 647–654.

Benjamini, Y. and Hochberg, Y. (1995) Controlling the false discovery rate—A practical and powerful approach to multiple testing, *J Roy Stat Soc B*, **57**, 289–300.

Bogaerts, J., Cardoso, F., Buyse, M. et al. (2006) Gene signature evaluation as a prognostic tool: Challenges in the design of the MINDACT trial, *Nat Clin Pract Oncol*, **3**, 540–551.

Bossuyt, P.M., Lijmer, J.G., and Mol, B.W. (2000) Randomised comparisons of medical tests: Sometimes invalid, not always efficient, *Lancet*, **356**, 1844–1847.

Buyse, M. and Michiels, S. (2013) Omics-based clinical trial designs, *Curr Opin Oncol*, **25**, 289–295.

Conforti, R., Boulet, T., Tomasic, G. et al. (2007) Breast cancer molecular subclassification and estrogen receptor expression to predict efficacy of adjuvant anthracyclines-based chemotherapy: A biomarker study from two randomized trials, *Ann Oncol*, **18**, 1477–1483.

de Graaff, J.C., Ubbink, D.T., Tijssen, J.G.P., and Legemate, D.A. (2004) The diagnostic randomized clinical trial is the best solution for management issues in critical limb ischemia, *J Clin Epidemiol*, **57**, 1111–1118.

Dunkler, D., Michiels, S., and Schemper, M. (2007) Gene expression profiling: Does it add predictive accuracy to clinical characteristics in cancer prognosis? *Eur J Cancer*, **43**, 745–751.

Early Breast Cancer Trialists' Collaborative Group (2012) Comparisons between different polychemotherapy regimens for early breast cancer: Meta-analyses of long-term outcome among 100,000 women in 123 randomised trials, *Lancet*, **379**, 432–444.

FDA (2014) Pathologic complete response in neoadjuvant treatment of high-risk early-stage breast cancer: Use as an endpoint to support accelerated approval. *Guidance for Industry*. www.fda.gov/downloads/drugs/guidancecompliance-regulatoryinformation/guidances/ucm305501.pdf (last accessed on November 2, 2014).

Fumagalli, D., Bedard, P.L., Nahleh, Z. et al. (2012) A common language in neoadjuvant breast cancer clinical trials: Proposals for standard definitions and endpoints, *Lancet Oncol*, **13**, e240–e248.

Hooper, R., Díaz-Ordaz, K., Takeda, A. et al. (2013) Comparing diagnostic tests: trials in people with discordant test results, *Stat Med*, **32**, 2443–2456.

Hsieh, F.Y., Bloch, D.A., and Larsen, M.D. (1998) A simple method of sample size calculation for linear and logistic regression, *Stat Med*, **17**, 1623–1634.

Ignatiadis, I., Singhal, S.K., Desmedt, C. et al. (2012) Gene modules and response to neoadjuvant chemotherapy in breast cancer subtypes: A pooled analysis, *J Clin Oncol*, **30**, 1996–2004.

Lu, B. and Gatsonis, C. (2013) Efficiency of study designs in diagnostic randomized clinical trials, *Stat Med*, **32**, 1451–1466.

Maglott, D., Ostell, J., Pruitt, K. D., and Tatusova, T. (2007) Entrez gene: Gene-centered information at NCBI, *Nucl Acids Res*, **35**, D26–D31.

Matsui, S., Simon, R., Qu, R. et al. (2012) Developing and validating continuous genomic signatures in randomized clinical trials for predictive medicine, *Clin Cancer Res* **18**, 6065–6073.

Michiels, S., Kramar, A., and Koscielny, S. (2011a) Multidimensionality of microarrays: Statistical challenges and (im) possible solutions, *Mol Oncol*, **5**, 190–196.

Michiels, S., Potthoff, R.F., and George, S.L. (2011b) Multiple testing of treatment-effect-modifying biomarkers in a randomized clinical trial with a survival endpoint, *Stat Med*, **30**, 1502–1518.

Paik, S. Shak, S., Tang, G. et al. (2004) A multigene assay to predict recurrence of tamoxifen-treated, node-negative breast cancer, *N Engl J Med*, **351**, 2817–2826.

Peterson, B. and George, S.L. (1993) Sample size requirements and length of study for testing interaction in a 2 × k factorial design when time-to-failure is the outcome [corrected], *Control Clin Trials*, **14**, 511–522.

Potthoff, R.F., Peterson, B.L., and George, S.L. (2001) Detecting treatment-by-centre interaction in multi-centre clinical trials, *Stat Med*, **20**, 193–213.

Rastogi, P., Anderson, S.J., Bear, H.D. et al. (2008) Preoperative chemotherapy: Updates of National Surgical Adjuvant Breast and Bowel Project Protocols B-18 and B-27, *J Clin Oncol*, **26**, 778–785.

Rodger, M., Ramsay, T., and Fergusson, D. (2012) Diagnostic randomized controlled trials: The final frontier, *Trials*, **13**, 137.

Rothwell, P.M. (2005) Treating individuals 2. Subgroup analysis in randomised controlled trials: Importance, indications, and interpretation, *Lancet*, **365**, 176–186.

Simon, R. (2012) Clinical trials for predictive medicine, *Stat Med*, **31**, 3031–3040.

Stewart, L.A. and Parmar, M.K. (1993) The results of a quantitative overview of chemotherapy in advanced ovarian cancer: What can we learn? *Bull Cancer*, **80**, 146–151.

Teutsch, S.M., Bradley, L.A., Palomaki, G.E. et al. (2009) The evaluation of genomic applications in practice and prevention (EGAPP) initiative: Methods of the EGAPP working group, *Genet Med*, **11**, 3–14.

Tibshirani, R. (1997) The lasso method for variable selection in the Cox model, *Stat Med*, **16**, 385–395.

Verweij, P.J. and Van Houwelingen, H.C. (1994) Penalized likelihood in Cox regression, *Stat Med*, **13**, 2427–2436.

von Minckwitz, G., Untch, M., Blohmer, J.U. et al. (2012) Definition and impact of pathologic complete response on prognosis after neoadjuvant chemotherapy in various intrinsic breast cancer subtypes, *J Clin Oncol*, **30**, 1796–1804.

Wang, R. and Lagakos, S.W. (2009) Inference after variable selection using restricted permutation methods, *Can J Stat*, **37**, 625–644.

Windeler, J. (2000) Prognosis—What does the clinician associate with this notion? *Stat Med*, **19**, 425–430.

Wirapati, P., Sotiriou, C., Kunkel, S. et al. (2008) Meta-analysis of gene expression profiles in breast cancer: Toward a unified understanding of breast cancer subtyping and prognosis signatures, *Breast Cancer Res*, **10**, R65.

Zhang, H.H. and Lu, W.B. (2007) Adaptive lasso for Cox's proportional hazards model, *Biometrika*, **94**, 691–703.

Zou, H. (2006) The adaptive lasso and its oracle properties, *J Am Stat Assoc*, **101**, 1418–1429.

Zou, H. and Hastie, T. (2005) Regularization and variable selection via the elastic net (vol. B 67, p. 301, 2005), *J Roy Stat Soc B*, **67**, 768–768.

Section IV

Analysis of High-Dimensional Data and Genomic Signature Developments

12

Statistical Issues in Clinical Development and Validation of Genomic Signatures

Shigeyuki Matsui

CONTENTS

12.1 Introduction

Advances in genomics and biotechnology have gradually uncovered the biological characteristics of diseases and the molecular heterogeneity among diseases with the same diagnosis. In particular, the recent establishment of high-throughput technologies, such as single-nucleotide polymorphism (SNP) arrays, exome sequencing, gene expression microarrays, and protein arrays, has allowed for the discovery of potential new genomic biomarkers and the development of composite genomic signatures that provide prognostic or predictive values for many diseases. For example, genomic signatures based on gene expression include the Oncotype-Dx (Paik et al. 2004) and MammaPrint (van't Veer et al. 2002) for recurrence risk classification of breast cancer patients, the Tissue of Origin Test for identifying tumor tissue of origin (Monzon et al. 2009), and the AlloMap test for rejection surveillance after cardiac transplantation (Pham et al. 2010). Genomic studies using high-throughput technologies have typically been conducted as an early phase of signature development and are followed by studies for clinical validation, including assessment of predictive accuracy, of the developed signatures. From past studies, we can identify various strategies for the development and clinical validation of genomic signatures that should be discerned at least from a statistical point of view.

The establishment of high-throughput technologies has also stimulated the application of data-driven analytical approaches to high-dimensional genomic data from high-throughput assays. In the development of genomic signatures, data-driven approaches are typically *supervised* in the sense that the information pertaining to a particular clinical variable of interest, such as response to a particular treatment and posttreatment survival outcomes, is utilized in analyzing genomic data. Specifically, two important statistical analyses can be identified: (1) screening relevant genomic features for subsequent studies and (2) building genomic classifiers or predictors for the clinical variable. The high dimensionality of genomic data has posed special challenges in extracting a small fraction of relevant signals in the presence of a large amount of noise variables. This has been addressed in the context of analysis of high-dimensional genomic data in a wide spectrum of research in biology and medicine (e.g., Speed 2003; McLachlan et al. 2004; Mayer 2011), and many statistical methods developed and discussed in these contexts are also applicable to the field of genomic signature development. However, it is important to adequately apply the two aforementioned statistical analyses to the established strategies for signature development and validation.

This chapter serves as an introduction to the other chapters, in particular, Chapters 13 through 17, possibly associated with developing and/or validating genomic signatures. In Section 12.2, we present the identified strategies for clinical development and validation of genomic signatures as well as statistical issues in these strategies. We offer some remarks on the assessment of clinical utility of signatures in Section 12.3 and on developing and validating predictive signatures in Section 12.4. Concluding remarks are presented in Section 12.5.

12.2 Strategies for Clinical Development and Validation of Genomic Signatures

The identified strategies are shown in Figure 12.1. We primarily consider two strategies, the standard strategy with use of an established clinical platform (strategy A), and that which uses a novel high-throughput platform for clinical applications (strategy B). We will discuss these strategies individually and review the statistical methods applicable to each. For the most part, our discussion of high-throughput technologies will refer to the development of gene expression signatures and use of DNA microarrays. The same underlying methodological principles will also apply to the development of genomic signatures based on other types of genomic data, such as somatic mutation data, SNP genotyping, copy number proofing, and proteomic profiling data.

Although various issues pertaining to availability and quality of appropriate clinical specimens, requirements for the analytical performance of the assays (see Chapter 3), and methods for preprocessing (including quantification and normalization) can impact the strategy for developing and validating genomic signatures across different assay platforms, we do not address these issues in this chapter. See McShane et al. (2013) for related and other criteria for using omics-based signatures in clinical trials.

12.2.1 Strategy A: The Standard Strategy with Established Clinical Platforms

Most high-throughput technologies to date have been used primarily as research tools, and therefore a conversion to platforms more applicable to clinical practice would be needed. For example, in measuring gene expression, quantitative polymerase chain reaction (PCR) assays can serve as this type of clinical platform. In comparison with high-throughput microarrays, many quantitative PCR assays are known to be highly specific, sensitive, and robust, but they can measure only small numbers of genes at one time in a single sample unlike the microarray platform (e.g., Erickson 2012). This may necessitate limiting the number of candidate genes when converting from the microarray platform into the clinical platform.

The standard strategy for developing genomic signatures is to base them on established clinical platforms, such as quantitative PCR. In order to take into account the possible limitations in the number of genes that can be investigated using the clinical platform, at least two approaches to signature development and validation can be considered. The most popular is to screen out a small number of relevant genes from a large pool of gene candidates in the earlier microarray study, and after conversion to a clinical platform, to build a classifier or predictor based on the selected genes using the data measured in the clinical platform. This strategy was adopted in developing the

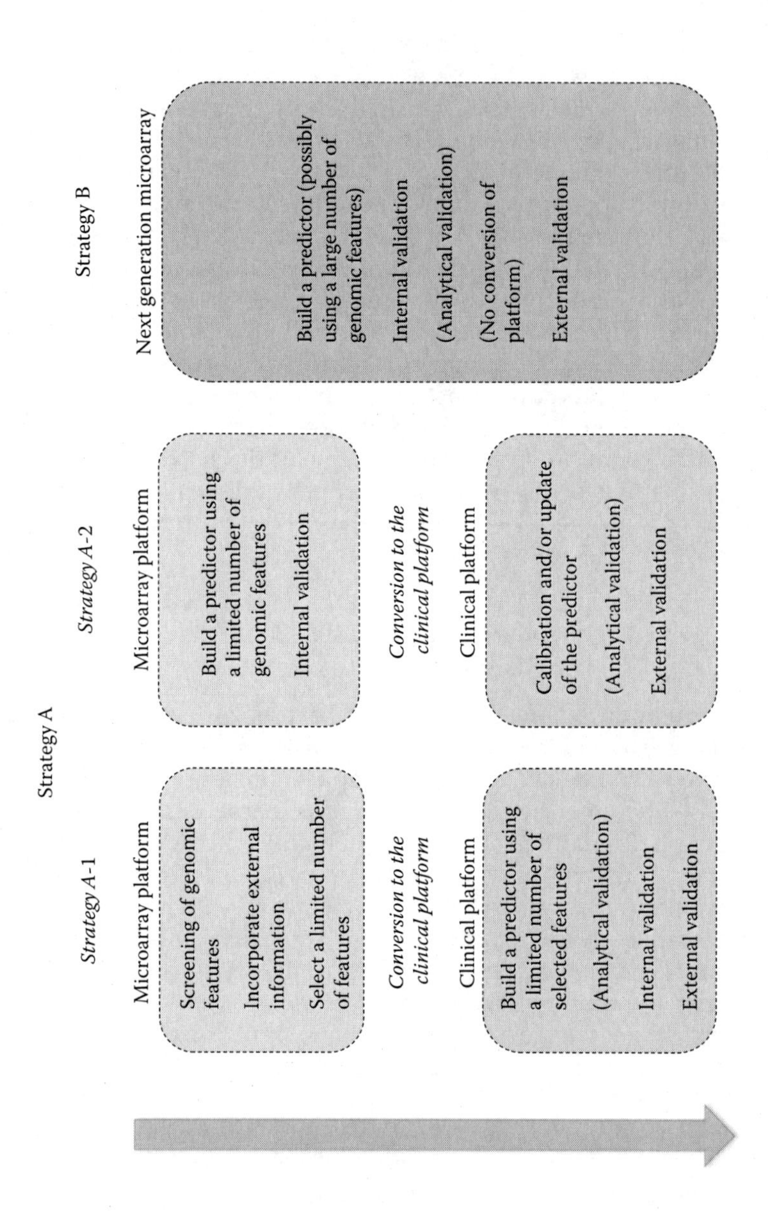

FIGURE 12.1
Strategies for clinical development and validation of genomic signatures.

Oncotype Dx signature for recurrent risk classification of breast cancer (Paik et al. 2004) and the AlloMap signature for rejection surveillance after cardiac transplantation (Pham et al. 2010). We refer to this approach as strategy A-1. Another possible strategy would be to build a predictor under the restriction of using a small number of genes in the microarray study, and, after conversion to a clinical platform, to perform some calibration and/or update for the constructed predictor using the data measured in the clinical platform. We refer to this approach as strategy A-2. In the following sections, we review the statistical methods for strategies A-1 and A-2.

12.2.1.1 Strategy A-1: Gene Screening with Microarrays and Prediction Using Clinical Platforms

With this approach, screening of relevant genes is conducted in an earlier clinical study with microarrays. The most popular approach for gene screening is to apply multiple testing methodologies that conduct separate statistical tests for each gene to test the null hypothesis of no association with the clinical variable. Another approach is to apply the ranking and selection methodologies that are used to rank genes based on the magnitude of the association or effect sizes, and then select a given number of top-ranking genes with the largest effect sizes; this may be appropriate given the limitation in the number of selected genes that can be investigated in subsequent studies using the clinical platform. The details of these methodologies are provided in Chapter 13.

In developing gene expression signatures, possible nonlinearity between signal intensity and transcript concentrations (particularly at the low and high ends of concentrations), as well as the necessary scale changes involved in the switch from the microarray platform to the PCR platform, could largely impair the ability to reproduce gene rankings established in a microarray study in a subsequent study based on the PCR platform. The use of distribution-free, nonparametric statistics, such as the Mann–Whitney–Wilcoxon statistic, to measure the association between each gene's expression and the clinical variable, can be advantageous because the invariance property of these statistics for a scale transformation of gene expression data could minimize the impact of both the nonlinearity and the scale change on the reproducibility of gene ranking (Matsui and Oura 2009).

Advantages of the multiple testing and gene ranking approaches relate to the ease with which the output from these analyses can be interpreted based on the marginal association between single genes and the clinical variable. Importantly, these approaches are usually complemented by the incorporation of external information from biological perspectives (such as annotation regarding gene function categories and partial information regarding genetic pathways) and knowledge from previous, similar screening studies. Typically, biologists and statisticians cooperatively narrow the list down to a subset of genes of limited size that can be investigated in subsequent studies utilizing the clinical platform.

These univariate approaches are often criticized because they fail to consider plausible correlations among genes in gene screening. Because of these correlations, as well as the random variation in gene expression, there is no guarantee that a set of selected genes is optimal in terms of predictive accuracy. One rationale for employing the univariate approaches would be the selection of genes strongly associated with the clinical variable that are essential for achieving significantly high predictive accuracy (Hess et al. 2011; Matsui and Noma 2011). Again, the relative ease in incorporating external information from biological perspectives and previous correlative studies can be advantageous in identifying a relevant gene list for improving predictive accuracy by incorporating biologically relevant genes as well as obtaining biologically interpretable predictors.

When candidate genes selected in the microarray study pass through to a subsequent study with the clinical platform, a predictor will be built using the data on these genes measured in the clinical platform. Because the number of genes at this stage is much smaller than that in the microarray study, standard methodologies for classification or prediction (e.g., Ripley 1996; Hastie et al. 2009), where the number of variables (genes) is relatively small compared to the number of samples, would be applicable. One may also consider an application of black box systems from ensemble methods, such as bagging and random forests (e.g., Hastie et al. 2009). For these methods, the variability in the final predictions caused by random components must be assessed and adequately controlled, as it is expected that the same set of observed genomic variables should lead to a consistent final test result (McShane et al. 2013).

12.2.1.2 Strategy A-2: Prediction with Microarrays and Calibration or Updating with Clinical Platforms

In this strategy, a prediction analysis is conducted in an earlier study with microarrays. Owing to the restriction on the number of genes that can be evaluated in subsequent studies with the clinical platform, gene selection would be mandatory in the prediction analysis. Several filtering methods have been proposed. The simplest, but most common approach is univariate filtering based on marginal association between each gene and the clinical variable, as described in Section 12.2.1.1. More complex, computationally demanding multivariate methods have also been developed (Saeys et al. 2007). Recent studies found that the performance of univariate filtering methods was comparable to that of multivariate methods for microarray datasets with small sample sizes (Lai et al. 2006; Lecocke and Hess 2007). Another approach is to apply a prediction method that involves feature selection. An example is the lasso, a regularized regression method with a penalty term that comprises the sum of the absolute value of the elements of the parameter vector (Tibshirani 1996). Typically, many regression parameters are estimated to be zero, that is, it provides a means for variable selection.

Before the predictor or classifier built in the microarray study is calibrated or updated in the subsequent clinical platform study, it must be ensured that the scale used to measure genomic data in the microarray platform can be adequately transformed into that used in the clinical platform. A calibration is to assess association between a genomic score in the prediction model calculated using genomic data measured in the microarray platform and that using genomic data measured in the clinical platform (with some scale change). If necessary, one may develop a model (such as a linear model) using the score obtained in the clinical platform as a single covariate to more fit to that obtained in the microarray platform.

If the predictive accuracy based on the (calibrated) score is proven to be poor in independent samples, one may consider a model updating that involves changing the weight assigned to each gene in the prediction model, as well as changing the cut-off point using in making classifications, using genomic data measured in the clinical platform for these samples (see Moons et al. 2012 for a more details about model updating). One may argue that the model updating is always warranted because of possible overestimation for weights or regression coefficients for selected genes under high dimensions. It is important to note that the predictive accuracy of an updated model should be assessed using additional independent samples (see Section 12.2.3).

12.2.2 Strategy B: Strategy with Novel High-Throughput Platforms for Clinical Application

Recent advances in biotechnology have gradually allowed the development of novel high-throughput platforms for clinical application. As an early endeavor in this direction, in developing the MammaPrint signature for recurrence risk classification of breast cancer, a custom microarray was developed to allow clinical application of a prediction system based on the expressions of 70 genes that was developed in an earlier study with experimental microarrays (van't Veer et al. 2002). More recently, in developing the Tissue of Origin Test for identifying tumor tissue of origin, a new microarray platform was developed to measure gene expressions of a pool of more than 1000 genes (Monzon et al. 2009). This new platform can work with formalin-fixed, paraffin-embedded tissue specimens that may contain degraded RNA, the clinical standard for tissue fixation and processing for the purpose of diagnostic histology and long-term storage. The advent of such new high-throughput assays may permit the development of genomic signatures with the same (high-throughput) platform, for all processes related to the development and analytical/clinical validation of genomic signatures, as well as the assessment of the medical utility of the signature or the new treatment under development. From the perspective of statistical analysis, this would remove the limitations currently required in developmental strategies based on standard clinical platforms regarding the number of genes used in building predictors.

When building a predictor using high-dimensional genomic data, where the number of variables (genes) is much greater than the number of samples, traditional regression modeling is ineffective. Conventional approaches that ensure that all variables are included would fail in estimation or result in overfitted models with poor prediction ability. Some sort of dimension reduction or regularization is needed. For details on the related techniques in regression modeling or classification, see Chapter 14 for class prediction and Chapter 15 for survival time prediction. Here, we make a few comments on dimension reduction and prediction modeling under high dimensions.

Filtering methods for dimension reduction, such as those based on a univariate approach in Section 12.2.1.2 in terms of limiting the number of genes for signature development in strategy A, can also effectively contribute to accurate prediction, because a large proportion of genes would be noise and would thus be useless in this regard. In this approach, the number of top genes selected can be regarded as a tuning parameter and determined on the basis of predictive accuracy. Again, as noted in Section 12.2.1.2, computationally intensive, multivariate filtering methods that takes correlations between genes into account can also be considered (Saeys et al. 2007), although comparative studies have not convincingly demonstrated the advantage of these methods (Lai et al. 2006; Lecocke and Hess 2007).

Concerning the building of prediction models, several studies have reported that simple methods that ignore correlations between genes, such as diagonal linear discriminant analysis, compound covariate predictors, and *k*-nearest neighbors, performed well in terms of prediction accuracy for microarray datasets with small to moderate sample sizes in comparison with more complex methods that incorporate correlations and also interactions between genes (Ben-Dor et al. 2000; Dudoit et al. 2002; Dudoit and Fridlyand 2003; Shi et al. 2010; Emura et al. 2012). These findings reflect the difficulty in extracting an additional relevant signal from the joint distribution across genes under the presence of huge numbers of noise variables.

Complex (multivariate) filtering methods and prediction models are more prone to collecting noises and (over-)fitting them. This is the fundamental difficulty in the prediction analysis using high-dimensional genomic data. As such, some kind of restriction on the complexity of prediction model building is generally crucial under high dimensions.

12.2.3 Clinical Validation of Genomic Signatures

12.2.3.1 Assessment of Predictive Accuracy of Genomic Signatures

The main task in the clinical validation of genomic signatures is the assessment of the predictive accuracy of the developed predictor. Predictive accuracy depends on the training set and the definition of what is to be predicted. It is best if the intended clinical use of the classifier or predictor is defined in advance and that this is reflected in the selection of the training samples and the definition of the objective of prediction. Measures of predictive accuracy include the proportion of correct classifications, sensitivity, specificity for two-class prediction (see Chapter 14) and Kaplan–Meier curves between risk groups, time-dependent ROC curves, the Brier scores, and concordance index for predicting survival times (see Chapter 15). In strategy A (A-1 and A-2), predictive accuracy is assessed in the clinical platform, while in strategy B it is evaluated in the high-throughput platform. Unbiased estimation of the predictive accuracy is particularly important, particularly when the number of candidate variables (genes) available for use in the predictor is much greater than the number of samples available for analysis. In this section, unless otherwise noted, we focus mainly on the assessment of predictive accuracy in such high-dimensional situations, including prediction analysis in the microarray studies in strategies A-2 and B. The same methodological principle would also be useful in other situations with lower dimensions (particularly when using complex prediction models with many parameters), such as prediction analysis using a limited number of variables in the clinical platform in strategy A-1.

In high-dimensional situations, one must focus clearly on the objective of accurate prediction and not confuse this objective with that of achieving biological insight or ensuring that all variables included are essential, or that the model is *correct* (George 2008; Simon 2008). For example, a prognostic genomic signature might contain a gene that is only representative for a group of highly correlated prognostic genes. With slightly different data, a different gene from that group might be selected. Therefore, the signature will be rather unstable with different interpretations, while prediction performance may not be affected much (Schumacher et al. 2012). As such, there might exist many *solutions* of predictor with comparable predictive accuracy for high dimensions. For example, Fan et al. (2006) found that several prognostic signatures developed for breast cancer had little overlap of the component genes, but showed comparable predictive accuracy. According to a numerical calculation in the framework of ranking and selection, top genes obtained from multiple univariate analyses will be highly instable, even for very large sample sizes, such as several hundreds of samples (Matsui et al. 2008). Reproducibility of the gene list among similar correlative studies can be critical in elucidating underlying biological mechanisms, but it can mislead in the assessment of genomic signatures for predictive medicine.

12.2.3.2 Internal Validation

Assessment of predictive accuracy includes internal and external validation. The purpose of internal validation is to assess predictive accuracy for the study population from which the predictor was built. Resampling techniques are useful, particularly when the sample size is relatively small (Molinaro et al. 2005; Jiang and Simon 2007). Such techniques include cross-validation

(Stone 1974), bootstrap (Efron 1983), and the 0.632 estimator (Efron and Gong 1983; Efron and Tibshirani 1997).

The cross-validation is one of the most popular methods. In a K-fold cross-validation, all the study samples are divided into K nonoverlapping and approximately equal sized subsets, and all subsets successively serve as test samples. More specifically, in each fold of cross-validation, one particular subset is regarded as a test set, and a predictor built from the remaining samples as a training set is used to make a prediction for all samples in the test set. Thus, after the completion of all rounds (folds) of cross-validation, a prediction is obtained for all of the study samples, and an average of prediction results is calculated as an estimate of predictive accuracy for the study samples.

The number of folds K can by any integer from 2 to the number of samples n. Leave-one-out cross-validation is a special case with $K=n$. For a smaller value of K, the predictive accuracy will be more underestimated as fewer samples are used for training the prediction model, but the variance of the estimate deceases as training sets become more different from each other. $K=5$ or 10 are one compromise between minimizing the bias and variance (e.g., Hastie et al. 2009). According to a simulation study for high-dimensional data with small sample sizes (Molinaro et al. 2005), leave-one-out cross-validation had the smallest bias and mean square error for linear and diagonal discriminant analysis, as well as 5- and 10-fold cross-validation, but differences among resampling methods were reduced as the number of sample available increased.

When using resampling techniques, it is critical that all aspects of model building, including gene selection, are reperformed for each fold in resampling (Ambroise and McLachlan 2002; Simon et al. 2003). A violation of this principle may lead to a serious overestimation of predictive accuracy (that may yield an incorrect recognition that the genomic signature is so promising). When performing a gene selection using the entire samples before a cross-validation, any test sets in the cross-validation have already been used as one component of the prediction model building and thus no longer serve as an independent test set. Again, in a valid cross-validation, all components of the prediction model building, including gene selection, are performed from scratch in each fold of cross-validation. In this complete cross-validation, the selected gene set and built predictor may vary across the folds of cross-validation, but the estimated predictive accuracy can be interpreted as that for a predictor that would be obtained from adopting the whole prediction algorithm (including gene selection) to the entire study samples, which will be further assessed in the future (external) validation studies. Violation of complete cross-validation is one of major flaws in many published prediction analyses using genomic data, in addition to the use of resubstitution estimates of predictive accuracy that is to apply the predictor to the training set from which it was built (Dupuy and Simon 2007; Subramanian and Simon 2010).

When gene selection and prediction models are optimized based on cross-validated predictive accuracy, the optimization process should be included in the cross-validation procedure (through invoking an inner loop of cross-validation), or an independent validation set will be needed in order to provide an unbiased estimate of the predictive accuracy (Dudoit and Fridlyand 2003; Wessels et al. 2005; Varma and Simon 2006). However, if the cross-validated predictive accuracy measures that do not incorporate the optimization process are relatively insensitive to selection of the tuning parameters used in the optimization, this bias may not be large. Confidence intervals for cross-validated predictive accuracy (or predictive error) can be calculated, but the length of the intervals is generally wide, reflecting high variation of cross-validated predictive accuracy estimates (Jiang et al. 2008). It is also important to establish that the predictive accuracy is statistically higher than that expected when there is no relationship between the genomic data and the clinical variable. A permutation procedure with repetition of all aspects of cross-validation analysis, including gene selection, after permuting the label of the clinical variable, is proposed to assess the statistical significance of cross-validated predictive accuracy (Radmacher et al. 2002).

When the model-building process is complex and not easily specified in an algorithmic manner, typically through incorporating external information from biological perspectives and previous correlative studies, an independent validation set would be needed (Simon et al. 2004). Typically, a split-sample approach to the entire study samples is a simple and effective way to have such a validation set (in addition to a training set), when the number of samples is relatively large. Some authors have provided a formula for determining sample sizes for the training and validation sets in two-class prediction problems (Dobbin and Simon 2007).

One limitation of resampling methods for internal validation is high variance in estimating predictive accuracy. In cross-validation (with $K < n$), the estimation result can largely depend on the partition used in it. Repeating the cross-validation analysis with different random partitions and averaging over the repetitions will reduce the variance (e.g., Braga-Neto and Dougherty 2004). For two-class prediction, a model-based estimate of predictive accuracy (such as the proportion of correct classifications, sensitivity, or specificity) in a diagonal linear discriminant analysis can be obtained with much less variance based on unbiased estimates of effect sizes and correlations across selected genes that can be derived from a hierarchical mixture modeling of genomic data (Matsui and Noma 2011; see also Chapter 13).

12.2.3.3 External Validation

External validation is performed using an independent set of samples, outside of the study population used for prediction model building, possibly from a more relevant population for the clinical application of the predictor. For example, in the development of the Oncotype Dx, the predictive accuracy of the developed predictor (the recurrence score based on 21 genes to classify 3 recurrence risk groups) was assessed in a PCR-based platform for an independent cohort from another clinical trial (Paik et al. 2004). The predictive accuracy of the 70-gene based MammaPrint classifier was assessed using independent patient cohorts from five European institutions (Buyse et al. 2006).

For the assessment of predictive accuracy, a completely specified predictor or signature is needed. Complete specification of the signature includes not just the list of component genes, but also the mathematical form used to combine genomic data for the genes used in the signature, weights for the relative importance of the genes, and cut-off values when making classifications (Simon 2008). More strictly, all the steps from collecting specimens to obtaining a final prediction result should be specified, including data preprocessing steps, such as overall data quality assessments, exclusion of unreliable measurements, data normalization, and calculation of intermediate summary gene-level statistics (e.g., from probe-level intensity values in microarray data) (McShane et al. 2013). Changes in any steps based on the data in a validation study may necessitate another independent validation study.

Generally, the most rigorous external validation for prognostic biomarkers requires that differs in investigator, location, and time period from those in the original prediction modeling (Justice et al. 1999; Altman and Royston 2000). For genomic signatures, there are many potential sources of variation in real-world conditions, not incorporated in experimental studies for developing predictors, including prospective tissue handling, assay drift, and reagent batch effects within an array laboratory, as well as interlaboratory array variation (Simon 2006). See McShane et al. (2013) for more discussions and guidelines.

Sample size calculation is an important issue in assessing external, clinical validation of a genomic signature. Required sample sizes may largely depend on various factors, including characteristics of the disease, the intended purpose of using the signature (or the criteria for *success* in using the signature; see Altman and Royston 2000 for a discussion), the prevalence of the clinical event of interest in prediction (e.g., progression/death or response to treatment), the distribution of prediction results (or score values) obtained by applying the signature, and the true predictive accuracy of the signature and so forth, in the intended population for clinical application. Some authors reported that substantial sample sizes are required for external validation of prognostic biomarkers (Vergouwe et al. 2005; Peek et al. 2007). Generally, prospective studies are more prone to encounter many challenges in collecting sufficient numbers of samples. A prospective–retrospective analysis (Simon et al. 2009; see also Chapters 1 and 8) that plans a prospective analysis using archived specimens in the past clinical trials or observational cohort studies can be a practical approach for assessing external validation of genomic signatures, which was originally proposed for assessing clinical utility of genomic signatures. Several conditions are needed for appropriately conducting this approach (Simon et al. 2009; see also Chapter 8). As one of such conditions, substantial data on the analytical validity of the signature must exist to ensure that results obtained from the archived specimens will closely resemble those that would have been obtained from analysis of specimens collected in real time. Assays should be conducted blinded to the clinical data.

12.2.3.4 Added Predictive Value of Prognostic Genomics Signatures

In clinical validation of a prognostic genomic signature, it is important to assess the added predictive value of the signature to established, clinical prognostic factor(s). When the genomic signature is based on a single composite score (such as a weighted linear function of genomic data across component genes), a standard multivariate model (such as a logistic model for binary outcomes and Cox proportional hazards model for survival time outcomes) with this genomic score and clinical factor(s) as covariates is frequently fit to a validation set. In this approach, it should be noted that the statistical significance for the regression coefficient of the genomic score after adjustment for the clinical factor(s) provides no implication on the added *predictive* value of the signature (Altman and Royston 2000; Pepe et al. 2004). A more appropriate approach is to compare estimated predictive accuracy between a multivariate model with both the genomic score and clinical factors and that only with the clinical factors. Again, resampling techniques, such as cross-validation, are useful for this end. In each round of cross-validation, after a subset of the validation set is left out for a test set, two prediction models with and without the genomic score are fitted to the remaining samples in the validation set. The two fitted models are then applied to the test set and assessed on the basis of an appropriate measure of predictive accuracy (as described in Section 12.2.3.1) for comparison.

This approach can also be applied to internal validation. Simon et al. (2011) compared cross-validated log-rank statistic (as a predictive measure in risk stratification) for a combined model and that for a model only using clinical factors, and proposed to assess the statistical significance of the difference between the two cross-validated statistics using a permutation method that permutes the genomic data. The null hypothesis considered is that the genomic data are independent of survival outcomes and clinical covariates. When the clinical information is well represented by a single discrete score, such as the International Prognostic Index (IPI) Score for risk stratification in lymphoma, a permutation of genomic data within each category of the clinical score (Matsui 2006) may allow considering the null hypothesis that genomic data is conditionally independent of survival given the clinical score.

See Boulesteix and Sauerbrei (2011) for more discussions about the assessment of added predictive values of genomic data in both internal and external validation of prognostic signatures. It should be noted that the accuracy assessment for the prediction model with both genomic score and established clinical factors *per se* will be meaningful for many situations where the genomic score has a potential to be used in conjunction with the clinical factors, rather than instead of them (Buyse et al. 2006).

12.3 Assessment of Clinical Utility

Assessment of clinical validity of genomic signature, as discussed so far, is different from that of clinical utility that aims to establish that patient benefit is improved by using genomic signatures (see Chapter 1).

One simple way to evaluate clinical utility of a prognostic signature is to compare the new strategy of using the signature in determining patients' treatments with that of not using the signature in determining treatments, that is, the marker strategy design, in clinical trials, although it generally suffers from a serious lack of efficiency because of a substantial overlap in the number of patients receiving the same treatment within the two strategies being compared (see Chapters 1, 9, and 11). See Chapter 11 for more discussions about evaluation of clinical utility of prognostic signatures.

The marker strategy design is also considered for evaluating clinical utility of predictive signatures or biomarkers. An example is a randomized trial for recurrent ovarian cancer that compares the strategy of determining treatment based on tumor chemosensitivity (predictive) assays with a strategy of using physician's choice of chemotherapy based on standard practice (Cree et al. 2007). Another example is a randomized trial for non–small cell lung cancer that compares a strategy of using a standard treatment (cisplatin + docetaxel) exclusively with a biomarker-based strategy in which patients diagnosed to be resistant to the standard treatment based on the biomarker are treated with an experimental treatment (gemcitabine + docetaxel) and the rest are treated with the standard treatment (Cobo et al. 2007). Again, these studies can be very inefficient. In the development of new treatments, clinical utility of a companion predictive signature for a particular new treatment can be considered through evaluating clinical utility of the new treatment with aid of the companion signature. To this end, enrichment and all-comers (or randomize-all) clinical trial designs are more appropriate (see Chapters 1 and 8 through 10).

12.4 Clinical Development and Validation of Predictive Signatures

We provide some remarks on the development and validation of predictive genomic signatures in the context of clinical trials. Again, a predictive signature is often designated as a companion biomarker in the development of a particular new treatment. When the molecular target of the new treatment is clear and the genomic alternation that leads to the deregulation of the target and the nature of this alteration (e.g., somatic point mutation or gene amplification) are known, a reliable biomarker may be identified. When such a biomarker is available at an early stage of clinical development, such as at a phase II trial, it can be designed so that it allows assessment of the clinical validity of the biomarker (see Chapters 5 and 6), possibly followed by a phase III trial with the enrichment design based on this biomarker (see Chapter 8). More commonly, however, our understanding of the treatment target(s) and the nature of the genomic alteration related to a particular target is far from complete. When several candidate predictive biomarkers are available, the phase II design can be tailored to incorporate these biomarkers so as to assess their validity and determine the best of them or their combinations or signatures.

In more extreme situations where genomic data with a large number of candidate genomic biomarkers are available in phase II trials, these trials can incorporate data-driven approaches to developing genomic signatures described in Section 12.2. For example, in a single-arm phase II trial with an endpoint of treatment response, for example, tumor shrinkage in oncology, relevant biomarkers can be screened out by comparing genomic data between the two classes of responders and nonresponders using methods described in Chapter 13 and two-class prediction methods described in Chapter 14 are applicable. A randomized phase II trial of the treatment versus its control, with the endpoint of occurrence of a disease event or change, such as disease-free survival, can also be tailored to incorporate the development of predictive signatures. For such situations, treatment by gene interactions should be detected to develop predictive signatures for identifying a subset of patients for whom the outcome when receiving the treatment would be better than that when receiving the control.

Incorporating the development of predictive signatures in phase II trials will generally require larger sample sizes than those required under standard phase II trials without use of the biomarker. The building of two-class prediction models for responders and nonresponders can suffer from a serious lack of power for small numbers of responders as frequently observed in many phase II trials (Pusztai et al. 2007). Dobbin and Simon (2007) suggested at least 20–30 responders in developing genomic signatures. Signature development based on treatment by gene interactions in randomized phase II trials would also encounter a limitation in efficiency in terms of general lack of power in detecting statistical interactions. In addition, a sufficient number of additional samples would be needed for clinical validation or assessing the predictive accuracy of the developed signature, irrespective of which of the strategies in Figure 12.1 is chosen.

Another approach to the clinical development and validation of predictive biomarkers is to use archived specimens from previously conducted clinical trials for *other*, but similar treatments. Again, the prospective–retrospective approach as described in Section 12.2.3.3 is also applicable for this purpose (Simon et al. 2009; see also Chapters 1 and 8).

A companion predictive signature will be eventually incorporated in evaluating the clinical utility of the new treatment in confirmatory randomized clinical trials. As described in Chapter 1 of this volume, there are several possible scenarios for which different approaches to design and analysis of clinical trials are considered.

When an analytically and clinically validated predictive signature is available at the initiation of a definitive phase III trial for the treatment, enrichment designs or all-comers (or randomize-all) designs with prestratification based on the signature are relevant (see Chapters 8 through 10). As noted in Section 12.2.3.3, the signature needs to be completely specified at this stage.

When a reliable predictive signature or biomarker is unavailable before initiating the phase III trial, as is more common in the clinical development of therapeutics, one approach is to archive pretreatment specimens and to design and analyze the randomized phase III trial in such a way that both developing a companion signature and testing treatment efficacy based on the developed signature are possible and validly conducted. The adaptive signature design (Freidlin and Simon 2005) and cross-validated adaptive signature design (Freidlin et al. 2010), and the continuous adaptive signature design (Matsui et al. 2012) have been proposed for this purpose. These designs are the topic of Chapters 16 and 17 of this volume. Clinical validation of predictive genomic signatures in phase III trials is covered by Chapter 11.

Another approach is to develop a predictive signature using archived specimens from a past pivotal trial for other, but similar treatments as discussed previously. In the prospective–retrospective analysis approach (see Chapter 1), the developed signature can be used for defining the prospective subgroup analysis that spends some of the 5% type I error reserved in the phase III trial to evaluate efficacy of the treatment under testing. Another possibility is to develop a predictive signature using archived specimens from a failed pivotal trial for the same treatment that showed no treatment effect for the entire patient population. The developed signature from such an analysis can provide useful information for designing a second confirmatory trial of the same treatment, possibly with an enrichment design with small sample sizes. The prospective–retrospective approach can also limit the indication for a treatment when some of clinical trials were positive overall for the treatment, as in the *KRAS* colorectal cancer situation with anti *EGFR* antibodies (Karapetis et al. 2008).

12.5 Conclusions

Recent advances in genomic and biotechnology have stimulated further research of biostatistical and bioinformatics methodologies for the clinical development and validation of new genomic signatures that are useful for selecting the right treatments for the right patients. The established heterogeneity of disease based on genomic signatures then warrants the development of new methodologies for the design and analysis of clinical trials that can establish the clinical utility of new treatments and their companion signatures, and help realize the vision of reliable personalized or predictive medicine.

References

Altman, D.G. and Royston, P. 2000. What do we mean by validating a prognostic model? *Stat Med* 19: 453–473.

Ambroise, C. and McLachlan, G.J. 2002. Selection bias in gene extraction on the basis of microarray gene-expression data. *Proc Natl Acad Sci USA* 99: 6562–6566.

Ben-Dor, A., Bruhn, L., Friedman, N. et al. 2000. Tissue classification with gene expression profiles. *J Comput Biol* 7: 559–583.

Boulesteix, A.L. and Sauerbrei, W. 2011. Added predictive value of high-throughput molecular data to clinical data and its validation. *Brief Bioinform* 12: 215–229.

Braga-Neto, U.M. and Dougherty, E.R. 2004. Is cross-validation valid for small-sample microarray classification? *Bioinformatics* 20: 374–380.

Buyse, M., Loi, S., van't Veer, L. et al. on behalf of the TRANSBIG Consortium. 2006. Validation and clinical utility of a 70-gene prognostic signature for patients with node-negative breast cancer. *J Natl Cancer Inst* 98: 1183–1192.

Cobo, M., Isla, D., Massuti, B. et al. 2007. Customizing cisplatin based on quantitative excision repair cross-complementing 1 mRNA expression: A phase III trial in non-small-cell lung cancer. *J Clin Oncol* 25: 2747–2754.

Cree, I.A., Kurbacher, C.M., Lamont, A., Hindley, A.C., Love, S.; TCA Ovarian Cancer Trial Group. 2007. A prospective randomized controlled trial of tumour chemosensitivity assay directed chemotherapy versus physician's choice in patients with recurrent platinum-resistant ovarian cancer. *Anticancer Drugs* 18: 1093–1101.

Dobbin, K. and Simon, R. 2007. Sample size planning for developing classifiers using high dimensional data. *Biostatistics* 8: 101–117.

Dudoit, S. and Fridlyand, J. 2003. Classification in microarray experiments. In Speed T.P. (ed.) *Statistical Analysis of Gene Expression Microarray Data*, pp. 93–158. Boca Raton, FL: Chapman & Hall/CRC.

Dudoit, S., Fridlyand, J., and Speed, T.P. 2002. Comparison of discrimination methods for the classification of tumors using gene expression data. *J Am Stat Assoc* 97: 77–87.

Dupuy, A. and Simon, R.M. 2007. Critical review of published microarray studies for cancer outcome and guidelines on statistical analysis and reporting. *J Natl Cancer Inst* 99: 147–157.

Efron, B. 1983. Estimating the error rate of a prediction rule: Improvement on cross-validation. *J Am Stat Assoc* 78: 316–331.

Efron, B. and Gong, G. 1983. A leisurely look at the bootstrap, the Jackknife, and cross-validation. *Am Stat* 37: 36–48.

Efron, B. and Tibshirani, R. 1997. Improvements on cross-validation: The.632+ bootstrap method. *J Am Stat Assoc* 92: 548–560.

Emura, T., Chen, Y.H., and Chen, H.Y. 2012. Survival prediction based on compound covariate under Cox proportional hazard models. *PLoS One* 7: e47627.

Erickson, H.S. 2012. Measuring molecular biomarkers in epidemiologic studies: Laboratory techniques and biospecimen considerations. *Stat Med* 31: 2400–2413.

Fan, C., Oh, D.S., Wessels, L. et al. 2006. Concordance among gene-expression-based predictors for breast cancer. *N Engl J Med* 355: 560–569.

Freidlin, B., Jiang, W., and Simon, R. 2010. The cross-validated adaptive signature design. *Clin Cancer Res* 16: 691–698.

Freidlin, B. and Simon, R. 2005. Adaptive signature design: An adaptive clinical trial design for generating and prospectively testing a gene expression signature for sensitive patients. *Clin Cancer Res* 11: 7872–7878.

George, S.L. 2008. Statistical issues in translational cancer research. *Clin Cancer Res* 14: 5954–5958.

Hastie, T., Tibshirani, R., and Friedman, J. 2009. *The Elements of Statistical Learning: Data Mining, Inference and Prediction*, 2nd ed. New York: Springer.

Hess, K.R., Wei, C., Qi, Y. et al. 2011. Lack of sufficiently strong informative features limits the potential of gene expression analysis as predictive tool for many clinical classification problems. *BMC Bioinformatics* 12: 463.

Jiang, W. and Simon, R. 2007. A comparison of bootstrap methods and an adjusted bootstrap approach for estimating the prediction error in microarray classification. *Stat Med* 26: 5320–5334.

Jiang, W., Varma, S., and Simon, R. 2008. Calculating confidence intervals for prediction error in microarray classification using resampling. *Stat Appl Genet Mol Biol* 7: Article 8.

Justice, A.C., Covinsky, K.E., and Berlin, J.A. 1999. Assessing the generalizability of prognostic information. *Ann Intern Med* 130: 515–524.

Karapetis, C.S., Khambata-Ford, S., Jonker, D.J. et al. 2008. K-ras mutations and benefit from cetuximab in advanced colorectal cancer. *N Engl J Med* 359: 1757–1765.

Lai, C., Reinders, M.J., van't Veer, L.J., and Wessels, L.F. 2006. A comparison of univariate and multivariate gene selection techniques for classification of cancer datasets. *BMC Bioinformatics* 7: 235.

Lecocke, M. and Hess, K. 2007. An empirical study of univariate and genetic algorithm-based feature selection in binary classification with microarray data. *Cancer Inform* 2: 313–327.

Matsui, S. 2006. Predicting survival outcomes using subsets of significant genes in prognostic marker studies with microarrays. *BMC Bioinformatics* 7: 156.

Matsui, S. and Noma, H. 2011. Estimation and selection in high-dimensional genomic studies for developing molecular diagnostics. *Biostatistics* 12: 223–233.

Matsui, S. and Oura, T. 2009. Sample sizes for a robust ranking and selection of genes in microarray experiments. *Stat Med* 28: 2801–2816.

Matsui, S., Simon, R., Qu, P., Shaughnessy, J.D. Jr, Barlogie, B., and Crowley, J. 2012. Developing and validating continuous genomic signatures in randomized clinical trials for predictive medicine. *Clin Cancer Res* 18: 6065–6073.

Matsui, S., Zeng, S., Yamanaka, T., and Shaughnessy, J. 2008. Sample size calculations based on ranking and selection in microarray experiments. *Biometrics* 64: 217–226.

Mayer, B. 2011. *Bioinformatics for Omics Data: Methods and Protocols*. New York: Humana Press.

McLachlan, G.J., Do, K.-A., and Ambroise, C. 2004. *Analyzing Microarray Gene Expression Data*. Hoboken, NJ: John Wiley & Sons.

McShane, L.M., Cavenagh, M.M., Lively, T.G. et al. 2013. Criteria for the use of omics-based predictors in clinical trials: Explanation and elaboration. *BMC Med* 11: 220.

Molinaro, A.M., Simon, R., and Pfeiffer, R.M. 2005. Prediction error estimation: A comparison of resampling methods. *Bioinformatics* 21: 3301–3307.

Monzon, F.A., Lyons-Weiler, M., Buturovic, L.J. et al. 2009. Multicenter validation of a 1,550-gene expression profile for identification of tumor tissue of origin. *J Clin Oncol* 27: 2503–2508.

Moons, K.G., Kengne, A.P., Grobbee, D.E. et al. 2012. Risk prediction models: II. External validation, model updating, and impact assessment. *Heart* 98: 691–698.

Paik, S., Shak, S., Tang, G. et al. 2004. A multigene assay to predict recurrence of tamoxifen-treated, node-negative breast cancer. *N Engl J Med* 351: 2817–2826.

Peek, N., Arts, D.G., Bosman, R.J., van der Voort, P.H., and de Keizer, N.F. 2007. External validation of prognostic models for critically ill patients required substantial sample sizes. *J Clin Epidemiol* 60: 491–501.

Pepe, M.S., Janes, H., Longton, G., Leisenring, W., and Newcomb, P. 2004. Limitations of the odds ratio in gauging the performance of a diagnostic, prognostic, or screening marker. *Am J Epidemiol* 159: 882–890.

Pham, M.X., Teuteberg, J.J., Kfoury A.G. et al. 2010. Gene-expression profiling for rejection surveillance after cardiac transplantation. *N Engl J Med* 362: 1890–1900.

Pusztai, L., Anderson, K., and Hess, K.R. 2007. Pharmacogenomic predictor discovery in phase II clinical trials for breast cancer. *Clin Cancer Res* 13: 6080–6086.

Radmacher, M.D., McShane, L.M., and Simon, R. 2002. A paradigm for class prediction using gene expression profiles. *J Comput Biol* 9: 505–511.

Ripley, B.D. 1996. *Pattern Recognition and Neural Networks*. New York: Cambridge University Press.

Saeys, Y., Inza, I., and Larrañaga, P. 2007. A review of feature selection techniques in bioinformatics. *Bioinformatics* 23: 2507–2517.

Schumacher, M., Hollander, N., Schwarzer, G., Binder, H., and Sauerbrei W. 2012. Prognostic factor studies. In Crowley J.J. and Hoering A. (eds.) *Handbook of Statistics in Clinical Oncology*, 3rd ed. Boca Raton, FL: CRC Press, pp. 415–469.

Shi, L., Campbell, G., Jones, W.D. et al. 2010. The MicroArray Quality Control (MAQC)-II study of common practices for the development and validation of microarray-based predictive models. *Nat Biotechnol* 28: 827–838.

Simon, R. 2006. Development and evaluation of therapeutically relevant predictive classifiers using gene expression profiling. *J Natl Cancer Inst* 98: 1169–1171.

Simon, R. 2008. The use of genomics in clinical trial design. *Clin Cancer Res* 14: 5984–5993.

Simon, R., Radmacher, M.D., Dobbin, K., and McShane, L.M. 2003. Pitfalls in the use of DNA microarray data for diagnostic and prognostic classification. *J Natl Cancer Inst* 95: 14–18.

Simon, R.M., Korn, E.L., McShane, L.M., Radmacher, M.D., Wright, G.W., and Zhao, Y. 2004. *Design and Analysis of DNA Microarray Investigations*. New York: Springer.

Simon, R.M., Paik, S., and Hayes, D.F. 2009. Use of archived specimens in evaluation of prognostic and predictive biomarkers. *J Natl Cancer Inst* 101: 1446–1452.

Simon, R.M., Subramanian, J., Li, M.C., and Menezes, S. 2011. Using cross-validation to evaluate predictive accuracy of survival risk classifiers based on high-dimensional data. *Brief Bioinform* 12: 203–214.

Speed, T. 2003. *Statistical Analysis of Gene Expression Microarray Data*. Boca Raton, FL: Chapman & Hall/CRC Press.

Stone, M. 1974. Cross-validatory choice and assessment of statistical predictions. *J R Stat Soc B* 36: 111–147.

Subramanian, J. and Simon, R. 2010. Gene expression-based prognostic signatures in lung cancer: Ready for clinical use? *J Natl Cancer Inst* 102: 464–474.

Tibshirani R. 1996. Regression shrinkage and selection via the lasso. *J R Stat Soc B* 58: 267–288.

van't Veer, L.J., Dai, H., van de Vijver, M.J. et al. 2002. Gene expression profiling predicts clinical outcome of breast cancer. *Nature* 415: 530–536.

Varma, S. and Simon, R. 2006. Bias in error estimation when using cross-validation for model selection. *BMC Bioinformatics* 7: 91.

Vergouwe, Y., Steyerberg, E.W., Eijkemans, M.J., and Habbema, J.D. 2005. Substantial effective sample sizes were required for external validation studies of predictive logistic regression models. *J Clin Epidemiol* 58: 475–483.

Wessels, L.F., Reinders, M.J., Hart, A.A. et al. 2005. A protocol for building and evaluating predictors of disease state based on microarray data. *Bioinformatics* 21: 3755–3762.

13

Univariate Analysis for Gene Screening: Beyond the Multiple Testing

Hisashi Noma and Shigeyuki Matsui

CONTENTS

13.1 Introduction

This chapter provides an overview of the statistical methods used in genome-wide screening of relevant genomic features or genes. The gene screening can help in deeper understanding of disease biology at the molecular level, possibly leading to discovery of new molecular targets for developing new treatments. In many gene screening studies, a particular biological or clinical phonotypic variable, such as those representing different types of disease, prognosis, or responsiveness to a treatment, is associated with genomic data for a group of samples. The most common approach to such a gene screening study is to apply multiple univariate analysis based on separate statistical tests for individual genes to test the null hypothesis of no association with the clinical variable (Parmigiani et al. 2003; Simon et al. 2003; Speed 2003; McLachlan et al. 2004).

One major limitation of the multiple testing in gene screening studies is related to the diversion from the multiple testing methodologies employed in confirmatory studies where strict control of false positives is critical. Although the adaptations of these methodologies to exploratory, gene screening studies are meaningful in terms of the use of less stringent criteria for false positives, such as false discovery rate (FDR), relatively less attention has been directed toward the control of true positives. In particular, a framework that facilitates the choice of an appropriate threshold point for gene screening, taking the balance between true positive and false positive into account, would be more relevant for gene screening analysis. Useful analytical tools in such a framework include a receiver operating characteristics (ROC) curve analysis that plots an estimated true-positive rate (or power) versus FDR. Importantly, this type of analysis can directly contribute to the sample size determinations of future screening studies, as current screening studies generally suffer from serious lack of power.

The gene screening can also contribute to identifying genes that are useful for developing genomic signatures in subsequent studies with an established clinical platform, such as a quantitative polymerase chain reaction (PCR) platform (see Strategy A-1 in Chapter 12 of this volume). Although discovery of a novel gene simply associated with a clinical variable is relevant for understanding disease biology, this does not necessarily contribute to developing signatures with good accuracy in predicting the clinical variable. Another, but more relevant criterion is to select a gene with a strong association or large effect size that would generally more contribute to improving predictive accuracy significantly over that of existing clinical diagnostics (e.g., Hess et al. 2011; Matsui and Noma 2011b). This warrants the estimation of effect sizes, in addition to the assessment of statistical significance. Estimates of effect sizes may also be helpful in interpreting biological or clinical significance of selected genes in understanding disease biology. In addition, in two-class prediction, we can assess predictive or classification accuracy for a subset of genes using unbiased estimates of gene-specific effect sizes and correlations among genes (see Section 13.5). This type of analysis can bridge a gap between multiple univariate analysis and prediction analysis.

Empirical Bayes approaches with hierarchical mixture models can provide a relevant framework for gene screening analysis. An advantage of using such model-based approaches is that, through borrowing the strength across genes, they can provide more efficient multiple tests in comparison to traditional multiple tests without information sharing across genes. More importantly, with empirical Bayes approaches, we can accurately estimate the strength of *signal* contained in the data, represented by parameters such as the proportion of *nonnull* genes that are associated with the clinical variable and the effect size distribution for nonnull genes. Based on the estimates of these parameters, we can derive various analytical tools useful for gene screening, including the ROC curve and estimates of effect sizes for individual genes, as well as classification accuracy based on a subset of selected genes. The empirical Bayes estimation can work well for high-dimensional genomic data with a large quantity of parallel data structures. This is in contrast to other analyses in genomic studies, such as multiple testing or classification/prediction, as they generally suffer from serious false positives or overfitting problems in high dimensions.

This chapter is organized as follows. We outline multiple testing and related model-based methods in Section 13.2. We then focus on empirical Bayes approaches with hierarchical mixture models and effect size estimation in Section 13.3. We present ROC curve analysis and sample size determination in Section 13.4, and the assessment of classification accuracy in Section 13.5. A brief note on the framework for ranking and selection is provided in Section 13.6. We present concluding remarks in Section 13.7.

The majority of our discussion in this chapter will refer to the development of gene expression signatures and use of high-throughput DNA microarrays. Many of the underlying methodological principles will also apply to other types of genomic data, such as single-nucleotide polymorphism genotyping, copy number proofing, and proteomic profiling data. For illustration, we will use the following two examples of microarray gene expression studies in oncology.

13.1.1 Breast Cancer Example

Because invasion into axillary lymph nodes is the most important prognostic factor in breast cancer, diagnosis of lymph node status is important for the accurate prediction of disease course and recurrence of breast cancer. Huang et al. (2003) collected 89 tumor samples from breast cancer patients to compare their gene expressions on the basis of clinical parameters and outcomes. Among the 89 samples, the distributions of lymph node status, with numbers of positive nodes in parentheses, were 19 (0), 52 (1–3), and 18 (>10). The authors first correlated gene expression data with the status of lymph node metastasis in 37 tumor samples, including 19 that were lymph node–negative and 18 with at least 10 positive nodes. The gene expression data for each sample comprised the normalized signal intensity values from 12,625 probe sets.

13.1.2 Prostate Cancer Example

Setlur et al. (2008) constructed complementary DNA-mediated annealing, selection, ligation, and extension assay panels for discovery of molecular signatures relevant to prostate cancer in archived biopsy samples from 455 patients. They prioritized 6144 transcriptionally informative genes based on the results of previous studies. The purpose of this study was to identify the gene signature of the transmembrane protease, serine 2-v-ets erythroblastosis virus E26 oncogene homolog (TMPRSS2-ERG) fusion, which is known to be associated with the aggressiveness of prostate cancer. Before building partitioning and classification models of TMPRSS2-ERG fusion as attempted in Setlur et al. (2008), we focused on screening those genes associated with the status of TMPRSS2-ERG fusion using 103 of the samples with TMPRSS2-ERG fusion and 352 of the other samples.

13.2 Multiple Testing and Related Model-Based Methods

We suppose a two-class comparison based on normalized expression data (log signals from oligonucleotide arrays or log-ratios from two-color spotted cDNA arrays). Let n be the total number of samples, and n_1 and n_2 be the number of samples in classes 1 and 2, respectively, so that $n = n_1 + n_2$. For a pool of m genes, separate statistical tests are conducted for each gene to compare expression levels between the two classes. Typically, for gene j, the two-sample t-statistic is calculated, $T_j = \left(\hat{\mu}_j^{(1)} - \hat{\mu}_j^{(2)}\right) / (\tau_{n,\phi}\hat{\sigma}_j)$ $(j = 1,\ldots, m)$. Here $\hat{\mu}_j^{(1)}$ and $\hat{\mu}_j^{(2)}$ are the mean expression levels for classes 1 and 2, respectively, and $\hat{\sigma}_j$ is a pooled estimate of the within-class standard deviation for gene j $(j = 1,\ldots, m)$. The sample size term $\tau_{n,\phi}^2 = n/(n_1 n_2)$ involves the proportion of class 1, $\phi = n_1/n$, such that $\tau_{n,\phi}^2 = 1/\{n\phi(1-\phi)\}$. Let p_j denote a p-value from the test for gene j $(j = 1,\ldots, m)$. The results of the m tests can be summarized as a contingency table as shown in Table 13.1. Note that whether the null or alternative status is true is unknown for each gene.

13.2.1 False Discovery Rate (FDR)

A long-standing definition of statistical significance for multiple hypothesis tests involves the probability of making one or more Type I errors among the family of hypothesis tests, called the *family-wise error rate* (FWER), defined as

$$\text{FWER} = \Pr(V \geq 1).$$

TABLE 13.1

Possible Outcomes from m Hypothesis Tests

	Significant	Not Significant	Total
Null true	V	U	m_0
Alternative true	S	T	m_1
	R	W	m

The FWER has traditionally been employed in clinical trials with the aim of confirming the efficacy of treatments (e.g., Westfall and Young 1993). The Bonferroni procedure is the simplest approach to control the FWER. More efficient procedures can be developed by using multivariate permutation methods that permute the class labels to take correlation between genes into account (Westfall and Young 1993; Dudoit and vander Laan 2007). However, the criterion of controlling the FWER is generally very conservative for testing a large number of hypotheses in genome-wide screening.

Soric (1989) proposed another framework for quantifying the statistical significance of multiple hypothesis tests based on the proportion of Type I errors among all hypothesis tests declared statistically significant. Specifically, Benjamini and Hochberg (1995) defined the FDR as

$$\mathrm{FDR} = E\left[\frac{V}{R \vee 1}\right] = E\left[\frac{V}{R}\middle| R > 0\right]\Pr(R > 0), \tag{13.1}$$

where $R \vee 1 = \max(R, 1)$. The effect of $R \vee 1$ in the denominator of the first expectation is to set $V/R = 0$ when $R = 0$. The FDR offers a less stringent criterion for false positives than the FWER, thus a more acceptable criterion for gene screening. There are some variants of the FDR, including the *positive false discovery rate* (pFDR) and the *marginal false discovery rate* (mFDR) (Benjamini and Hochberg 1995; Storey 2002, 2003);

$$\mathrm{pFDR} = E\left[\frac{V}{R}\middle| R > 0\right], \quad \mathrm{mFDR} = \frac{E[V]}{E[R]}.$$

Note that $\mathrm{pFDR} = \mathrm{mFDR} = 1$ whenever all null hypotheses are true, whereas FDR can always be made arbitrarily small because of the extra term $\Pr(R > 0)$. However, in general, when the number of hypothesis tests m is particularly large, as is the case in genome-wide screening, the FDR measures are all similar, and thus, the distinction between these measures is not crucial (Storey 2002, 2003; Storey and Tibshirani 2003; Tsai et al. 2003).

13.2.2 Control and Estimation of the FDR

Two major FDR-based approaches have been proposed. The first one is to fix the acceptable FDR level beforehand and find a data-dependent threshold, so that the FDR is less than or equal to a prespecified level. This approach is called *FDR control* (Benjamini and Hochberg 1995; Shaffer 1995). Benjamini and Hochberg (1995) proposed the following algorithm to control the FDR at the level of α. For the ordered p-values of the m-tests, $p_{(1)} \le \cdots \le p_{(m)}$, the quantity $\hat{k} = \max\{1 \le k \le m; p_{(k)} \le \alpha \cdot k/m\}$ is calculated, and then the null hypotheses corresponding to $p_{(1)} \le \cdots \le p_{(k)}$ are rejected. We refer to this method as the BH method. For other algorithms for FDR control, see Benjamini and Liu (1999), Benjamini and Hochberg (2000), and Benjamini and Yekutieli (2001).

The second approach is to fix the p-value threshold at a particular value and then form an appropriate point estimate of the FDR whose expectation is greater than or equal to the true FDR at that particular threshold (Storey 2002, 2003; Storey et al. 2004). This approach is more flexible in practice, because it is often difficult to specify the level of FDR before exploratory gene screening analysis. Let FDR(t) denote the FDR when calling null hypotheses significant whenever $p_j \le t$, for $j=1, 2,\ldots, m$. For $t \in (0, 1)$, we also define random variables $V(t)$ and $R(t)$ based on the notation in Table 13.1 as the number of false positives and the number of significant null hypotheses, respectively. Using these terms, we have

$$\mathrm{FDR}(t) = E\left[\frac{V(t)}{R(t) \vee 1}\right].$$

For fixed t, Storey (2002) provided a conservative point estimator of FDR(t),

$$\tilde{\mathrm{FDR}}(t) = \frac{\tilde{m}_0(\lambda)\cdot t}{[R(t) \vee 1]},$$

where $\tilde{m}_0(\lambda)$ is an estimate of m_0, the number of true null hypotheses. Specifically, $\tilde{m}_0(\lambda) = \{m - R(\lambda)\}/(1-\lambda)$ using a tuning parameter λ. This is a reasonable estimate when most of the p-values near 1 are null. When the p-values corresponding to the true null hypotheses are distributed on Uniform(0, 1), $E[\tilde{m}_0(\lambda)] \ge m_0$. Storey and Tibshirani (2003) provided a method for selecting a parameter-free m_0 estimator by smoothing over $\tilde{m}_0(\lambda)$. We refer to this FDR-estimation method as the ST method. Other estimators of m_0 or $\pi = m_0/m$ have been proposed to estimate FDR(t) in an unbiased manner (Langaas et al. 2005; Pounds 2006; see also Sections 13.2.3 and 13.3).

In conventional single hypothesis testing, it is common to report p-values as a measure of statistical significance. Storey (2002, 2003) proposed the *q-value* for an FDR-based measure of statistical significance that can be calculated simultaneously for multiple tests. Intuitively, it seems that the q-value should capture the FDR incurred when the significance threshold is set at the p-value itself (monotonically varies corresponding to the p-value). However, unlike Type I error rates in single hypothesis testing, the FDR does not necessarily monotonically increase with an increasing significance threshold. For accommodating this property, the q-value is defined to be the minimum pFDR at which the test is called significant, $q\text{-value}(t) = \min_{t \ge p_j} p\mathrm{FDR}(t)$. For estimating the q-value, a naïve plug-in estimate is formulated as $\hat{q}\text{-value}(t) = \min_{t \ge p_j} \hat{\mathrm{FDR}}(t)$ when m is large.

Multiple testing methods generally suffer from serious lack of power in high dimensions. One promising analytical approach for improving the power of multiple testing is to borrow the strength across genes (see Sections 13.2.3 and 13.3). Another direction is to use an optimal test that maximizes the expected number of true positives for a given expected number of false positives called the *optimal discovery procedure* (Storey 2007; Noma and Matsui 2012). However, the most effective approach for controlling power or true positives would be determination of the number of biological replicates at the design stage of gene screening studies (see Section 13.4 for sample size determination).

13.2.3 Model-Based Approach

The model-based approach utilizes information sharing across genes by assuming exchangeability across comparable genes and particular data structures across genes. One commonly assumed structure is a finite mixture model with two components; one of these represents *null* genes with no association with the clinical variable and the other represents *nonnull* genes with association. As an example of mixture models for gene-level summary statistics, we consider modeling of the statistic, $Y_j = \left(\hat{\mu}_j^{(1)} - \hat{\mu}_j^{(2)}\right)/\hat{\sigma}_j$ that estimates the standardized mean difference between the two classes, $\delta_j = \left(\mu_j^{(1)} - \mu_j^{(2)}\right)/\sigma_j$, as the effect-size parameter. We assume the following mixture model for the distribution of Y_j,

$$f(y) = \pi f_0(y) + (1-\pi) f_1(y), \tag{13.2}$$

where f_0 and f_1 are the density functions of Y for null and nonnull genes, respectively, and null or nonnull genes occur with prior probabilities of π or $1 - \pi$, respectively.

Under this model, a *Bayesian FDR* can be defined (Efron and Tibshirani 2002). Specifically, when detecting nonnull genes with negative effects $\delta_j < 0$, the FDR measure for a threshold y is defined as

$$\begin{aligned} \text{FDR}(y) &= \frac{\pi F_0(y)}{F(y)} \\ &= \text{Prob}\{\text{gene } j \text{ is null} \mid Y_j \le y\}, \end{aligned} \tag{13.3}$$

where F_0 and F are the cumulative distribution functions (CDFs) corresponding to f_0 and f, respectively. For large $R = \#\{Y_j \le y\}$, the FDR(y) will be close to the original FDR defined in (13.1) (Genovese and Wasserman 2002; Storey 2003). As a related quantity, the *local* FDR at point y can be defined as $\ell\text{FDR}(y) = \pi f_0(y)/f(y) = \text{Prob}\{\text{gene } j \text{ is null} \mid Y_j = y\}$ (Efron et al. 2001; Efron and Tibshirani 2002). These quantities are connected as

$$\mathrm{FDR}(y) = \frac{\int_{-\infty}^{y} \ell\mathrm{FDR}(y) f(y)\,dy}{\int_{-\infty}^{y} f(y)\,dy}$$

$$= E_f\{\ell\mathrm{FDR}(y) \mid Y \leq y\}. \tag{13.4}$$

In other words, FDR(y) is a conditional average of ℓFDR(y) with respect to f for $\{Y \leq y\}$.

Various model-based methods have been proposed. Some methods have led to modified statistics using more stable estimates of the variance component. Baldi and Long (2001) considered a Bayesian model with a conjugate inverse gamma prior for a gene-specific variance of gene expression, and yielded a modified t-statistic for gene j with a variance component that combines the naïve variance estimate $\hat{\sigma}_j^2$ and a variance estimate from genes whose expression levels are similar to those of gene j. Lönnstedt and Speed (2002) considered an empirical Bayes method with a similar hierarchical model, and defined a log odds on the posterior probability of nonnull for each gene as a statistic for gene ranking. Smyth (2004) extended their approach in the context of general linear models. Other related model-based methods include those of Wright and Simon (2003), Cui et al. (2005), and Tong and Wang (2007).

The popular significance analysis of microarrays (SAM) method (Tusher et al. 2001) employs another modified t-statistic with a different variance component, $T_j^* = \left(\hat{\mu}_j^{(1)} - \hat{\mu}_j^{(2)}\right) / \left(\tau_{n,\phi}\hat{\sigma}_j + c_0\right)$. The constant c_0 is chosen to make the coefficient of variation of T_j^* approximately constant as a function of $\hat{\sigma}_j$ without specifying a particular parametric model for information sharing across genes. In estimating the FDR, a permutation method that permutes the class labels is applied to obtain a distribution of T_j^* under the complete null hypothesis of $m_0 = m$, thus yielding a conservative estimate of the FDR.

Efron et al. (2001) and Efron and Tibshirani (2002) proposed an empirical Bayes nonparametric method. They modeled a gene-level score, $Z_j = \Phi^{-1}(F_{t,n-2}(T_j))$, where $F_{t,n-2}$ is the CDF of a Student's t-distribution with $n-2$ degrees of freedom and Φ is the standard normal CDF. They assumed the mixture model for the Z-score, $h(z) = \pi h_0(z) + (1 - \pi)h_1(z)$. The marginal distribution $h(z)$ is estimated directly from the frequency distribution of z_j's based on a Poisson regression. Specifically, for binned counts of m z-values with L bins, the counts $b_k = \{\#z_j \text{ in bin } k\}$ $(k = 1,\ldots, L)$ are used to obtain the estimate $\hat{\mathbf{h}} = (\hat{h}_1,\ldots,\hat{h}_L)$ of $h(z)$ at the L bin midpoints, where $\hat{\mathbf{h}}$ is the discretized maximum likelihood estimate of $h(z)$ in the seven-parameter exponential family defined by the natural spline basis. The null distribution h_0 is specified by $N(0, 1^2)$ as the *theoretical* null distribution or by $N(\eta_0, \tau_0^2)$ as an *empirical* null distribution. Some procedures have been proposed to estimate the empirical null distribution (Efron 2010). Then, these estimates are used to estimate the ℓFDR(z) and FDR(z) in (13.4). The aforementioned procedures can be implemented in the R package `locfdr` (Efron 2010) or `fdrtool` (Strimmer 2008; see Table 13.2). We refer to this FDR estimation method as the Locfdr method.

Other methods for modeling gene-level statistics include that of McLachlan et al. (2006), who proposed a normal mixture model of another score, $S_j = \Phi^{-1}(1 - P_j)$ using a two-sided p-value, $P_j = 2\{1 - F_{t,n-2}(|T_j|)\}$, when one wishes for only large positive values of the score that are consistent with large effect sizes, without regard to the sign of the effect size δ_j. Matsui and Noma (2011a,b) proposed an empirical Bayes method with semiparametric hierarchical mixture models for Y_j and S_j (see also Section 13.3). Alternatively, some authors considered direct specification of the p-value, for example, a uniform distribution as a theoretical null and a beta distribution as a nonnull distribution (Pounds and Morris 2003).

Another category of model-based approaches is modeling inside the matrix of gene expression levels. Although such an approach can be more efficient, it requires more careful attention to the details of the data to minimize model misspecification, compared with the approaches to modeling gene-level statistics, such as Y or Z scores.

Many empirical Bayes methods have been proposed. Newton et al. (2001) employed a hierarchical gamma–gamma model in two-class comparison. Kendziorski et al. (2003) extended it to multiple class comparisons, and provided the option of using a hierarchical lognormal-normal model. These methods assume a constant coefficient of variation across genes, but this restriction can be relaxed (Lo and Gottardo 2007). Bhowmick et al. (2006) also introduced another empirical Bayes method based on a Laplace mixture model as a long-tailed alternative to the normal distribution. Newton et al. (2004) developed a more flexible approach using a semiparametric hierarchical mixture model.

Full Bayesian methods have also been proposed. Lewin et al. (2007) and Lönnstedt and Britton (2005) discussed Bayesian parametric mixture modeling. Gottardo et al. (2006) developed a robust method based on a t-distribution for the error distribution to account for outliers caused by experimental and preprocessing steps in microarray studies. Do et al. (2005) developed a nonparametric Bayesian method based on Dirichlet process mixture models. Unstructured prior models, which do not assume mixture models with the null/nonnull two-component structure, have been proposed (Lewin et al. 2006; Bochkina and Richardson 2007). Lewin et al. (2006) adopted an unstructured prior and assumed *interval null hypothesis*; they regarded genes with small effect sizes as nondifferential or null genes and used the posterior probability of nonnull for gene selection. For other Bayesian methods, see Do et al. (2006) and Dey et al. (2011).

13.2.4 Illustration

We applied multiple t-tests to the breast and prostate cancer datasets. Figure 13.1 shows histograms of two-sided p-values. For both datasets, there

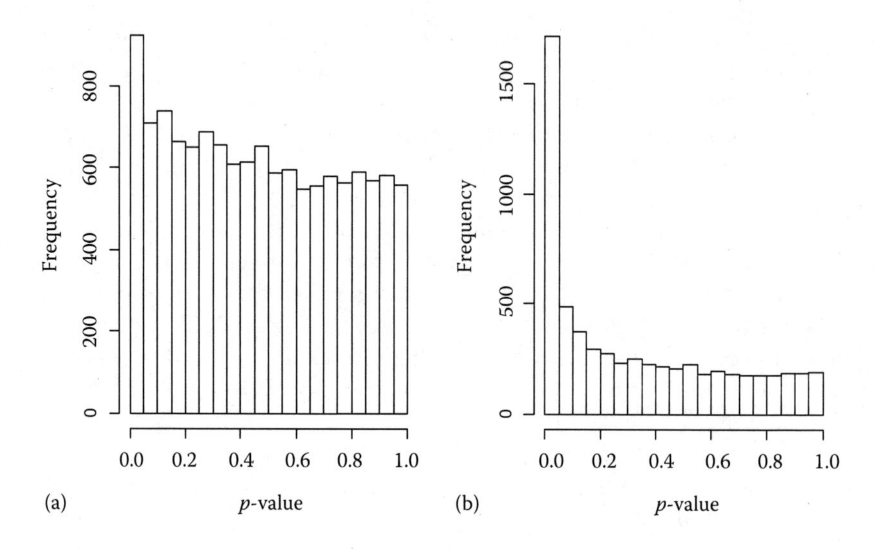

FIGURE 13.1
Histograms of two-sided p-values from multiple t-tests for (a) the breast cancer dataset and (b) the prostate cancer dataset.

was a peak at small p-values close to zero, indicating the presence of nonnull genes. The peak was clearer for the prostate cancer dataset. The estimate of the proportion of null genes, $\tilde{\pi} = \tilde{m}_0/m$, by Storey and Tibshirani (2003) (see Section 13.2.2) was 0.89 for the breast cancer dataset and 0.60 for the prostate cancer dataset, indicating a large proportion of nonnull genes for the prostate cancer dataset. This could be partly explained by the fact that the set of 6144 genes on microarrays was selected based on previous studies (Setlur et al. 2008).

The results of applying the FDR-based methods, BH, ST, SAM, and Locfdr, at FDR levels of 5% and 10%, are summarized in Table 13.2. For the breast

TABLE 13.2

Results of Multiple Testing: Numbers of Significant Genes Controlling FDR at 5% and 10%

	FDR Levels	BH[a]	ST[b]	SAM[c]	Locfdr[d]
Breast cancer	5%	0	3	44	3
	10%	5	5	81	5
Prostate cancer	5%	964	1213	973	1215
	10%	1294	1666	1442	1675

[a] `p.adjust` in `stats` package (involved as a default in R software).
[b] `qvalue`: http://www.bioconductor.org/packages/release/bioc/html/qvalue.html.
[c] `samr`: http://cran.r-project.org/web/packages/samr/index.html.
[d] `fdrtool`: http://cran.r-project.org/web/packages/fdrtool/index.html.

cancer dataset, the numbers of significant genes were generally small among all methods, except for SAM. For the prostate cancer dataset, we had much larger numbers of significant genes compared with those for the breast cancer dataset. This was also indicated by the power analysis (see Section 13.4.1). The ST and Locfdr methods detected larger numbers of genes than the other methods.

13.3 Empirical Bayes Estimation of Effect Sizes

Hierarchical mixture modeling and empirical Bayes estimation facilitate assessment of the parameters representing the relevant signal contained in the genomic data, namely, the proportion of nonnull genes and the effect size distribution for nonnull genes. We again assume the mixture model (13.2) for the gene-level statistic Y,

$$f(y) = \pi f_0(y) + (1-\pi) f_1(y),$$

and the theoretical null $N(0, \tau_{n,\phi}^2)$ for f_0. For the nonnull component, f_1, we assume the following hierarchical structure:

$$Y_j \mid \delta_j \sim N(\delta_j, \tau_{n,\phi}^2) \text{ and } \delta_j \sim g_1. \quad (13.5)$$

In the first level, given a gene-specific mean δ_j, Y_j follows a normal distribution. In the second level, the gene-specific δ_j follows a distribution g_1. Let γ_j be the indicator variable for null/nonnull status for gene j, such that $\gamma_j = 1$ if gene j is nonnull and $\gamma_j = 0$ otherwise. Note that γ_j is unknown and has the prior $P(\gamma_j = 1) = 1 - \pi$. When restricting the introduction of the effect size parameter to only nonnull genes (i.e., $\gamma_j = 1$), the posterior distribution is calculated for the nonnull genes,

$$f(\delta \mid \gamma_j = 1, y_j = y) = \frac{\varphi((\delta - y)/\tau_{n,\phi}) g_1(\delta)}{f_1(y)},$$

where $\varphi(.)$ is the density function of the standard normal distribution. As an estimate of the effect size δ_j, the posterior mean is a natural choice,

$$E(\delta \mid \gamma_j = 1, y_j = y) = \int \delta f(\delta \mid \gamma_j = 1, y_j = y) d\delta.$$

In addition, the posterior probability of being nonnull is expressed as

$$P(\gamma_j = 1 \mid y_j = y) = \frac{(1-\pi) f_1(y)}{f(y)},$$

which corresponds to one minus the local FDR, $1 - \ell\mathrm{FDR}(y)$. As a conjugation of these two posterior indices, we have the following posterior mean:

$$E(\delta \mid y_j = y) = P(\gamma_j = 1 \mid y_j = y) E(\delta \mid \gamma_j = 1, y_j = y).$$

The posterior indices can be estimated by plug-in by the estimates of hyperparameters π and g_1:

$$e_j = \hat{E}(\delta \mid \gamma_j = 1, y_j = y), \ell_j = \hat{P}(\gamma_j = 1 \mid y_j = y),$$

$$w_j = \hat{E}(\delta \mid y_j = y) = \ell_j e_j.$$

The estimate w_j adjusts for two different errors in gene selection from thousands of genes (Matsui and Noma 2011b). One type of error is the incorrect selection of null genes, and ℓ_j is used to incorporate this error. The other is overestimation of effect sizes, and the shrinkage estimate e_j is used for adjusting this bias.

As to the specification of the prior distribution g_1, we can assume either parametric or nonparametric forms. When the information on the form of g_1 is limited, the latter choice would be more reasonable. Irrespective of the type of the prior distribution, the hyperparameters can be estimated via an expectation maximization (EM) algorithm. When specifying a nonparametric g_1, its estimate can be obtained as that supported by fixed discrete mass points, as in the *smoothing-by-roughening* approach by Shen and Louis (1999) (see Matsui and Noma 2011a,b). Another empirical Bayes estimation approach is proposed by Efron (2009). See Matsui and Noma (2011b) for differences between these two approaches.

13.3.1 Illustration

For the breast cancer and prostate cancer datasets, we fit the hierarchical mixture model (13.2) and (13.5) with a nonparametric prior for g_1 by applying the smoothing-by-roughening approach (Matsui and Noma 2011a,b). The estimate of the proportion of null genes π, $\hat{\pi}$, was 0.90 for the breast cancer dataset and 0.50 for the prostate cancer dataset, again indicating a larger population of nonnull genes for the prostate cancer dataset. Figure 13.2 shows the estimates of g_1, and Figure 13.3 provides the estimates of the marginal distribution, f, fitting well to the empirical distribution (histogram) of Y_j. For both datasets, the absolute effect size estimates were below 1 for almost all of the non null genes. For the breast cancer dataset, frequencies for negative effects were higher than those for positive effects. There was a single peak

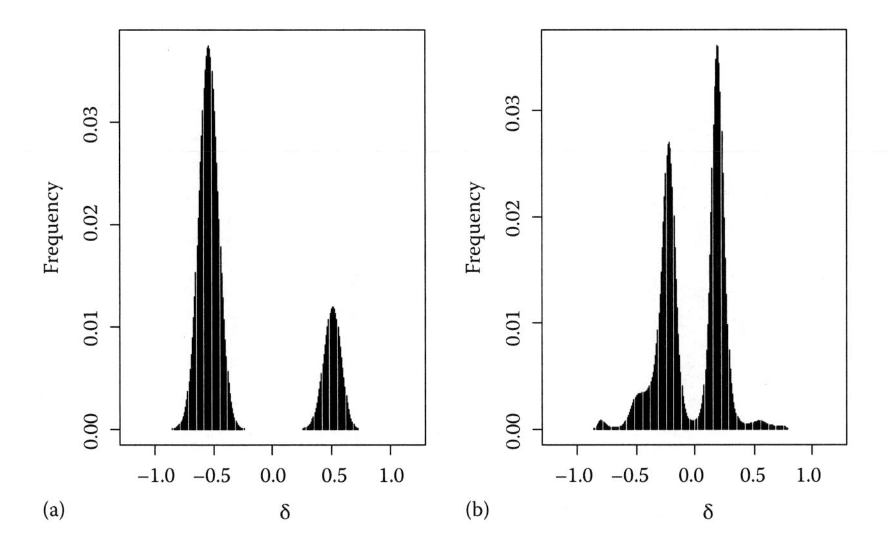

FIGURE 13.2
The nonparametric estimates of g_1 via the smoothing-by-roughing approach for (a) the breast cancer dataset and (b) the prostate cancer dataset.

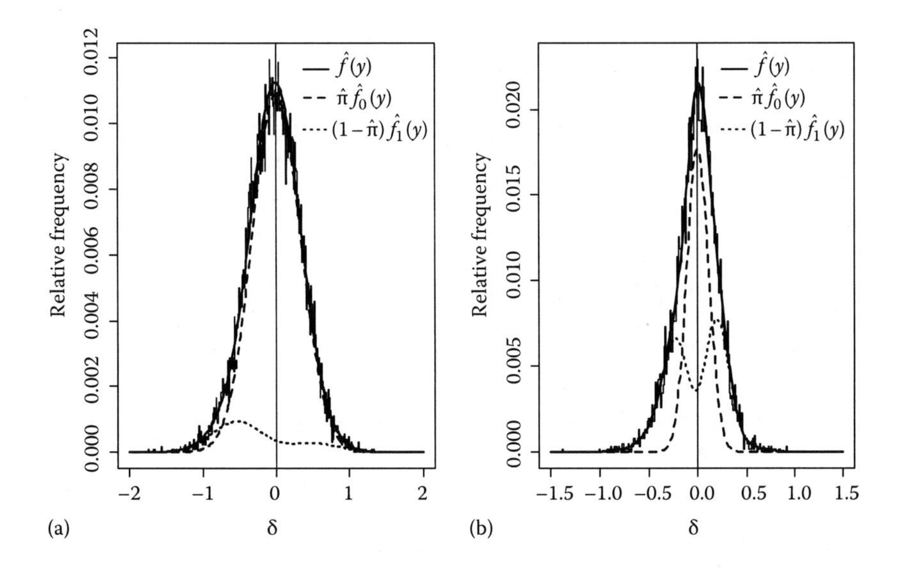

FIGURE 13.3
The estimates of the marginal distribution f and two components, πf_0 and $(1 - \pi)f_1$, for (a) the breast cancer dataset and (b) the prostate cancer dataset. The relative frequency is based on the mass points used in the smoothing-by-roughing approach.

TABLE 13.3

The Posterior Indices for Some of the Top-Ranking Genes for Breast Cancer Data and Prostate Cancer Data

Ranking	Probe	y_j	e_j	ℓ_j	w_j
Breast cancer data					
1	35428_g_at	−1.759	−0.618	0.996	−0.615
2	35622_at	−1.687	−0.613	0.993	−0.609
3	38151_at	−1.668	−0.611	0.993	−0.607
4	35707_at	−1.576	−0.605	0.988	−0.598
5	33406_at	−1.575	−0.605	0.988	−0.597
10	35834_at	−1.320	−0.589	0.951	−0.560
50	31573_at	−1.101	−0.575	0.857	−0.492
100	35156_at	−0.994	−0.568	0.773	−0.439
200	33292_at	−0.866	−0.560	0.636	−0.356
Prostate cancer data					
1	DAP2_5229	−1.386	−1.385	1.000	−1.385
2	DAP4_1042	−1.002	−0.802	1.000	−0.802
3	DAP2_5076	−0.925	−0.789	1.000	−0.789
4	DAP4_3958	−0.920	−0.788	1.000	−0.788
5	DAP4_0109	−0.898	−0.782	1.000	−0.782
10	DAP4_4250	−0.836	−0.755	1.000	−0.755
50	DAP4_0122	−0.669	−0.566	1.000	−0.566
100	DAP1_5823	−0.587	−0.481	1.000	−0.481
200	DAP1_5260	0.515	0.384	0.999	0.384

around −0.5 for negative effects and around 0.5 for positive effects. For the prostate cancer dataset, frequencies were more comparable between positive and negative effects, but the effect size estimates were more variable than those for the breast cancer dataset. Interestingly, there were multiple peaks or clusters of top genes for both negative and positive intervals of δ.

Table 13.3 summarizes posterior means as effect size estimates for top-ranking genes with the greatest values of the estimate. The posterior mean w_j entails shrinkage toward zero, compared with the naïve effect size estimate y_j. The magnitude of shrinkage was larger for the breast cancer dataset. One possible explanation for this result is the small sample size ($n=37$) compared with the prostate cancer dataset ($n=455$).

13.4 ROC Curve Analysis and Sample Size Determination

We consider a screening rule to select genes with $|Y_j| \geq c$ for a given threshold c (>0) to detect nonnull genes irrespective of the sign of effect size δ_j.

Under the hierarchical mixture models (13.2) and (13.5), the Bayesian FDR in (13.3) for a threshold c is estimated by

$$\hat{\mathrm{FDR}}(c) = \frac{\hat{\pi}\{F_0(-c) + 1 - F_0(c)\}}{\hat{F}(-c) + 1 - \hat{F}(c)},$$

where F_0 and F_1 are the CDFs of f_0 and f_1, respectively, and $\hat{F} = \hat{\pi}F_0 + (1-\hat{\pi})\hat{F}_1$ (Matsui and Noma 2011a). As an index regarding true positives in gene screening, the expected proportion of true positives or average power for all the m_1 differential genes is commonly used (e.g., Jung 2005; Shao and Tseng 2007):

$$\Psi(c) = F_1(-c) + 1 - F_1(c).$$

Note that this is an *overall* power index in that it reflects the intent to detect all of the m_1 differential genes with $\delta \neq 0$. However, in many real-life genome-wide screening studies, it would generally be difficult to achieve high levels of the overall power, $\Psi(c)$, for acceptable sample sizes. One compromise would be to consider that selection of the top nonnull genes with the largest effect sizes, which are generally deemed to be more relevant for signature development, precedes selection of the other nonnull genes with smaller effect sizes. Specifically, for the prespecified levels of effect size that one is likely to detect, η_1 (<0) and η_2 (>0) in the negative and positive intervals of δ, respectively, we consider the *partial power* for top genes with $\delta \leq \eta_1$ or $\delta \geq \eta_2$:

$$\Psi_P(c;\eta_1,\eta_2) = \frac{\int_{|u|\geq c}\int_{\delta\leq\eta_1,\delta\geq\eta_2} g_1(\delta)\varphi_{\delta,\tau_{n,\phi}^2}(u)\,d\delta du}{\int_{\delta\leq\eta_1,\delta\geq\eta_2} g_1(\delta)\,d\delta},$$

where $\varphi_{\delta,\tau_{n,\phi}^2}(\cdot)$ is the density function of the normal distribution with mean δ and variance $\tau_{n,\phi}^2$. The quantities η_1 and η_2 can represent biologically significant levels of effect size. Alternatively, they can be percentiles of the estimated effect size distribution $\hat{g}_1$ (e.g., the 10th and 90th percentiles of $\hat{g}_1$ for η_1 and η_2, respectively) or some points that segregate clusters of top genes as illustrated in the prostate cancer dataset (see Figure 13.2b). The overall and partial power indices can be estimated by plug-in by the estimates of hyperparameters π and g_1. A confidence interval for the FDR and power indices can be constructed by using a parametric bootstrap method (Matsui and Noma 2011a). The estimated ROC curves serve as a useful tool for determining an appropriate threshold point c that takes the balance of FDR and power into account.

The ROC analysis can also serve as an effective tool for determining the sample sizes of future gene screening studies. In designing a new, similar or full-scale study with sample size n^* and an arbitrary value of the sample size ratio between two classes ϕ^*, we can estimate power curves by changing from $\tau^2_{n,\phi}$ to $\tau^2_{n^*,\phi^*}$ in calculating the power curves based on the parameter estimates $\hat{\pi}$ and $\hat{g}_1$. One may search for n^* and ϕ^* that provide a desirable ROC curve with high values of power $\Psi(c)$ or $\Psi_p(c; \eta_1, \eta_2)$ for acceptably small values of FDR.

In sample size determination, accurate assessment of the *signal* contained in the data, represented by π and g_1, is crucial, because these parameters can greatly impact the sample size estimates. In many cases, given an estimate of π, such as $\tilde{\pi}$, a proportion of $(1 - \tilde{\pi})$ genes with the largest values of $|Y|$ is used to estimate g_1. However, this naive estimate using only top genes can be subject to serious overestimation due to random variation. In contrast, the framework of empirical Bayes hierarchical modeling in Section 13.3 can provide more accurate estimates of these parameters, and thus improve the performance of other methods of sample size determination (Dobbin and Simon 2005; Pawitan et al. 2005; Tsai et al. 2005; Shao and Tseng 2007; Tong and Zhao 2008).

13.4.1 Illustration

Estimated ROC curves with overall and partial power indices are given in Figure 13.4. Generally, the power indices for the prostate cancer dataset were greater than those for the breast cancer dataset. This can be explained by the

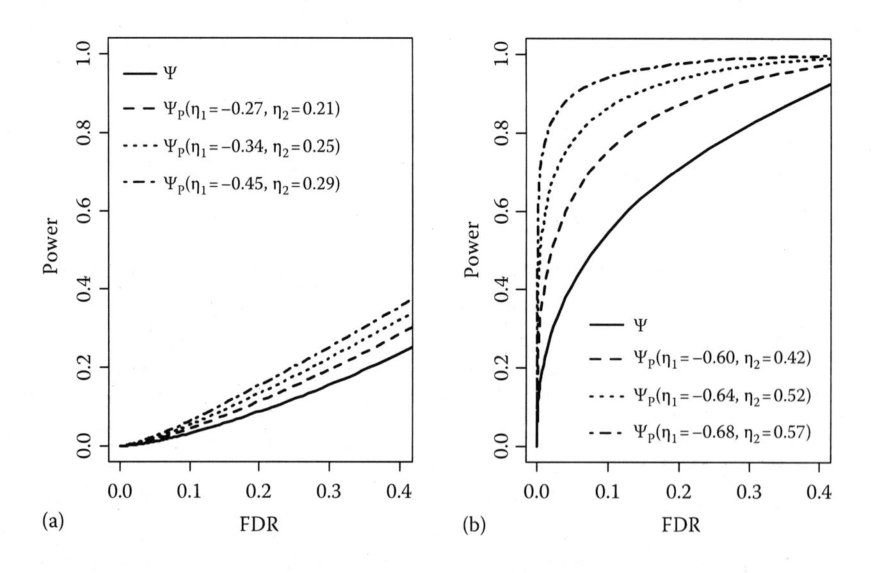

FIGURE 13.4
Plots of overall power Ψ and three plots of partial power Ψ_p for various values of the threshold c for (a) the breast cancer data and (b) the prostate cancer data.

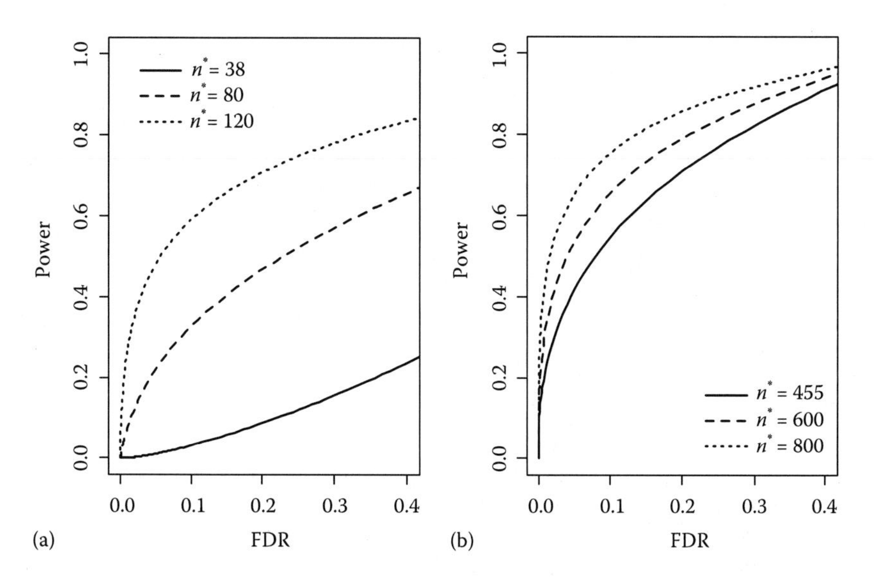

FIGURE 13.5
Plots of overall power under various sample sizes when $\phi^* = \phi$ for (a) the breast cancer data when $n^* = 38$ (=n), 80, and 120, and (b) the prostate cancer data when $n^* = 455$ (=n), 600, and 800.

larger sample size ($n = 455$) and larger estimated proportion of nonnull genes ($1 - \hat{\pi} = 0.5$) for the prostate cancer dataset. As expected, we achieved higher partial power when restricting our interest to top genes with larger effect sizes in the tail of the effect size distribution $\hat{g}_1$. Restricting to top genes impacted partial power relatively minimally for the breast cancer dataset. This can be explained by a relatively small dispersion of $\hat{g}_1$ as seen in Figure 13.2a.

With regard to sample size estimation for a future gene screening study with sample size n^* with the proportion of class 1 equal to ϕ^*, Figure 13.5 shows how the overall power improves by increasing n^* when fixing the proportion of class 1 as $\phi^* = \phi$. For the breast cancer dataset, a substantial improvement in power is expected when increasing the sample size from 38 to 80 or more. On the other hand, improvement in power is expected to be relatively small for the prostate cancer dataset. We can expect improvement of nearly 55%–75% at an FDR of 10% by increasing n^* from 455 to 800, but the size $n^* = 800$ seems to be unrealistically large for current gene screening studies using microarrays.

13.5 Assessment of Classification Accuracy

When candidate genes that may pass through to the clinical platform are identified, possibly incorporating biological perspectives and knowledge from previous correlative studies, it is worthwhile to assess whether classification or prediction using a candidate subset of selected genes is in fact promising or worth using in progression to subsequent phases of genomic signature development. A wide variety of standard classification or prediction methods (e.g., Hastie et al. 2009) are applicable for relatively small numbers of the variable (gene) after gene selection. However, with this approach, an independent test sample would generally be needed to assess the accuracy of prediction.

For binary classification, a misclassification rate can be estimated based on shrinkage estimates w_j of the standardized effect size δ_j of selected genes in the framework of the empirical Bayes approach with the hierarchical models in Section 13.3 (Efron 2009; Matsui and Noma 2011b). Let Ω represent a gene set for which one would like to assess the prediction ability. For an individual sample i, the gene expression data from m genes consist of $X_i = (X_{i1}, X_{i2}, \ldots, X_{im})$. We use the standardized expression levels, $Z_{ij} = (X_{ij} - \hat{\mu}_j)/\hat{\sigma}_j$, for gene j in Ω, where $\hat{\mu}_j = \left(\hat{\mu}_j^{(1)} - \hat{\mu}_j^{(2)}\right)/2$. Then, for a new sample i^*, we consider the following diagonal linear discriminant classifier:

$$C_{i^*} = \sum_{j \in \Omega} w_j Z_{i^* j}.$$

The sample is assigned to class 1 if $C_{i^*} > 0$ and to class 2 otherwise. The probability of correct classification (PCC) is estimated as

$$\hat{\text{PCC}} = \Phi\left(\frac{\mathbf{w}'\mathbf{w}}{2\sqrt{\mathbf{w}'\mathbf{R}\mathbf{w}}}\right), \quad (13.6)$$

where

w is a column vector of the coefficient w_j

R is an estimate of the within-class correlation matrix of expression levels for all genes in Ω

Efron (2009) considered prediction using top genes with the greatest effect sizes based on (13.6). The shrunken centroids procedure (Tibshirani et al. 2002) is another approach using a shrinkage estimate, where the shrinkage size is determined on the basis of cross-validated predictive accuracy. One advantage of using the empirical Bayes approach with (13.6) is its smaller estimation error, compared with highly variable, cross-validated prediction analyses. Another important advantage of the approach with (13.6) is that we can estimate the predictive accuracy of any gene sets, possibly those selected on the basis of biological perspectives. In contrast, cross-validated prediction analyses cannot handle complex gene selection processes incorporating biological information, because it needs some defined algorithm for gene selection, typically, selection of top-ranking genes (Simon et al. 2003).

Lastly, as internal validation, the empirical Bayes method with (13.6) directly estimates predictive accuracy when a completely specified classifier C_{i^*} with a particular weight **w** (estimated using the entire dataset) for a given set of genes is applied to the entire study samples. In contrast, the standard classification approach entails sample splitting for training and testing, but accuracy estimates are usually interpreted as those pertaining to the classifier that would be obtained through applying the same feature selection and classification algorithms to the entire samples for convenience.

13.5.1 Illustration

Figure 13.6 shows $\hat{PCC}$ based on the (shrinkage) effect-size estimates w_j shown in Table 13.3 for top-ranked genes. The estimated predictive accuracy was generally insensitive to the number of selected genes when 20 or more genes were used for prediction. The predictive accuracy for the prostate cancer dataset was slightly better than for the breast cancer dataset. For example, using the top 50 genes, $\hat{PCC}=0.74$ for the breast cancer dataset and $\hat{PCC}=0.80$ for the prostate cancer dataset. Of note, comparable cross-validated estimates of PCC (or misclassification rate) were obtained by applying various machine learning methods for the prostate cancer dataset (see Chapter 14).

The estimation approach with (13.6) allows for the evaluation of gene subsets selected on the basis of biological perspectives. For the breast cancer

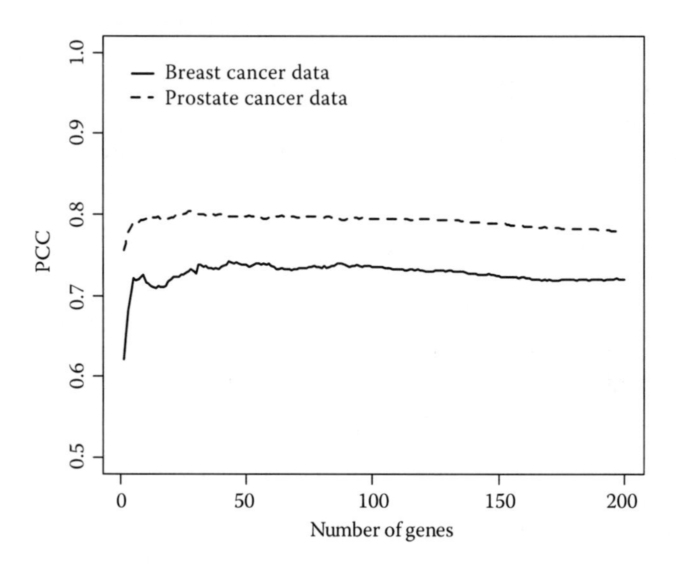

FIGURE 13.6
Plots of PCC estimates versus number of selected top-ranked genes for the breast cancer and prostate cancer datasets.

dataset, after an initial screening of top genes, we selected 35 genes with different functional aspects possibly involved in the metastatic process of breast cancer, including cell–cell signaling, cell death, cell growth, cell proliferation, kinase activity, metabolism, signal transduction, and regulation of transcription. For this set of genes, $\widehat{PCC}$ was calculated as 0.73. One may also include other interesting metastatic genes reported in previous correlative studies of breast cancer.

13.6 Gene Ranking and Selection

As gene ranking has been commonly performed as an essential part of the output of gene screening analysis, assessment of gene ranking methods is particularly important. For two-class comparison, some studies have reported that gene ranking based on the fold change, which corresponds to the difference in mean expression levels between two classes, is *reproducible* among gene rankings based on various univariate statistics for real datasets from several microarray studies (e.g., MAQC Consortium 2006). However, a reproducible gene ranking does not necessarily have to be *accurate* in selecting genes with larger effect sizes. Actually, some simulation studies have shown that gene ranking based on simple univariate statistics, such as the fold change, is not necessarily accurate, particularly in small or moderate sample settings (Noma et al. 2010; Noma and Matsui 2013).

Recently, more accurate methods based on hierarchical mixture models such as (13.2) and (13.5) have been proposed (Noma et al. 2010; Noma and Matsui 2013). These methods considered several criteria of ranking accuracy in the framework of empirical Bayes ranking and selection (Laird and Louis 1989; Lin et al. 2006), including minimizing mean squared errors of estimation for ranks of effect size parameters and maximizing sensitivity in selecting a fixed number of nonnull genes with the largest effect sizes. The ranking and selection framework, which is used to rank genes based on effect sizes and to select a *fixed* number of top-ranking genes with the largest effect sizes, can be a more relevant approach to incorporate the limitation in the number of genes that can be investigated in subsequent studies based on established clinical platforms (Pepe et al. 2003; Matsui et al. 2008).

13.7 Concluding Remarks

In this chapter, we have discussed various statistical methods for gene screening in the context of genomic signature development. The high dimensionality of genomic data has posed special difficulties in extracting a small fraction of relevant signals in the presence of a large quantity of noise variables. We have therefore stressed the importance of assessing the strength of signals contained in the genomic data, represented by parameters such as the proportion of nonnull genes and the effect size distribution for nonnull genes, for the design and analysis of successful gene screening studies. Hierarchical mixture modeling and empirical Bayes estimation can provide an effective framework for this assessment. In addition, various useful tools for gene screening analysis can be derived from this framework. From these perspectives, we can recognize the gene screening analysis as *estimation and selection,* rather than just applying multiple tests.

With the empirical Bayes approach with hierarchical mixture models, it would be worthwhile to clarify the strength of the signals in past gene screening studies. This is to quantitatively assess the promise of genomic signature development and provide a useful guidance for designing and analyzing future gene screening studies.

References

Baldi, P. and Long, A.D. 2001. A Bayesian framework for the analysis of microarray expression data: Regularized *t*-test and statistical inferences of gene changes. *Bioinformatics* 17: 509–519.

Benjamini, Y. and Hochberg, Y. 1995. Controlling the false discovery rate—A practical and powerful approach to multiple testing. *Journal of the Royal Statistical Society, Series B* 57: 289–300.

Benjamini, Y. and Hochberg, Y. 2000. On the adaptive control of the false discovery rate in multiple testing with independent statistics. *Journal of Educational and Behavioral Statistics* 25: 60–83.

Benjamini, Y. and Liu, W. 1999. A step-down multiple hypothesis procedure that controls the false discovery rate under independence. *Journal of Statistical Planning and Inference* 82: 163–170.

Benjamini, Y. and Yekutieli, D. 2001. The control of the false discovery rate in multiple testing under dependency. *Annals of Statistics* 29: 1165–1188.

Bhowmick, D., Davison, A.C., Goldstein, D.R., and Ruffieux, Y. 2006. A Laplace mixture model for identification of differential expression in microarray experiments. *Biostatistics* 7: 630–641.

Bochkina, N. and Richardson, S. 2007. Tail posterior probability for inference in pairwise and multiclass gene expression data. *Biometrics* 63: 1117–1125.

Cui, X.G., Hwang, J.T.G., Qiu, J., Blades, N.J., and Churchill, G.A. 2005. Improved statistical tests for differential gene expression by shrinking variance components estimates. *Biostatistics* 6: 59–75.

Dey, D.K., Ghosh, S., and Mallick, B.K. (eds.) 2011. *Bayesian Modeling in Bioinformatics*. Boca Raton, FL: CRC Press.

Do, K.-A., Müller, P., and Tang, F. 2005. A Bayesian mixture model for differential gene expression. *Journal of the Royal Statistical Society, Series C* 54: 627–644.
Do, K.-A., Müller, P., and Vannucci, M. (eds.) 2006. *Bayesian Inference for Gene Expression and Proteomics*. New York: Cambridge University Press.
Dobbin, K. and Simon, R. 2005. Sample size determination in microarray experiments for class comparison and prognostic classfication. *Biostatistics* 6: 27–38.
Dudoit, S. and van der Laan, M.J. 2007. *Multiple Testing Procedures with Applications to Genomics*. New York: Springer.
Efron, B. 2009. Empirical Bayes estimates for large-scale prediction problems. *Journal of the American Statistical Association* 104: 1015–1028.
Efron, B. 2010. *Large-Scale Inference: Empirical Bayes Methods for Estimation, Testing, and Prediction*. New York: Cambridge University Press.
Efron, B. and Tibshirani, R. 2002. Empirical Bayes methods and false discovery rates for microarrays. *Genetic Epidemiology* 23: 70–86.
Efron, B., Tibshirani, R., Storey, J.D., and Tusher, V. 2001. Empirical Bayes analysis of a microarray experiment. *Journal of the American Statistical Association* 96: 1151–1160.
Genovese, C. and Wasserman, L. 2002. Operating characteristics and extensions of the false discovery rate procedure. *Journal of the Royal Statistical Society, Series B* 64: 499–517.
Gottardo, R., Raftery, A.E., Yeung, K.Y., and Bumgarner, R.E. 2006. Bayesian robust inference for differential gene expression in microarrays with multiple samples. *Biometrics* 62: 10–18.
Hastie, T., Tibshirani, R., and Friedman, J. 2009. *The Elements of Statistical Learning: Data Mining, Inference, and Prediction*, 2nd ed. New York: Springer.
Hess, K.R., Wei, C., Qi, Y. et al. 2011. Lack of sufficiently strong informative features limits the potential of gene expression analysis as predictive tool for many clinical classification problems. *BMC Bioinformatics* 12: 463.
Huang, E., Cheng, S.H., Dressman, H. et al. 2003. Gene expression predictors of breast cancer outcomes. *Lancet* 361: 1590–1596.
Jung, S.H. 2005. Sample size for FDR-control in microarray data analysis. *Bioinformatics* 21: 3097–3104.
Kendziorski, C.M., Newton, M.A., Lan, H., and Gould, M.N. 2003. On parametric empirical Bayes methods for comparing multiple groups using replicated gene expression profiles. *Statistics in Medicine* 22: 3899–3914.
Laird, N.M. and Louis, T.A. 1989. Empirical Bayes ranking methods. *Journal of Educational Statistics* 14: 29–46.
Langaas, M., Lindqvist, B.H., and Ferkingstad, E. 2005. Estimating the proportion of true null hypotheses, with application to DNA microarray data. *Journal of the Royal Statistical Society, Series B* 67: 555–572.
Lönnstedt, I. and Britton, T. 2005. Hierarchical Bayes models for cDNA microarray gene expression. *Biostatistics* 6: 279–291.
Lönnstedt, I. and Speed, T. 2002. Replicated microarray data. *Statistica Sinica* 12: 31–46.
Lewin, A., Bochkina, N., and Richardson, S. 2007. Fully Bayesian mixture model for differential gene expression: Simulations and model checks. *Statistical Applications in Genetics and Molecular Biology* 6: Article 36.
Lewin, A., Richardson, S., Marshall, C., Glazier, A., and Altman, T. 2006. Bayesian modeling of differential gene expression. *Biometrics* 62: 1–9.

Lin, R., Louis, T.A., Paddock, S.M., and Ridgeway, G. 2006. Loss function based ranking in two-stage, hierarchical models. *Bayesian Analysis* 1: 915–946.

Lo, K. and Gottardo, R. 2007. Flexible empirical Bayes models for differential gene expression. *Bioinformatics* 23: 328–335.

MAQC Consortium. 2006. The MicroArray Quality Control (MAQC) project shows inter- and intraplatform reproducibility of gene expression measurements. *Nature Biotechnology* 24: 1151–1161.

Matsui, S. and Noma, H. 2011a. Estimating effect sizes of differentially expressed genes for power and sample-size assessments in microarray experiments. *Biometrics* 67: 1225–1235.

Matsui, S. and Noma, H. 2011b. Estimation and selection in high-dimensional genomic studies for developing molecular diagnostics. *Biostatistics* 12: 223–233.

Matsui, S., Zeng, S., Yamanaka, T., and Shaughnessy, J. 2008. Sample size calculations based on ranking and selection in microarray experiments. *Biometrics* 64: 217–226.

McLachlan, G.J., Bean, R.W., and Jones, L.B.T. 2006. A simple implementation of a normal mixture approach to differential gene expression in multiclass microarrays. *Bioinformatics* 22: 1608–1615.

McLachlan, G.J., Do, K.-A., and Ambroise, C. 2004. *Analyzing Microarray Gene Expression Data*. Hoboken, NJ: Wiley.

Newton, M.A., Kendziorsk, C.M., Richmond, C.S., Blattner, F.R., and Tsui, K.W. 2001. On differential variability of expression ratios: Improving statistical inference about gene expression changes from microarray data. *Journal of Computational Biology* 8: 37–52.

Newton, M.A., Noueiry, A., Sarkar, D., and Ahlquist, P. 2004. Detecting differential gene expression with a semiparametric hierarchical mixture method. *Biostatistics* 5: 155–176.

Noma, H. and Matsui, S. 2012. The opitimal discovery procedure in multiple significance testing: An empirical Bayes approach. *Statistics in Medicine* 31: 165–176.

Noma, H. and Matsui, S. 2013. Empirical Bayes ranking and selection methods via semiparametric hierarchical mixture models in microarray studies. *Statistics in Medicine*: 32: 1904–1916.

Noma, H., Matsui, S., Omori, T., and Sato, T. 2010. Bayesian ranking and selection methods using hierarchical mixture models in microarray studies. *Biostatistics* 11: 281–289.

Parmigiani, G., Garrett, E.S., Irizarry, R.A., and Zeger, S.L. 2003. *The Analysis of Gene Expression Data: Methods and Software*. New York: Springer.

Pawitan, Y., Michiels, S., Koscielny, S., Gusnanto, A., and Ploner, A. 2005. False discovery rate, sensitivity and sample size for microarary studies. *Bioinformatics* 21: 3017–3024.

Pepe, M.S., Longton, G., Anderson, G.L., and Schummer, M. 2003. Selecting differentially expressed genes from microarray experiments. *Biometrics* 59: 133–142.

Pounds, S. 2006. Estimation and control of multiple testing error rates for microarray studies. *Briefings in Bioinformatics* 7: 25–36.

Pounds, S. and Morris, S.W. 2003. Estimating the occurrence of false positives and false negatives in microarray studies by approximating and partitioning the empirical distribution of p-values. *Bioinformatics* 19: 1236–1242.

Setlur, S.R., Mertz, K.D., Hoshida, Y. et al. 2008. Estrogen-dependent signaling in a molecularly distinct subclass of aggressive prostate cancer. *Journal of the National Cancer Institute* 100: 815–825.

Shaffer, J. 1995. Multiple hypothesis testing. *Annual Review of Psychology* 46: 561–584.

Shao, Y. and Tseng, C.-H. 2007. Sample size calculation with dependence adjustment for FDR-control in microarray studies. *Statistics in Medicine* 26: 4219–4237.

Shen, W. and Louis, T.A. 1999. Empirical Bayes estimation via the smoothing by roughening approach. *Journal of Computational and Graphical Statistics* 8: 800–823.

Simon, R.M., Korn, E.L., McShane, L.M. et al. 2003. *Design and Analysis of DNA Microarray Investigations*. New York: Springer.

Smyth, G. 2004. Linear models and empirical Bayes methods for assessing differential expression in microarray experiments. *Statistical Applications in Genetics and Molecular Biology* 3: Article 3.

Soric, B. 1989. Statistical discoveries and effect-size estimation. *Journal of the American Statistical Association* 84: 608–610.

Speed, T. 2003. *Statistical Analysis of Gene Expression Microarray Data*. Boca Raton, FL: Chapman & Hall/CRC.

Storey, J.D. 2002. A direct approach to false discovery rates. *Journal of the Royal Statistical Society, Series B* 64: 479–498.

Storey, J.D. 2003. The positive false discovery rate: A Bayesian interpretation and the q-value. *Annals of Statistics* 31: 2013–2035.

Storey, J.D. 2007. The optimal discovery procedure: A new approach to simultaneous significance testing. *Journal of the Royal Statistical Society, Series B* 69: 347–368.

Storey, J.D., Taylor, J.E., and Siegmund, D. 2004. Strong control, conservative point estimation and simultaneous conservative consistency of false discovery rates: A unified approach. *Journal of the Royal Statistical Society, Series B* 66: 187–205.

Storey, J.D. and Tibshirani, R. 2003. Statistical significance for genomewide studies. *Proceedings of the National Academy of Sciences of the United States of America* 100: 9440–9445.

Strimmer, K. 2008. FDR tool: A versatile R package for estimating local and tail area-based false discovery rates. *Bioinformatics* 24: 1461–1462.

Tibshirani, R., Hastie, T., Narasimhan, B., and Chu, G. 2002. Diagnosis of multiple cancer types by shrunken centroids of gene expression. *Proceedings of the National Academy of Sciences of the United States of America* 99: 6567–6572.

Tong, T. and Wang, Y. 2007. Optimal shrinkage estimation of variances with applications to microarray data analysis. *Journal of the American Statistical Association* 102: 113–122.

Tong, T. and Zhao, H. 2008. Practical guidelines for assessing power and false discovery rate for a fixed sample size in microarray experiments. *Statistics in Medicine* 27: 1960–1972.

Tsai, C.-A., Hsueh, H.-M., and Chen, J.J. 2003. Estimation of false discovery rates in multiple testing: Application to gene microarray data. *Biometrics* 59: 1071–1081.

Tsai, C.-A., Wang, S.J., Chen, D.T., and Chan, J.J. 2005. Sample size for gene expression microarray experiments. *Bioinformatics* 21: 1502–1508.
Tusher, V.G., Tibshirani, R., and Chu, G. 2001. Significance analysis of microarrays applied to the ionizing radiation response. *Proceedings of the National Academy of Sciences of the United States of America* 98: 5116–5121.
Westfall, P.H. and Young, S.S. 1993. *Resampling-Based Multiple Testing*. New York: Wiley.
Wright, G. and Simon, R. 2003. A random variance model for detection of differential gene expression in small microarray experiments. *Bioinformatics* 19: 2448–2455.

14

Statistical and Machine-Learning Methods for Class Prediction in High Dimension

Osamu Komori and Shinto Eguchi

CONTENTS

14.1 Introduction

In recent years, the rapid progress in molecular biology and biotechnology has enabled widespread and increasing use of high-throughput technologies. These technologies, which exhaustively monitor the characteristics of biological specimens at the molecular level, include genome-wide single-nucleotide polymorphism typing, gene-expression microarrays, and protein mass spectrometry. One mission for statistics and bioinformatics is to develop novel data-learning methodologies for pattern recognition and prediction or classification through extracting useful information from these high-dimensional genomic data, and to contribute to the medical science and healthcare development through applications of these methodologies.

Traditional statistical data-learning methods, such as Fisher's linear discriminant analysis (LDA) and logistic discriminant analysis, are not directly applicable to high-dimensional genomic data with small sample sizes. In effect, the dimension p of data, the number of genomic features available, becomes much higher than the sample size n. In the statistical literature, there are very few methods that work well in this setting of $p \gg n$. Traditionally, statistical methods are discussed in the context of asymptotic properties, where n goes to ∞ for a fixed p. However, this discussion is useless for the setting of $p \gg n$. This situation motivates consideration of new ideas and approaches for developing prediction methods that might be used to tackle this problem, such as regression analysis with L_1 regularization (Efron et al. 2004; Zou and Hastie 2005; Zou et al. 2007). On the other hand, the community of machine learning has been engaged in active research in boosting methods, support vector machines (SVMs), and kernel methods in reproducing kernel Hilbert space (Hastie et al. 2009). These machine-learning methods are algorithmic and not based on stochastic models (Breiman 2001). They are more specialized to prediction or classification problems. This is in contrast to statistical data-learning methods that also allow making inference about the underlying mechanisms behind the data.

However, we must recognize that such emerging solutions for the $p \gg n$ problem are far from complete, probably reflecting the limitation of our human perception and recognition when the number of genomic features increases exponentially. Nevertheless, addressing this problem will help to promote personalized medicine through identification, association, and prediction regarding phenotypes, such as disease subtype, prognosis, treatment responsiveness, and adverse reaction. In particular, effective statistical methods and their applications for these aims are urgently required in oncology and other disease fields.

In this chapter, we outline several machine-learning approaches to the analysis of high-dimensional genomic data. We provide an overview of novel methods, such as boosting, SVMs, kernel methods, least absolute shrinkage and selection operator (Lasso), and related methods. Finally, we summarize current problems and describe an outlook for the future.

14.2 Framework of Classification

14.2.1 Classifier

Statistical pattern recognition is a direct representation for our brain to make prediction in an instinctive way. The framework is simple such that there are a vector for p features in the p-dimensional real number space $x \in \mathbb{R}^p$ and a class label or response y. Here, as a simplest problem, we confine ourselves to a two-class prediction where y is binary with values $\{-1, +1\}$. A function h of x to predict y is called a classifier. When x and y are viewed as an input and output, respectively, the classifier is also called a learner in the machine-learning community. This is typically given by a function $F(x, y)$,

$$h(x) = \underset{y \in \{-1,+1\}}{\operatorname{argmax}} \; F(x, y),$$

where $\operatorname{argmax}_{y \in \{-1, +1\}} F(x, y)$ denotes a maximizer of $F(x, y)$ with respect to y. That is, $h(x)$ takes -1 or 1. For example, $F(x, y)$ could be a log ratio of two probability densities for $y=-1$ and $y=+1$ in the LDA. When we conventionally define a discriminant function $F(x)=F(x, +1) - F(x, -1)$, the classifier reduces to

$$h(x) = \operatorname{sign} F(x), \tag{14.1}$$

where sign $F(x)$ denotes the sign of $F(x)$. Both Fisher's linear discriminant function and the logistic discriminant function have a linear form

$$F(x) = \beta^{T} x + \beta_0, \tag{14.2}$$

where β denotes a vector of parameters and β^T denotes a transpose of $\beta \in \mathbb{R}^p$.

Here Fisher's linear discriminant function is derived by the probability density functions given class label y, while the logistic discriminant function is directly given by the maximum likelihood for the probability density functions of y given x. Note that, in these discussions, the conventional setting with $p<n$ is supposed. The classifier in (14.1) can be generalized to incorporate various values of threshold for classification,

$$h_c(x) = \operatorname{sign}\{F(x) - c\}, \tag{14.3}$$

where c is a threshold value. This is to classify as $y=+1$ if $F(x)>c$ and $y=-1$ otherwise. Actually, we build the classifier h, including determination of the form of F and the parameters in F (such as β and β_0 in [14.2]) and the threshold value for classification in h_c (such as c in [14.3]) using the data from a collection of samples, called training set.

14.2.2 Assessment of Classification Performance

Classification accuracy of the built classifier can be unbiasedly assessed using an independent set of samples, called test set. When making a classification for each of n test samples using the discriminant function F and a

TABLE 14.1

Classification Results by Discriminant Function F and a Threshold c

Class Label	$F(x) > c$ (Positive)	$F(x) \leq c$ (Negative)	Total
$y = +1$	s_1	s_0	n_+
$y = -1$	r_1	r_0	n_-
Total	n_p	n_n	n

threshold c, classification results are typically summarized by the observed true class labels as a 2×2 contingency table in Table 14.1. As a simplest measure of classification accuracy, the proportion of correct classification or that of miss classification are calculated as $\text{PCC} = (s_1 + r_0)/n$ or $1 - \text{PCC} = (s_0 + r_1)/n$, respectively. We call the latter as the error rate for simplicity. The PCC is composed of the two measures, sensitivity, $Se = s_1/n_+$, and specificity, $Sp = r_0/n_-$, such that $\text{PCC} = (n_+ Se + n_- Sp)/n$.

When considering various values of threshold c for classification in (14.3), the sensitivity and specificity can be expressed as

$$Se(c) = \frac{1}{n_+} \sum_{i=1}^{n} I(F(x_i) > c) I(y_i = +1) \tag{14.4}$$

$$Sp(c) = 1 - \frac{1}{n_-} \sum_{i=1}^{n} I(F(x_i) > c) I(y_i = -1) \tag{14.5}$$

respectively. Apparently, there is a trade-off between them when changing the value of c. The ROC curve is defined as a plot of the pairs $(1 - Sp, Se)$ on the unit square as c moves in the real number space $\mathbb{R}$, $\text{ROC}(F) = \{(1 - Sp(c), Se(c)) | c \in \mathbb{R}\}$ (Green and Swets 1966; Dorfman and Alf 1969; Hanley and McNeil 1982). As a threshold-free measure of classification accuracy, the area under the ROC curve (AUC) is defined as

$$\overline{\text{AUC}}(F) = \frac{1}{n_- n_+} \sum_{i=1}^{n_-} \sum_{j=1}^{n_+} I(F(x_{+j}) > F(x_{-i})), \tag{14.6}$$

where $\{x_{-i}: i = 1, \ldots, n_-\}$ and $\{x_{+j}: j = 1, \ldots, n_+\}$ are samples for $y = -1$ and $y = +1$. Since the ROC is a curve in the unit square, its maximum value of AUC is 1, where the samples are completely separable without any misclassification. Interestingly it is equivalent to c-statistic or Mann–Whitney U statistic for $F(x)$ (Bamber 1975). The AUC has a probabilistic interpretation when both n_- and n_+ go to infinity (Bamber 1975) as

$$\text{AUC}(F) = P(F(x_+) > F(x_-)). \tag{14.7}$$

If we consider a subset of $\{x_{-i}: i = 1,\ldots, n_-\}$ such as $S_- = \{i \mid c_1 < F(x_{-i}) < c_2\}$ for some threshold values c_1 and c_2, then the partial AUC (McClish 1989) is defined as

$$\overline{\text{pAUC}}(F) = \frac{1}{n_- n_+} \sum_{i \in S_-} \sum_{j=1}^{n_+} I(F(x_{+j}) > F(x_{-i})). \tag{14.8}$$

This measure reflects different implications of *Se* and *Sp* and puts more weight on a specific range of *Sp* determined by c_1 and c_2 . In disease screening, classification with high values of *Sp* that keep false-positive rates low is generally considered more practical (Pepe 2003). We can encounter similar situations in medicine, for example, in identifying patients with a high risk of developing a relatively rare, but very serious adverse event for an effective treatment. In these cases, it would be reasonable to use pAUC for maximizing *Se* for high values of *Sp*.

14.2.3 Optimal Discriminant Function

We can consider an optimal discriminant function $F^*(x)$, which minimizes the error rate as well as maximizes sensitivity, specificity, and AUC. For a population of test samples, let $r(x, y)$ be a distribution of the data (x, y) with a decomposition

$$r(x,y) = p(y \mid x) q(x), \tag{14.9}$$

where $p(y|x)$ is a conditional distribution of y given x and $q(x)$ is a marginal distribution of x.

Then, a classifier h taking values −1 or +1 has the (expected) error rate

$$\text{err}(h) = E\{I(y \neq h(x))\},$$

where E denotes the expectation with respect to the distribution (14.9). It is known that the Bayes rule

$$h^*(x) = \text{sign}\, F^*(x), \tag{14.10}$$

where

$$F^*(x) = \frac{1}{2} \log \left\{ \frac{p(+1|x)}{p(-1|x)} \right\}, \tag{14.11}$$

minimizes the error rate (Eguchi and Copas 2006). That is, $\operatorname{argmin}_h \operatorname{err}(h) = h^*$. This property is called the Bayes risk consistency (Breiman 2000; Lugosi and Vayatis 2004). Both Fisher's linear discriminant function and the logistic discriminant function aim to satisfy the Bayes risk consistency. Inverting (14.11) leads to

$$p(y \mid x) = \frac{\exp\{yF^*(x)\}}{\exp\{F^*(x)\} + \exp\{-F^*(x)\}}. \tag{14.12}$$

If $F^*(x)$ is a linear discriminant function, then (14.12) has the same form as a logistic linear model.

In addition to the error rate, we can consider the exponential loss

$$L_{\exp}(F) = E[\exp\{-yF(x)\}]. \tag{14.13}$$

Interestingly, by solving the Euler equation, we find that the optimal discriminant function to minimize the exponential loss has the same form as (14.11). In fact, the exponential loss is used in a boosting method, AdaBoost (Freund and Schapire 1997) (see Section 14.3.1). Also, the AUC-based optimal function has the explicit form as

$$\arg\max_F \operatorname{AUC}(F) = F^*,$$

representing that the discriminant function F^* is also optimal in terms of AUC. Moreover, F^* is shown to be optimal in terms of sensitivity and specificity. These properties come from an application of the Neyman–Pearson fundamental lemma in the theory of hypothesis testing (Eguchi and Copas 2002; McIntosh and Pepe 2002).

14.3 Machine-Learning Methods

14.3.1 Boosting

14.3.1.1 AdaBoost

The key concept of boosting is to combine various weak learners, which are slightly better than random guessing, to produce a flexible (nonlinear) and powerful discriminant function $F(x)$. The typical example of a weak learner used in AdaBoost (Freund and Schapire 1997) is called a stump, which consists of one component of $x = (x_1, \ldots, x_p)^T$ as

$$f(x,k,c)=\begin{cases}+1 & \text{if } x_k > c\\ -1 & \text{if } x_k \le c,\end{cases} \tag{14.14}$$

where $1 \le k \le p$ and c is a threshold in the range of data points. If we assume x to be a vector of expression data from p genes in a microarray experiment, then the stump in (14.14) is a simplest learner that focuses on only a single (the kth) gene and puts aside the continuous nature of the data through using a threshold. However, the simplicity of each learner can be regarded as an advantage, because less assumption is posed, thus flexible in capturing underlying complex data structures. As such, through effectively combining such weak learners, the boosting is expected to produce a flexible and powerful discriminant function. In the AdaBoost, the weighted sum of stumps selected from many genes with a variety of threshold values, the set of all the stumps $\{f(x, k, c): 1 \le k \le p, c \in \mathbb{R}\}$, is expected to sufficiently capture the overall characteristics of the total genes.

In the algorithm of AdaBoost, the values of k and c and the weight of stump α are sequentially chosen to minimize the exponential loss in (14.13). For a given number of iteration T, the discriminant function is given by

$$F(x)=\sum_{t=1}^{T}\alpha_t f(x,k_t,c_t). \tag{14.15}$$

The number T is typically determined by cross-validation. By decomposing $F(x)$ according to k, it can be expressed in an additive model (Friedman et al. 2000):

$$F(x)=\sum_{t\in S_1}\alpha_t f(x,k_t,c_t)+\cdots+\sum_{t\in S_p}\alpha_t f(x,k_t,c_t) \tag{14.16}$$

$$=F_1(x_1)+\cdots+F_p(x_p), \tag{14.17}$$

where $S_l = \{t: k_t = l\}$. The function $F_k(x_k)$, called a coordinate function (Friedman et al. 2000), is useful to observe how each component x_k contributes to classification in the combined function F. This kind of boosting that attaches importance to the interpretability of the resultant discriminant function $F(x)$ is called *statistical boosting* (Mayr et al. 2014), and has been paid much attention recently.

14.3.1.2 Boosting for AUC

The AdaBoost algorithm can be modified to sequentially maximize the AUC. To cope with the sum of noncontinuous function $I(F(x_{+j}) > F(x_{-i}))$ in AUC (see [14.6]), an optimization method is proposed through applying a grid search for coefficients of an linear discriminant function (Pepe and Thompson 2000; Pepe et al. 2006). However, this technique is feasible only in the case of low dimensionality. For high-dimensional settings with $p > n$, an approximate function that smooths the AUC is proposed (Ma and Huang 2005; Wang et al. 2007). One of them is based on the standard normal distribution function $\Phi(\cdot)$:

$$\overline{\text{AUC}}_\sigma(F) = \frac{1}{n_- n_+} \sum_{i=1}^{n-} \sum_{j=1}^{n+} \Phi\left(\frac{F(x_{+j}) - F(x_{-i})}{\sigma} \right).$$

The smaller value of σ means the better approximation of the AUC. The relationship between the approximated AUC and the original AUC is discussed by Komori (2011) to justify the approximation of the AUC. A similar updating algorithm to that of AdaBoost can be employed to have a discriminant function $F(x)$ (Komori 2011).

14.3.1.3 Boosting for pAUC

The AdaBoost algorithm can also be modified to sequentially maximize the pAUC. A method for maximization of the pAUC based on a few variables is firstly proposed by Pepe and Thompson (2000). To accommodate a large number of variables, an approximate function of the pAUC is considered in a similar way to that of the AUC described earlier in order to select useful variables for maximization of the pAUC (Wang and Chang 2011). Komori and Eguchi (2010) proposed a boosting algorithm based on natural cubic splines as weak learners for maximizing pAUC.

14.3.2 Support Vector Machine

In the SVM, we assume a hyperplane $\{x \in \mathbb{R}^p : \beta^T x + \beta_0 = 0\}$ that distinguishes between observations of $y = -1$ and those of $y = +1$ (Hastie et al. 2009). If the two classes are completely separable, the distance between the hyperplane and one observation x_i with class label y_i is calculated as $y_i(\beta^T x_i + \beta_0)/\|\beta\|$, where $\|\ \|$ is the Euclidean norm. Then, the optimal hyperplane in terms of classification accuracy is determined such that the minimum distance to the hyperplane across all observations is maximized. It is generally called the maximization of the margin regarding the hyperplane.

For a more general case where the two classes are not completely separable, we introduce slack variables $\xi = (\xi_1, \ldots, \xi_n)^T$ and maximize the margin reformulated as

$$(\hat{\beta}, \hat{\beta}_0, \hat{\xi}) = \underset{\beta, \beta_0, \xi}{\arg\min} \left[\frac{1}{2} \|\beta\|^2 + \gamma \sum_{i=1}^{n} \xi_i - \sum_{i=1}^{n} \alpha_i \{ y_i(\beta^T x_i + \beta_0) - (1 - \xi_i) \} - \sum_{i=1}^{n} \mu_i \xi_i \right], \tag{14.18}$$

under the constraints $\gamma > 0$ and $\alpha_i \geq 0, \mu_i \geq 0, \xi_i \geq 0$ for $i = 1,\ldots, n$ (Hastie et al. 2009). Here $\hat{\beta}, \hat{\beta}_0$, and $\hat{\xi}$ can be regarded as the estimators of β, β_0, and ξ, respectively, where ξ is a nuisance parameter of no interest. The constraints such that $y_i(\beta^T x_i + \beta_0) \geq 1 - \xi_i \geq 0$ are summarized into $\xi_i \geq \max\{0, 1 - y_i(\beta^T x_i + \beta_0)\}$. Moreover, the objective function in the right-hand side in (14.18) is minimized in terms of ξ_i when $\xi_i = \max\{0, 1 - y_i(\beta^T x_i + \beta_0)\}$, resulting in

$$(\hat{\beta}, \hat{\beta}_0) = \arg\min_{\beta, \beta_0} \left[\sum_{i=1}^{n} \max\{0, 1 - y_i(\beta^T x_i + \beta_0)\} + \frac{1}{2\gamma} \| \beta \|^2 \right]. \qquad (14.19)$$

The first term in the right-hand side is called *hinge loss* and the second one is called L_2 penalty. This provides another perspective of SVM, and we can consider some extensions through replacing the L_2 penalty with other penalty functions (Bradley and Mangasarian 1998; Fan and Li 2001). It is also worth mentioning that in formulating the SVM, we do not assume any stochastic structures discussed in Section 14.2.3, which means that the discriminant function derived from the SVM does not necessarily have the optimality properties such as the Bayes risk consistency. Another important direction for extension is that the idea of SVM in the original space $\mathcal{X}(=\mathbb{R}^p)$ can be easily extended to a more general space with higher dimensions, from which a nonlinear discriminant function can be easily constructed. The space for this extension is called the reproducing kernel Hilbert space $\mathcal{H}$ as explained in Section 14.3.3. Such an extension can improve the practical utility and classification accuracy of the SVM methods (Hua and Sun 2001; Guyon et al. 2002; Zhang et al. 2006; Henneges et al. 2009).

14.3.3 Kernel Methods

We consider a mapping Φ from the original space $\mathcal{X}$ to a space of functions $\mathcal{H}$. The mapping Φ is generated by a positive definite kernel so that $\mathcal{H}$ becomes the reproducing kernel Hilbert space, where the inner product is easily calculated by the positive definite kernel such as $\langle \Phi(x_i), \Phi(x_j) \rangle_{\mathcal{H}} = k(x_i, x_j)$. This property is called *kernel trick* (Schölkipf 2001). The following are some typical examples:

- Linear kernel: $k(x_i, x_j) = x_i^T x_j$
- Gaussian (radial basis) kernel: $k(x_i, x_j) = \exp(-\| x_i - x_j \|_2^2 / \sigma^2), \sigma > 0$
- Polynomial kernel: $k(x_i, x_j) = (x_i^T x_j + 1)^d, d = 1, 2, 3, \ldots$

The Lagrangian dual form of (14.18) has the form (Hastie et al. 2009)

$$(\hat{\beta}, \hat{\beta}_0) = \arg\max_{\beta, \beta_0} \left\{ \sum_{i=1}^{n} \alpha_i - \frac{1}{2} \sum_{i=1}^{n} \sum_{j=1}^{n} \alpha_i \alpha_j y_i y_j x_i^T x_j \right\}. \qquad (14.20)$$

Thus, we can replace the inner product $x_i^T x_j$ in the original space with $k(x_i, x_j)$ in $\mathcal{H}$, enabling us to extend the SVM in Section 14.3.2 to a more general setting. The same approaches can be applied to principal component analysis (Schölkipf et al. 1997), robust kernel principal component analysis (Huang et al. 2009), canonical correlation analysis (Melzera et al. 2003), dimensionality reduction (Fukumizu et al. 2004), and Fisher's discriminant analysis (Mika et al. 1999). As such, the kernel methods have a wide range of applicability in reality.

14.3.4 Lasso

We provide a simple overview for L_1 regularization, which is widely employed for prediction and variable selection for high-dimensional data. We focus on the original contribution for this progress, which is called the Lasso (Tibshirani 1996). Let us consider a linear model for the ith subject with a p-dimensional feature vector x_i $(i = 1, \ldots, n)$ by

$$y_i = x_i^T \beta + \beta_0 + \varepsilon_i, \tag{14.21}$$

where $\beta = (\beta_1, \ldots, \beta_p)^T$ and ε_i denotes the residual. Note that β_0 can be omitted if we standardize x_i, such that $\sum_{i=1}^{n} x_i / n = 0$, without loss of generality. Here we assume that $p \gg n$ and almost all components of β are zeros, but a small number of components are nonzeros. The Lasso is defined by minimization of the residual sum of squares in (14.21) under a constraint on the vector of regression coefficients β, $S_u^{(1)} = \left\{\beta : \sum_{k=1}^{p} |\beta_k| = u\right\}$, where u is a positive constant. It can be reformulated using the Lagrange multiplier λ (Tibshirani 1996) as

$$\hat{\beta} = \arg\min_{\beta} \left\{ (y - X\beta)^T (y - X\beta) + \lambda \sum_{k=1}^{p} |\beta_k| \right\}, \tag{14.22}$$

where $y = (y_1, \ldots, y_n)^T$ and X is a $n \times p$ matrix with ith row being x_i^T.

Note that there is a one-to-one correspondence between u and λ. The L_1 constraint space $S_u^{(1)}$ is a hypersquare in the p-dimensional Euclidean space. Alternatively, the contour surface of the residual sum of square $(y - X\beta)^T (y - X\beta)$ is equivalent apart from a constant to a hyperellipsoid

$$\left\{\beta : (\beta - \hat{\beta}_{\text{ols}})^T X^T X (\beta - \hat{\beta}_{\text{ols}}) = v\right\}, \tag{14.23}$$

where $\hat{\beta}_{\text{ols}}$ is the ordinary least squares estimator and v is also a positive constant.

As a result, the minimization in (14.22) is attained when the hypersquare $S_u^{(1)}$ touches the hyperellipsoid. This often occurs at a corner of $S_u^{(1)}$, for which some components of β are equal to zero. In this way, Lasso can automatically perform variable selection according to appropriate choices of λ (or u). This optimization algorithm is obtained by a little modification of least angle regression (LARS) in a forward-stage manner with geometrical understandings (Efron et al. 2004). The value of λ (or u) is typically determined via cross-validation. We note that the L_1 constraint is in contrast with the L_2 constraint $S_u^{(2)} = \left\{\beta : \sum_{k=1}^{p} \beta_k^2 = u\right\}$ in the sense that $S_u^{(1)}$ is hypersquare with 2^p vertices, whereas $S_u^{(2)}$ is hypersphere without any vertices or corners. Hence, the L_2 constraint will succeed in finding a reasonable shrinkage of the estimator toward a zero vector, but no effect for variable selection.

14.3.4.1 Other Lasso-Type Methods

Many variants of Lasso have been proposed by changing the objective function (residual sum of squares) or the L_1 penalty in (14.22). The adaptive Lasso is a sophisticated version of Lasso with a weighted L_1 penalty denoted as $\lambda \sum_{k=1}^{p} w_k |\beta_k|$ so that it detects more precisely truly nonzero components of β than the original Lasso through adjusting w_k for the kth gene appropriately, which is called an oracle propriety (Zou 2006). The elastic net efficiently combines the L_2 penalty $\lambda_2 \sum_{k=1}^{p} \beta_k^2$ with the L_1 penalty to allow for high correlations between variables, which is often the case in microarray data analysis (Zou et al. 2007). That is, it modifies the penalty term so as to be strictly convex, resulting in similar values of estimates of the regression coefficients for highly correlated variables. Thus, it can deal with the grouping effect in the modeling. The sparsity can be encouraged to the group of variables more explicitly instead of the individual variables in *grouped Lasso* (Yuan and Lin 2006) through modifying L_1 penalty as $\lambda \sum_{g=1}^{G} \| \beta_g \|_{K_g}$, so that the coefficient vector β_g in the gth group is penalized as a unit based on a positive definite matrix K_g and the norm $\| \beta_g \|_{K_g} = (\beta_g^{\mathrm{T}} K_g \beta_g)^{1/2}$. The matrix K_g is typically chosen as $K_g = I_{p_g}$ or $p_g I_{p_g}$, where I_{p_g} is the identity matrix with $p_g \times p_g$ and p_g is the dimensionality of β_g. Hence, the grouped Lasso can be considered to be intermediate between Lasso and adaptive Lasso when the weight p_g is different according to the groups ($g = 1, \ldots, G$). Besides, it can be also considered as a variant of elastic net, because the norm $\|\beta_g\|_{Kg}$ includes both L_1 and L_2 penalties. Apparently, the concept of grouping is applicable to nonparametric regression, where the groups of basis functions are L_1-penalized in *basis pursuit* (Zhanga et al. 2004) and the L_1-regularization is imposed on the orthogonal projection of a nonlinear function $f(x)$, instead of the linear function $x^{\mathrm{T}}\beta$, in *Cosso* (Lin and Zhang 2006).

The ideas of the extension of Lasso to the generalized linear model and the Cox proportional hazards model were proposed (Tibshirani 1996, 1997), where the objective function in (14.22) is replaced with the likelihood or partial likelihood for these models. The packages `glmpath` and `penalized` in `R` are provided for these models (Park and Hastie 2007; Goeman 2010). Moreover, a fast algorithm was proposed to deal with very large datasets based on cyclical coordinate descent methods (Friedman et al. 2010), offering `glmnet`. The grouped Lasso can also be extended to the logistic regression model, and its applications to breast cancer data (Kim et al. 2006) and splice site detection in DNA sequences (Meier et al. 2008) were provided. More details of Lasso as well as the other related methods are discussed in Clarke et al. (2009) and Hastie et al. (2009).

14.3.5 Comparison of Classification Methods

Based on real microarray gene expression or mass spectrometry proteomics data and simulated data, several classification methods, including a LDA, were compared (Dudoit et al. 2002; Manad et al. 2004; Hess et al. 2006; Dossat et al. 2007; Khondoker et al. 2013). The interest is to clarify *which method performs better in what circumstances*. In general, a simple (diagonal) linear discriminant function ignoring correlations between features (genes) performs well in small sample size n in real data analyses (Dudoit et al. 2002; Hess et al. 2006). The standard LDA, which takes the correlations into account, performed well under the case of $p/n < 0.5$ with p ranging 5–100, while the SVM with Gaussian kernel performed best under a setting of $p/n \geq 0.5$ in a comprehensive simulation study (Khondoker et al. 2013). The SVM with Gaussian kernel performed well in real datasets analysis with a wide range of p from 50 to more than 7000 (Pirooznia et al. 2008). The performance of slightly modified AdaBoost algorithm was comparable with SVM-based algorithm in microarray data analysis (Long and Vega 2003). Dettling and Bühlmann (2003) argued that the boosting algorithms could be suitable for application in clinical setting because of its simplicity to implement.

14.4 Application to Prostate Cancer Data

We illustrate the performances of AdaBoost, AUCBoost, SVM with linear kernel, SVM with radial basis kernel, and Lasso through their applications to a prostate cancer dataset (Setlur et al. 2008). We used the same dataset as Chapter 13, where 6144 transcriptionally informative genes from 455 prostate cancer patients were analyzed (see Section 13.1). We considered the prediction as to whether TMPRESS2-ERG fusion exists or not. Since this study is a classification for binary class, we employed the Lasso for generalized linear models (Goeman 2010), where the penalized log likelihood was optimized instead of the minimization of the residual sum of squares in the original Lasso (Tibshirani 1996).

To evaluate the performance of the prediction methods, we first divided the whole data randomly into a training dataset and a test dataset with a ratio of 2:1, that is, 303 and 152 patients, respectively. Then the prediction models for TMPRESS2-ERG fusion were constructed by the machine-learning methods only using the training dataset. The classification accuracy was evaluated by the AUC and error (misclassification) rate using the test data. To determine the values of tuning parameters, such as the iteration time T in AdaBoost and AUCBoost, a smoothing penalty in AUCBoost, and the bandwidth σ in radial basis kernel and the cost of constraints violation in SVM, and the shrinkage parameter λ in Lasso, we conducted a fivefold cross-validation for the training dataset. We chose such values that maximized a cross-validated AUC for AdaBoost, AUCBoost, and SVM and cross-validated log likelihood for Lasso (using `penalized` package (Goeman 2010) in `R` statistical software). To reduce the computational costs, we conducted a gene filtering before applying the machine-learning methods. In each fold of the cross-validation, we selected the top 100 or 500 genes ($p=100$ or $p=500$) with smallest two-sided p-values in two-sample Wilcoxon tests. The recursive feature elimination (Guyon et al. 2002) was used in SVM for variable selection. We also conducted predictions without the filtering process ($p=6144$). We repeated the whole analysis 100 times with different random sample splits into training and test sets to evaluate the distribution of the classification accuracy measures.

Figure 14.1 shows the results of AUCs and error rates calculated for the test datasets. As a whole, the filtering process led to better classification accuracy in terms of both AUC and error rate. The SVM with radial basis kernel and Lasso showed better performance than the others. We also see that the Lasso performed well regardless of the filtering process. The numbers of genes finally selected after applying the machine-learning methods are given in Figure 14.2. It is clear that SVM with linear kernel and radial kernel selected much more genes than the others, which might be one of the explanations on why they achieved the good classification accuracies. The most parsimonious method in terms of the number of selected genes with relatively good classification accuracy is AUCBoost, which might reflect the use of the smoothing penalty to prevent selection of redundant genes. Finally, the average error rates were generally comparable with or slightly smaller than those based on a diagonal linear discriminant classifier with empirical Bayes shrunken effect size estimates (see Figure 13.6).

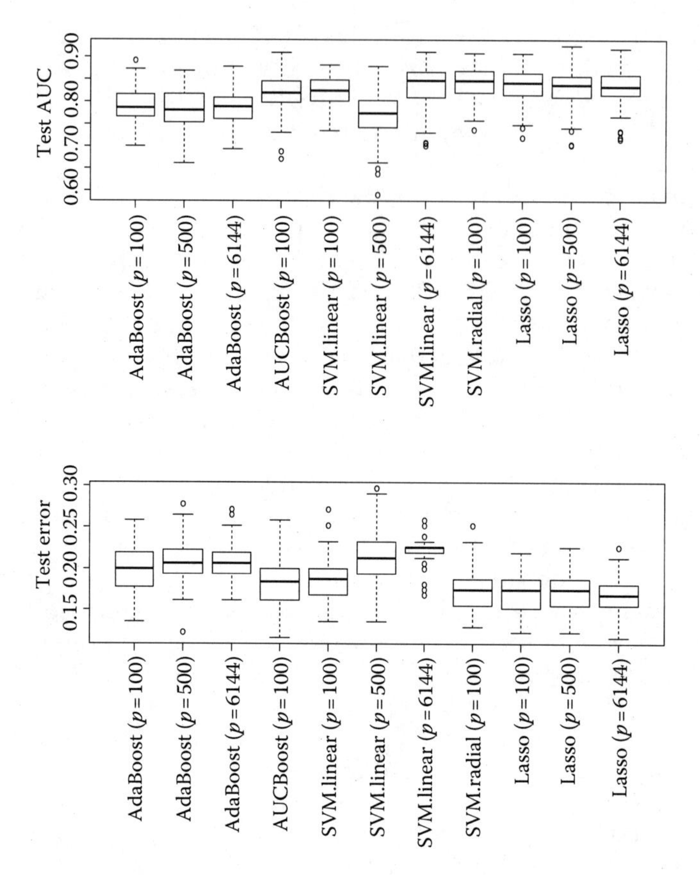

FIGURE 14.1
Boxplots of the AUCs (upper panel) and error rates (lower panel) by AdaBoost, AUCBoost, SVM with linear kernel, SVM with radial basis kernel, and Lasso for 100 test datasets. The filtering process is conducted to reduce the number of variables to $p=100$ and $p=500$ before applying the methods.

14.5 Discussion and Conclusions

Since the revolution in genomics and biotechnology at the end of twentieth century, there has been an urgent mission for biostatistics and bioinformatics to establish effective data-learning methods for analyzing high-dimensional genomic datasets. Promising approaches have arisen in the field of machine learning. In this chapter, we outlined the methods of boosting, SVMs, kernel methods, and Lasso, and discussed how these machine-learning methods aid in fulfilling the mission. However, many of these methods still remain under development.

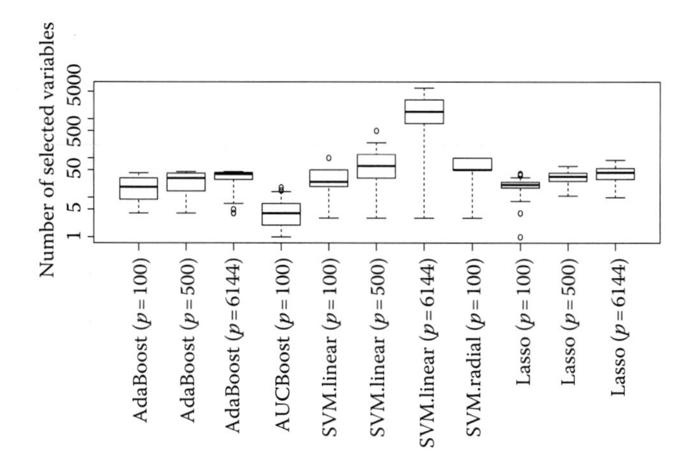

FIGURE 14.2
Boxplot of the number of variables selected by AdaBoost, AUCBoost, SVM with linear kernel, SVM with radial basis kernel, and Lasso based on the 100 training datasets. The filtering process is conducted to reduce the number of variables to $p=100$ and $p=500$ before applying the methods.

We discussed why it is difficult to extract relevant signals from high-dimensional genomic data. One reason is that genes are mutually linked in networks, so that their expression levels are strongly correlated, and many genes exhibit significant changes in expression. However, the study of gene networks in humans is not well established, because humans exhibit large amounts of complex genetic polymorphism. In addition, it is difficult to find one good solution reflecting signals in the presence of large amounts of noise in high-dimensional data. Another challenge is integration of various sources of biological data obtained from one individual. Gene polymorphism, transcription, and translation, which are typically measured by single-nucleotide polymorphisms, mRNA expression, and protein expression levels, respectively, have been usually monitored separately. Integration of these biological sources should give us new insights into the mechanisms underlying diseases or pathological abnormalities in individuals. We hope that this integration will promote the development of molecularly targeted treatments and various biomarkers toward personalized medicine in the near future.

From a statistical point of view, we must say that if biological and medical researches are conducted only in situations of $p \gg n$, the conclusions will not constitute robust and strong statistical evidence. Accordingly, signatures developed earlier to predict clinical phenotypes should be reconsidered through confirmatory clinical studies. For this purpose, we need to establish a framework for systematic development of signatures from discovery, prediction, and validation.

References

Bamber, D. The area above the ordinal dominance graph and the area below the receiver operating characteristic graph. *Journal of Mathematical Psychology*, 12:387–415, 1975.

Bradley, P.S. and Mangasarian, O.L. Feature selection via concave minimization and support vector machines. In *Proceedings of the 15th International Conference on Machine Learning*, Madison, Wisconsin, 1998.

Breiman, L. Some infinite theory for predictor ensembles. Technical Report 577, University of California, Berkeley, CA, 2000.

Breiman, L. Statistical modeling: The two cultures. *Statistical Science*, 16:199–231, 2001.

Clarke, B., Fokoue, E., and Zhang, H.H. *Principles and Theory for Data Mining and Machine Learning*. Springer, New York, 2009.

Dettling, M. and Bühlmann, P. Boosting for tumor classification with gene expression data. *Bioinformatics*, 19:1061–1069, 2003.

Dorfman, D.D. and Alf, E. Maximum-likelihood estimation of parameters of signal-detection theory and determination of confidence intervals—Rating-method data. *Journal of Mathematical Psychology*, 6:487–496, 1969.

Dossat, N., Mangé, A., Solassol, J. et al. Comparison of supervised classification methods for protein profiling in cancer diagnosis. *Cancer Informatics*, 3: 295–305, 2007.

Dudoit, S., Fridlyand, J., and Speed, T.P. Comparison of discrimination methods for the classification of tumors using gene expression data. *Journal of the American Statistical Association*, 97:77–87, 2002.

Efron, B., Hastie, T., and Johnstone, I. Least angle regression. *The Annals of Statistics*, 32:407–499, 2004.

Eguchi, S. and Copas, J. A class of logistic-type discriminant functions. *Biometrika*, 89:1–22, 2002.

Eguchi, S. and Copas, J. Interpreting Kullback-Leibler divergence with the Neyman-Pearson lemma. *Journal of Multivariate Analysis*, 97:2034–2040, 2006.

Fan, J. and Li, R. Variable selection via nonconcave penalized likelihood and its oracle properties. *Journal of the American Statistical Association*, 96:1348–1360, 2001.

Freund, Y. and Schapire, R.E. A decision-theoretic generalization of on-line learning and an application to boosting. *Journal of Computer and System Sciences*, 55:119–139, 1997.

Friedman, J., Hastie, T., and Tibshirani, R. Additive logistic regression: A statistical view of boosting. *The Annals of Statistics*, 28:337–407, 2000.

Friedman, J., Hastie, T., and Tibshirani, R. Regularization paths for generalized linear models via coordinate descent. *Journal of Statistical Software*, 33:1–22, 2010.

Fukumizu, K., Bach, F.R., and Jordan, M.I. Dimensionality reduction for supervised learning with reproducing kernel Hilbert spaces. *The Journal of Machine Learning Research*, 5:73–99, 2004.

Goeman, J.J. L_1 penalized estimation in the cox proportional hazards model. *Biometrical Journal*, 52:70–84, 2010.

Green, D.M. and Swets, J.A. *Signal Detection Theory and Psychophysics*. John Wiley & Sons, Inc., New York, 1966.

Guyon, I., Weston, J., Barnhill, S., and Vapnik, V. Gene selection for cancer classification using support vector machines. *Machine Learning*, 46:389–422, 2002.

Hanley, J.A. and McNeil, B.J. The meaning and use of the area under a receiver operating characteristic (ROC) curve. *Radiology*, 143:29–36, 1982.

Hastie, T., Tibshirani, R., and Friedman, J. *The Elements of Statistical Learning: Data Mining, Inference, and Prediction*, 2nd ed. Springer, New York, 2009.

Henneges, C., Bullinger, D., Fux, R. et al. Prediction of breast cancer by profiling of urinary RNA metabolites using support vector machine-based feature selection. *BMC Cancer*, 9:104, 2009.

Hess, K.R., Anderson, K., Symmans, W.F. et al. Pharmacogenomic prediction of sensitivity to preoperative chemotherapy with paclitaxel and fluorouracil, doxorubicin, and cyclophosphamide in breast cancer. *Journal of Clinical Ontology*, 24:4236–4244, 2006.

Hua, S. and Sun, Z. Support vector machine approach for protein subcellular localization prediction. *Bioinformatics*, 17:721–728, 2001.

Huang, S., Yeh, Y., and Eguchi, S. Robust kernel principal component analysis. *Neural Computation*, 21:3179–3213, 2009.

Khondoker, M., Dobson, R., Skirrow, C., Simmons, A., Stahll, D., and Initiative, A.D.N. A comparison of machine learning methods for classification using simulation with multiple real data examples from mental health studies. *Statistical Methods in Medical Research*, 2013. DOI: 10.1177/0962280213502437.

Kim, Y., Kim, J., and Kim, Y. Blockwise sparse regression. *Statistica Sinica*, 16:375–390, 2006.

Komori, O. A boosting method for maximization of the area under the ROC curve. *Annals of the Institute of Statistical Mathematics*, 63:961–979, 2011.

Komori, O. and Eguchi, S. A boosting method for maximizing the partial area under the ROC curve. *BMC Bioinformatics*, 11:314, 2010.

Lin, Y. and Zhang, H.H. Component selection and smoothing in multivariate nonparametric regression. *The Annals of Statistics*, 5:2272–2297, 2006.

Long, P.M. and Vega, V.B. Boosting and microarray data. *Machine Learning*, 52:31–44, 2003.

Lugosi, B.G. and Vayatis, N. On the Bayes-risk consistency of regularized boosting methods. *The Annals of Statistics*, 32:30–55, 2004.

Ma, S. and Huang, J. Regularized ROC method for disease classification and biomarker selection with microarray data. *Bioinformatics*, 21:4356–4362, 2005.

Manad, M.Z., Dysonb, G., Johnsona, K., and Liaoc, B. Evaluating methods for classifying expression data. *Journal of Biopharmaceutical Statistics*, 14:1065–1084, 2004.

Mayr, A., Binder, H., Gefeller1, O., and Schmid, M. The evolution of boosting algorithms—From machine learning to statistical modelling. *Methods of Information in Medicine*, arXiv:1403.1452, 2014.

McClish, D.K. Analyzing a portion of the roc curve. *Medical Decision Making*, 9:190–195, 1989.

McIntosh, M.W. and Pepe, M.S. Combining several screening tests: Optimality of the risk score. *Biometrics*, 58:657–664, 2002.

Meier, L., Geer, van de, S., and Buhlmann, P. The group lasso for logistic regression. *Journal of the Royal Statistical Society: Series B*, 70:53–71, 2008.

Melzera, T., Reitera, M., and Bischofb, H. Appearance models based on kernel canonical correlation analysis. *Pattern Recognition*, 36:1961–1971, 2003.

Mika, S., Fitscht, G., Weston, J., Scholkopft, B., and Mullert, K.-R. Fisher discriminant analysis with kernels. In *Proceedings of the 1999 IEEE Signal Processing Society Workshop*, Madison, Wisconsin, 1999.

Park, M.Y. and Hastie, T. L_1-regularization path algorithm for generalized linear models. *Journal of the Royal Statistical Society: Series B*, 69:659–677, 2007.

Pepe, M.S. *The Statistical Evaluation of Medical Tests for Classification and Prediction*. Oxford University Press, New York, 2003.

Pepe, M.S., Cai, T., and Longton, G. Combining predictors for classification using the area under the receiver operating characteristic curve. *Biometrics*, 62:221–229, 2006.

Pepe, M.S. and Thompson, M.L. Combining diagnostic test results to increase accuracy. *Biostatistics*, 1:123–140, 2000.

Pirooznia, M., Yang, J.Y., Yang, M.Q., and Deng, Y. A comparative study of different machine learning methods on microarray gene expression data. *BMC Genomics*, 9:S1–S13, 2008.

Schölkipf, B. The kernel trick for distances. *Advances in Neural Information Processing Systems*, 13:301–307, 2001.

Schölkipf, B., Smola, A., and Müller, K.-R. Kernel principal component analysis. *Artificial Neural Networks—ICANN'97*, 1327:583–588, 1997.

Setlur, S.R., Mertz, K.D., Hoshida, Y. et al. Estrogen-dependent signaling in a molecularly distinct subclass of aggressive prostate cancer. *Journal of the National Cancer Institute*, 100:815–825, 2008.

Tibshirani, R. Regression shrinkage and selection via the lasso. *Journal of Royal Statistical Society*, 58:267–288, 1996.

Tibshirani, R. The lasso method for variable selection in the cox model. *Statistics in Medicine*, 16:385–395, 1997.

Wang, Z. and Chang, Y.I. Markers selection via maximizing the partial area under the ROC curve of linear risk scores. *Biostatistics*, 12:369–385, 2011.

Wang, Z., Chang, Y.I., Ying, Z., Zhu, L., and Yang, Y. A parsimonious threshold-independent protein feature selection method through the area under receiver operating characteristic curve. *Bioinformatics*, 23:2788–1794, 2007.

Yuan, M. and Lin, Y. Model selection and estimation in regression with grouped variables. *Journal of the Royal Statistical Society: Series B*, 68:49–67, 2006.

Zhang, X., Lu, X., Shi, Q. et al. Recursive SVM feature selection and sample classification for mass-spectrometry and microarray data. *BMC Bioinformatics*, 7:197, 2006.

Zhanga, H.H., Wahbaa, G., Lina, Y. et al. Variable selection and model building via likelihood basis pursuit. *Journal of the American Statistical Association*, 99: 659–672, 2004.

Zou, H. The adaptive lasso and its oracle properties. *Journal of American Statistical Association*, 101:1418–1429, 2006.

Zou, H. and Hastie, T. Regularization and variable selection via the elastic net. *Journal of the Royal Statistical Society: Series B*, 67:301–320, 2005.

Zou, H., Hastie, T., and Tibshirani, R. On the "degrees of freedom" of the lasso. *The Annals of Statistics*, 35:2173–2192, 2007.

15

Survival Risk Prediction Using High-Dimensional Molecular Data

Harald Binder, Thomas Gerds, and Martin Schumacher

CONTENTS

15.1 Introduction

Prognostic models can link molecular measurements to clinical outcomes, that is, molecular measurements take the role of prognostic markers, which provide information on the likely course of disease of (untreated) individuals. Similarly, predictive models can incorporate molecular markers that provide information on the treatment effect with respect to the clinical outcome. If the outcome of interest is an event time, then the observation for each individual includes a time and status information. The status may either indicate that the individual experienced the event of interest, or that a competing event has occurred, or that the event time was censored. Event times are called *censored* if the individual was alive and event-free at the end of the study period. For example, for bladder cancer patients, the event of interest can be cancer-related death. Competing events are death due to other causes and censoring occurs for patients that survived until the end of the study period. Note that gradual inclusion into a study with a fixed duration in calendar time leads to follow-up periods of different lengths for the individual patients. Therefore, it may happen that censoring times are smaller than the overall study period.

A multitude of statistical techniques are available for time-to-event settings with a small number of covariates. Typically, it is required that the number of covariates is much smaller than the number of events. For comparing survival between a small number of groups of patients, prominent tools are the Kaplan–Meier method and the log-rank test. In the presence of competing risks, the Kaplan–Meier method can be biased and event probabilities (cumulative incidences) should be analyzed with the Aalen–Johansen method [1] instead. Groups can be compared with Gray's test [30]. For continuous covariates and more generally regression modeling, the Cox proportional hazards model is widely used. For more details and background on these methods, we refer textbooks on survival analysis [2,43,44,47].

Many methods of survival analysis have been adapted to high-dimensional settings with a large number of covariates. This is often needed for building risk prediction models based on molecular markers. It may appear straightforward to adapt some of the many techniques developed for class prediction (e.g., as reviewed in the previous chapter), by transforming the time-to-event into a binary response. For example, the status, such as *still alive* versus *death occurred*, at a landmark, say after 5 years, can be considered as a binary response and, for example, used to apply support vector machine (SVM) techniques. However, there are pitfalls when data are censored and for some patients the follow-up was shorter than the landmark, such that the status at the landmark is unknown [8]. However, in this case, so-called pseudovalue approaches can be used for constructing response variables for semiparametric binomial regression and machine learning [3,9,48,52].

In this chapter, we review techniques that can adequately deal with time-to-event outcomes when the aim is to determine the impact of molecular markers. Specifically, we will distinguish between techniques with implementations available that can deal with censoring in single event survival analysis, and techniques that also can deal with competing risks. Some of these techniques, such as specific regression modeling approaches, can provide prediction as well as an importance ranking of molecular quantities, but some will only provide prediction. We will not consider techniques that do not directly provide predictions for new patients. For example, this excludes univariate testing strategies from our presentation, as these do only provide lists of significant molecular features without a rule for risk prediction.

In addition to the modeling techniques, we also review measures of prediction performance and means for their estimation based on right censored data, and in the presence of competing risks. As a basis for this, we first review some concepts of time-to-event analysis, including competing risks. Before that, we describe an application that will be used for illustrating the techniques in the following.

15.2 Bladder Cancer Application

Dyrskjøt et al. [17] investigated gene expression from bladder cancer patients, for developing a prognostic signature. The preprocessed 1381 covariates from gene expression microarrays are publicly available from the Gene Expression Omnibus (GSE5479). In addition to these, age, sex, stage, and grade are available as potentially important clinical predictors. Treatment information is also provided and might be used for adjustment. The clinical and microarray information is available for 301 patients. The original analysis [17] considered progression or death from bladder cancer as the primary endpoint. This event (with corresponding time) was observed for 84 patients. The number of events corresponds to the effective sample size with respect to model building. While censored observations still contribute to the analysis, the number of events is the critical constraint on high-dimensional modeling. Censoring is present for 194 patients, and death from unknown causes was observed for further 33 patients. While the latter was treated similar to the censored observations in the original analysis, this might be more appropriately analyzed as a competing event type. Techniques for a competing risks analysis of this dataset were considered in [5], and we will use this dataset for illustration in the following.

15.3 Concepts and Models

In a time-to-event setting, observations will often be given in the form $(T_i, \Delta_i, \epsilon_i, X_i)$, $i=1,\ldots, n$. Here T_i is the observed time and Δ_i is the censoring indicator. Usually data are coded such that $\Delta_i=1$ means that an event was observed at T_i and $\Delta_i=0$ indicates that the event time was right censored at T_i. The event type $\epsilon_i \in \{1,\ldots, K\}$ allows to account for several (competing) events. The special case $K=1$ refers to conventional survival analysis where there are no competing risks. The covariate vector $X_i=(X_{i1},\ldots, X_{ip})'$ contains the molecular measurements, potentially in addition to clinical predictors. If p is greater than n, the setting is called high dimensional.

The aim is to use the data for building a risk prediction rule $\hat{r}(t \mid X)$ that uses covariate information X to predict the event risk, that is, the cumulative incidence of the event of interest. For example, $\hat{r}_1(t \mid X_i)$ can be an estimate of the probability that an event of type $\epsilon_i = 1$ occurs to patient i until time t.

In the case of a single event type, that is, $K = 1$, we will denote the cumulative incidence by $F(t)$ in the following. In this setting, a survival probability can be translated into a cumulative incidence and vice versa by the relation: $S(t|X) = 1 - F(t|X)$. While alternative targets for prediction may be considered, we will focus on risk prediction rules $\hat{r}(t \mid X)$ for the cumulative incidence.

The hazard function $h(t) = -d\log(F(t))$ describes the instantaneous risk of an event given that no event has occurred until time t. It is often possible to translate a regression model for the hazard function into a prediction rule. A widely used regression model is the Cox proportional hazards model

$$h(t \mid X) = h_0(t)\exp(X'\beta). \tag{15.1}$$

The model is characterized by a baseline hazard function $h_0(t)$ and a regression parameter vector $\beta = (\beta_1, \ldots, \beta_p)$. The Cox regression risk prediction rule is obtained based on the partial likelihood estimate $\hat{\beta}$ and the Breslow estimate $\hat{H}_0(t)$ for the cumulative baseline hazard $H_0(t) = \int_0^t h_0(s)\,ds$ and given by

$$\hat{r}(t \mid X) = 1 - \exp\left(-\hat{H}_0(t)\exp(X'\hat{\beta})\right).$$

15.3.1 Competing Risks

A competing risk analysis is indicated when there are time-dependent events that may change the risk of the event of interest. Death due to other causes is the classical example as it changes the future risk of any other event to zero. Also other nonfatal events can be considered in a competing risk analysis, for example, the risk of disease-related death may be significantly reduced when some patients receive a transplant. Nonfatal events can alternatively be incorporated as time-dependent predictors, for example, in an illness-death model. Practical implementation of such analyses in a low-dimensional setting is illustrated in [4], using the statistical environment *R*. In the following, we introduce the notation needed later on for explaining the analyses in high-dimensional settings.

With two competing risks, there are at least two cause-specific hazards, $h_k(t)$ for $k = 1, \ldots, K$, that describe the instantaneous risk of an event of type $\epsilon = k$, given that no event has occurred until t. Regression models $\hat{h}_k$ for each of the cause-specific hazard functions can be combined into a rule that predicts the cumulative incidence of an event of type 1:

$$\hat{r}_1(t \mid X) = \int_0^t \exp\left\{-\int_0^s \left[\hat{h}_1(u \mid X) + \cdots + \hat{h}_K(u \mid X)\right] du\right\} \hat{h}_1(s \mid X)\,ds.$$

For interpreting the effects of the covariates on the cumulative incidence, that is, on the risk of the event, models for all causes need to be considered jointly. This quickly becomes challenging in particular when there are more than two competing risks.

As an alternative, regression techniques can be applied that directly model the effect of covariates on the risk of an event of type 1. A suitable class of transformation models for this purpose is given by

$$\hat{r}_1(t \mid X) = \hat{F}_{1,0}(t)g(X'\hat{\beta}).$$

Here g is a link function and $\hat{F}_{1,0}(t)$ is a function that describes the risk when $X = (0,\ldots,0)'$. The most prominent example is perhaps the Fine–Gray regression model [21]. Note that this technique circumvents the need for modeling the hazard functions of the competing causes. However, instead one has to rely on a model for the censoring distribution. Also, the interpretation of the regression parameters depends on the link function that may become cumbersome [27].

15.3.2 Binomial Regression and Pseudovalues

The general idea of binomial regression in survival analysis is to analyze the binary event status at a sequence of times called landmarks. This is justified as even a complex time-to-event response is usually equivalently characterized by a time series of binary event status variables [16,41]. The relation can be exploited when the aim is to model event risk for a complex outcome and a high-dimensional predictor space. The basic idea for the handling of censored data is to replace the possibly unknown status of a patient at the landmarks by a pseudovalue. The pseudovalues are constructed such that their average across a sample of patients is an unbiased estimate of the average event risk at the landmark [3]. This technique requires a model for the censoring distribution [9]. The most simple censoring model is to assume that censoring is independent of all predictors. In this case, a pseudovalue for the event status is obtained based on a nonparametric estimate $\hat{F}_j(t)$ of the marginal cumulative incidence of an event of type j:

$$\text{Pseudo value (subject } i, \text{ landmark } t) = n\hat{F}_j(t) - (n-1)\hat{F}_j^i(t).$$

Here n is the sample size and $\hat{F}_j^i$ the nonparametric estimate obtained when the data of subject i are excluded. It is easy to verify that without censoring the pseudovalues obtained with the Aalen–Johansen estimate of F_1 are equal to the binary event status at t.

15.4 Techniques for Fitting Risk Prediction Rules

15.4.1 Overview of Approaches

As indicated earlier, there are two main approaches for linking high-dimensional molecular measurements to a time-to-event endpoint. For several machine learning approaches that were initially developed for classification, specifically for a binary endpoints, variants for time-to-event endpoints have been developed. As an alternative strategy, classical biostatistical techniques, which were originally developed for time-to-event endpoints in a low-dimensional setting, have been adapted for high-dimensional settings. While many of the classical biostatistical techniques are based on a regression model, machine learning approaches usually operate without an explicit model formulation. In subsequent sections of this chapter, we illustrate how probabilistic predictions can be obtained from regression and machine learning techniques for censored time-to-event data in high-dimensional settings.

Regularized regression techniques adapt classical regression modeling approaches for time-to-event endpoints to high-dimensional settings. One approach to regularize a regression model is provided by penalized likelihood techniques. These techniques attach a penalty term to the likelihood. Parameter estimates for regression models are then obtained by maximizing the penalized likelihood. Often the penalty term is additive in the elements of the parameter vector, and generally, it penalizes large values. Thus, each covariate can potentially only make a small contribution to the model and it becomes possible to simultaneously consider many covariates. Ridge regression [35] employs a quadratic penalty. It has been extended for the Cox regression for time-to-event endpoints [62], and was applied successfully to analyze high-dimensional gene expression data [37]. While it is very competitive in terms of prediction performance [12], the downside is that it does not perform variable selection. The lasso [57] penalizes the sum of the absolute values of the regression parameters, resulting in parameter estimates equal to zero for some covariates, that is, it performs variable selection. Finally, the elastic net combines the quadratic (ridge) and absolute (lasso) penalties. It has also been adapted for time-to-event endpoints [19]. While many adaptations of penalized likelihood approaches focus on the Cox proportional hazards model [28,58], accelerated failure time models [15,38,63] and additive risk models have also been considered [45,46]. Besides regularized regression, there are several other techniques, such as partial least squares and supervised principal components that perform some kind of dimension reduction before incorporating covariates into a Cox proportional hazards model. A general overview, that also contrasts these approaches with regularized regression, is given in [64]. A particular advantage of the lasso is that the resulting signature only depends on a small number of selected covariates, for example, in contrast to dimension reduction by principal components, where the result still depends on all covariates.

There are two popular classes of machine learning approaches [66], SVMs and ensemble techniques. Both have been adapted to time-to-event endpoints, and will be briefly reviewed in the following. In a classification setting, SVMs identify hyperplanes, via a kernel and arbitrary combinations of covariates, such that classes are separated in an optimal way. In simple settings, this approach is closely related to ridge regression [33]. SVMs have been adapted for the Cox proportional hazards model [20,60].

Ensemble approaches repeatedly apply a procedure to perturbations of the original data. For example, tree-based approaches have been adapted for time-to-event data and combined with resampling to obtain bagged survival trees [36]. Random survival forests [40] extend this idea by introducing further random variability into the tree building. The resulting approach is completely nonparametric, and will be considered as one alternative for data analysis in the following.

Boosting is another ensemble approach. Models are built in a sequence of boosting steps in which observations are reweighted according to the classification performance in the respective previous boosting step [22]. This can be seen as performing gradient descent in a function space [23]. Componentwise boosting incorporates variable selection into the boosting steps, and results can be obtained that are similar to those obtained with the lasso [14]. This indicates that componentwise boosting provides another way for regularized regression. The algorithm starts by setting all regression parameters to zero. In each boosting step, one element of the parameter vector is updated by a small amount. In contrast to stepwise variable selection approaches, all other elements are kept fixed. When there are strong correlations between covariates, such as with high-dimensional molecular measurements, solutions of stagewise approaches, such as componentwise boosting, are more stable than those from the lasso [32]. Componentwise likelihood-based boosting has been adapted for the Cox proportional hazards model. The methods allow that the parameters of a low-dimensional set of clinical covariates can be estimated in an unpenalized way. This enables comparison to models comprising only clinical covariates [7]. The latter approach has also been adapted for the Fine–Gray regression model in competing risks setting [5], and for different types of molecular data, such as single nucleotide polymorphism measurements [6]. It will be used for illustration in the following, and compared to random survival forests. A more detailed description of the algorithm is given in the Appendix.

15.4.2 Selecting the Tuning Parameters

Regardless of the specific approach that is used for linking high-dimensional covariate values to a time-to-event endpoint, there will always be tuning parameters that drive the performance of the resulting model. Tuning parameters that determine the flexibility of the model (degrees of freedom) have to be chosen carefully to avoid overfitting. In the present context, a model is considered *overfitting* if it extracts artifacts from the training data that are not useful for predicting new cases. For example, the number of boosting steps is a critical parameter for componentwise boosting. It determines the model complexity via the maximum number of covariates that have a nonzero effect.

Cross-validation is a powerful approach to control tuning parameters. Data is repeatedly split into training and test sets. Also bootstrap can be used to obtain training sets in the cross-validation steps in which case the individuals that are not sampled in the bootstrap set form the corresponding test set.

The value of a tuning parameter can then be chosen such that a suitable criterion is optimized across the splits. In the context of the Cox proportional hazards model, likelihood-based cross-validation was considered in [37]. Prediction performance is an alternative criterion [49]. Tuning parameter selection according to cross-validated prediction performance can also be used for approaches that do not explicitly provide a model and corresponding likelihood. For example, the performance of random survival forests can be improved by data-based selection of tree parameters [50].

Generally, cross-validation for selection of tuning parameters has to be distinguished from cross-validation used for internal validation of a risk prediction model. If cross-validation is used to evaluate prediction performance, as in Section 15.5, it is important that all model building steps, including variable selection and selection of tuning parameters, are repeated in each cross-validation step. Thus, this often requires a nested approach where cross-validation for the selection of the tuning parameters is repeated in each step of cross-validation for evaluating prediction performance. If this is not fully implemented, the prediction performance can be severely overestimated [61].

15.4.3 Boosting for the Bladder Cancer Application

Componentwise likelihood-based boosting has been adapted for Cox proportional hazards models. It can select important features from a large number of molecular markers and clinical predictors [7]. In competing risks settings, it can be applied to the cause-specific Cox models of all competing risks. In the following, these analyses will be contrasted with a corresponding boosting approach applied to the Fine–Gray regression model of the cause of interest, see [5].

An implementation of componentwise likelihood-based boosting for Cox models and Fine–Gray regression is provided in the package CoxBoost for the statistical environment *R*. The main tuning parameter is the number of boosting steps, that is, the number of updates for the estimated parameter vector $\hat{\beta}$ performed for one element in each boosting step, such that the partial log-likelihood increases the most. The number of boosting steps is typically selected by 10-fold cross-validation. The size of the updates, which are obtained from a penalized partial likelihood, is regulated by a penalty parameter. The value of this parameter is not critical, as long as it results in steps that are small enough. As a rule of thumb, the penalty should be set to $\sum I(\Delta_i = 1)(1/v - 1)$. This will result in updates roughly the size of v times the maximum partial likelihood estimate. Values $v \in [0.1; 0.01]$ result in steps of reasonable size, often corresponding to about 50–200 boosting steps selected by cross-validation. Naturally, the exact number of boosting steps that is selected by cross-validation will depend on the amount of information in the data. If there is little to no predictive information, even small values of v, such as $v = 0.01$, will result in selection of a number of steps close to zero.

In the bladder cancer application, Cox proportional hazards models can be fitted by boosting for the cause-specific hazard corresponding to progression or death from bladder cancer, and the cause-specific hazard corresponding to death from other causes. Fine–Gray regression modeling typically focuses on one primary event of interest. While Fine–Gray regression models can be fitted for each of the two event types in principle, it is worth noting that two separately fitted Fine–Gray models may result in inconsistent estimates of the cumulative incidence functions [4, p. 139]. Also, from a technical perspective, the proportional hazards assumption cannot hold for the cause-specific and the Fine–Gray models at the same time, that is, some of these models will be misspecified, but might nevertheless provide usable results [29]. Concerning interpretation, note that each cause-specific hazard model describes the effects of covariates on the biological mechanisms that drive the specific cause. In contrast, the Fine–Gray regression models describe the effects of the covariates on the prediction of the event, which also depends on the competing risks. Thus, for selection of covariates, it may be preferable to consider hazard models [42].

Figure 15.1 shows the coefficient paths for the two cause-specific hazard models, and the two Fine–Gray models, as obtained from componentwise likelihood-based boosting. Results are presented for illustrating selection of genes, that is, without considering prediction of cumulative incidences from both models. The clinical covariates have been incorporated as mandatory, that is, their effect is estimated by standard maximum partial likelihood techniques. Figure 15.1 only shows the estimates for the gene expression covariates, as they move from the initial value of zero toward nonzero values in the course of the boosting steps. The vertical lines indicate the number of boosting steps that have been selected by 10-fold cross-validation. Zero boosting steps were selected for the Fine–Gray model that corresponds to death from other causes (bottom right panel), indicating that reasonable prediction for the corresponding cumulative incidence cannot be obtained, at least by componentwise boosting. A much larger number of steps were

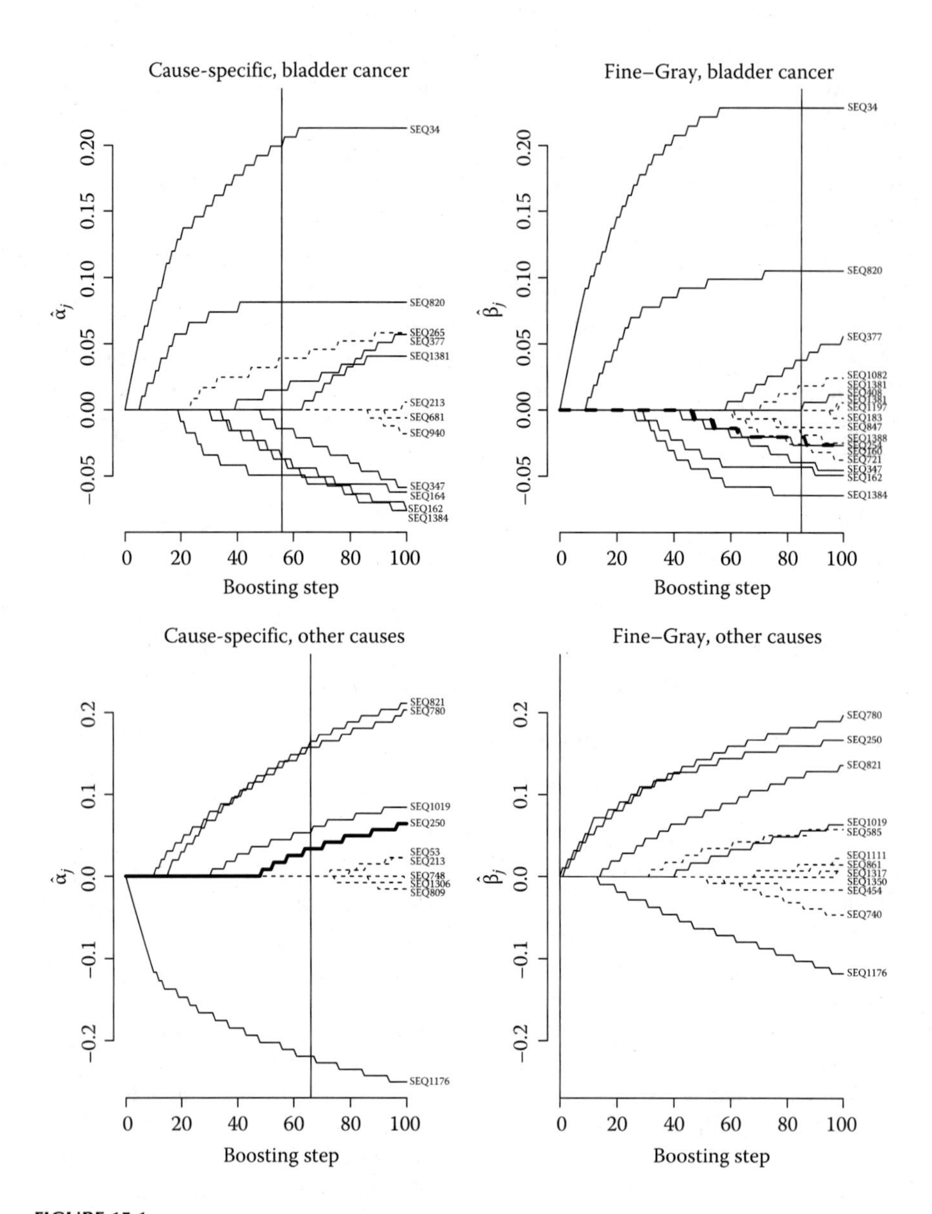

FIGURE 15.1
Coefficient paths from componentwise likelihood-based boosting, that is, parameter estimates in the course of the boosting steps, for the bladder cancer application. Estimates from Cox models for the cause-specific hazards are shown in the left panels, estimates for Fine–Gray models in the right panels. The top panels correspond to the event progression or death from bladder cancer, the bottom panels to death from other causes. Solid lines indicate those genes that are selected both in the respective model for the cause-specific hazard and the Fine–Gray model. The number of boosting steps that was selected by cross-validation is indicated by vertical lines. The gene SEQ250, which receives nonzero estimates in the top left panel as well as in the bottom right panel, is indicated by thick lines.

selected for the more interesting Fine–Gray model corresponding to the cumulative incidence for progression or death from bladder cancer (top right panel). Many of the genes that were assigned nonzero estimates by componentwise likelihood-based boosting also received nonzero estimates in the model for the corresponding cause-specific hazard (top left panel). This is no surprise, as the cause-specific hazard for progression or death from bladder cancer can reasonably be expected to drive the cumulative incidence for this event. Notably, there is one gene (SEQ250) that receives an estimate equal to zero in the model for the cause-specific hazard, but is assigned a nonzero estimate in the Fine–Gray model (highlighted by thick lines). This gene also has a nonzero effect in the model for the cause-specific hazard for death from other causes, but with opposite sign. A decreasing effect on the cause-specific hazard results in an increasing effect on the cumulative incidence for progression or death from bladder cancer.

15.4.4 Random Survival Forests

Like random forest [13], random survival forest is an ensemble method with excellent prediction performance [40]. It also implements efficient algorithms that can provide lists of the top variables in high-dimensional settings [39]. The method works with a large number of bootstrap samples obtained by resampling or subsampling the original data. A survival tree (or a competing risk tree) is fitted using the data of each bootstrap sample. The forest then consists of the ensemble of survival trees obtained in all bootstrap samples. In order to predict a new patient, the patient's covariates are dropped down each tree. The prediction is obtained as a suitably weighted average of the outcome of those learning data patients that share the terminal node of the trees with the new case. Several parameters are used to optimize the performance of the forest. The most important parameters are the following:

1. *split-function*: It is used to decide between possible splits in tree growing. This defaults to the log-rank test for survival endpoints without competing risks and to an efficient modification of Gray's test for situations with competing risks.
2. *ntree*: the number of bootstrap samples used to build the forest.
3. *mtry*: the number of variables tried to identify the best split of each mother node.
4. *nsplit:* for random splitting of continuous variables, the number of random split points.

For the purpose of illustration, we applied random survival forest to the bladder cancer data [17]. Specifically, we fitted a forest with 1000 competing risk trees. We included all clinical variables and the expression array and set *mtry* to 37 (the default) and *nsplit* to 10.

15.5 Evaluating Risk Prediction Rules

Prediction rules will often be assessed and compared with respect to prediction performance. In addition to good prediction performance, a useful prediction rule should distinguish the relative importance of the molecular covariates. Many aspects of variable selection in survival analysis resemble that of settings with binary or continuous response as discussed in the previous chapters. Here we focus on the aspects of evaluating prediction performance that are specific for time-to-event data. For a more general overview of approaches for assessing the performance of risk prediction models see, for example, [24]. We do not illustrate all approaches that have been proposed. In particular, we will not consider approaches based on the area under the time-dependent receiver operating characteristic (ROC) curve ([34]; see [11] for a discussion and comparison), which have recently also been adapted for competing risks settings [10,51].

Evaluation of prediction performance has two main aspects. First, a measure of prediction performance is needed. Second, in an internal or external validation approach [56], this measure needs to be applied to and summarized across the data of the test set(s) in order to simulate the application of the risk prediction rule in future patients. Note that the performance of a risk prediction rule in the same dataset that was used to develop the rule generally has no useful interpretation for prediction.

15.5.1 Assessing the Distinction between Risk Groups

Consider the situation where a prediction model distinguishes only two groups of patients (high risk and low risk). The following discussion can be generalized to multiple risk groups. The aim is to assess the predictive performance of the model. Suppose further that we have an independent validation set and thus can apply external validation.

Frequently, Kaplan–Meier curves are plotted for the two groups and compared in this situation. Simon et al. [55] adapted this approach for a setting without validation set, by proposing a resampling approach for estimating the Kaplan–Meier curves as they would be expected for two risk groups when applying a risk prediction rule to new individuals. However, note that Kaplan–Meier curves computed in the two risk groups do not quantify the predictive performance. The reason is that the graph displays the average survival of all individuals that are predicted to be in the high- and low-risk groups, and does not display the variability of individual predictions with risk groups. For the same reason, it does not seem to help to compute a log-rank test or a Gray test in order to assess the prediction performance. A more suitable approach is based on personalized residuals as described in Section 15.5.2.

15.5.2 Prediction Error Curves

For each individual, the Brier score is the squared difference between the predicted event probability and the true event status which is 0 if no event occurred and 1 if the event occurred. The expected Brier score of a risk prediction rule is the average of the patient-individual Brier scores. Alternative names for the expected Brier scores are prediction error and mean squared error, and its square root can be interpreted as the expected distance between the predicted risk and the true event status. Since, both the event status and the prediction are time dependent, the expected Brier score is also a function of time.

To estimate the expected Brier score in survival analysis, censoring has to be taken into account. Specifically, the empirical Brier score

$$\overline{err}(t,\hat{r}) = \frac{1}{n}\sum_{i=1}^{n}(N_i(t) - \hat{r}(t \mid X_i))^2 W_i(t;\hat{G})$$

will evaluate the risk prediction rule $\hat{r}(t \mid X_i)$ with respect to the true status $N_i(t)$ (0 indicating that no event has occurred, and 1 that an event [of interest] has occurred). A prediction error curve is obtained by following the Brier score over time. Using notation $I(\cdot)$ for the indicator function, taking value 1 if its argument is true, and 0 otherwise, the weights are given by

$$W_i(t;\hat{G}) = \frac{I(T_i \le t)\delta_i}{\hat{G}(T_i - \mid X_i)} + \frac{I(T_i > t)}{\hat{G}(t \mid X_i)}.$$

The weights are based on a working model $\hat{G}$ for the conditional censoring distribution given covariates. It can be shown that the empirical Brier score is a consistent estimate of the expected Brier score if the working model is correctly specified. In high-dimensional settings, often a simple model is imposed, which assumes that the censoring mechanism does not depend on the covariates. In this case, the nonparametric Kaplan–Meier estimate $\hat{G}(t)$ is used to estimate the weights. Gerds and Schumacher [26] adapted the Efron and Tibshirani [18] .632+ resampling estimate of prediction performance to time-to-event settings. This approach has been illustrated in high-dimensional applications [54], and extended to competing risks settings [5,53].

15.5.3 Concordance Index

A widely used measure of prediction accuracy is the concordance index [31]. For applications with right censored data, a time-truncated version can be estimated using appropriate weights [25,59]. The concordance index measures the discrimination ability, that is, how well the model can distinguish a high-risk patient from a low-risk patient. In survival analysis, the truncated concordance index is interpreted as the ability of the risk prediction model to correctly rank pairs of patients where at least one of the patients has an event before the truncation time. By *correctly rank*, we mean that the patient who has the event earlier receives the higher predicted event risk. In the presence of competing risks, there are multiple concordance indices, one for each of the competing events. Also the estimation technique needs to be modified accordingly, see [65] for details.

Being a rank statistic like the area under the ROC curve, the concordance index is insensitive to monotone transformations of the predicted risk, and hence, it does not assess the calibration of the risk prediction rule. Therefore, for a complete evaluation of prediction performance, the concordance index is often accompanied by a calibration plot, which compares the predicted risk with the average outcome. Note also that the expected Brier score is not insensitive to transformations of risks and can be used to assess the calibration of a risk prediction rule.

15.5.4 Performance in the Bladder Cancer Application

The left panel of Figure 15.2 shows prediction error curves and discrimination curves for different models that predict the cumulative incidence of progression or death from bladder cancer in the bladder cancer application.

As a reference for interpretation, we show the prediction error curve of the Aalen–Johansen estimator, which ignores all covariates. We also show the prediction error curve of a Fine–Gray regression model, which only uses the clinical covariates. The prediction error is small in the beginning, where few events occur; it increases subsequently, and will become smaller again, in principle, when most of the individuals have experienced an event. However, the time points at which the prediction error curves can be estimated are limited due to end of follow-up (censoring). Figure 15.2 shows that in this dataset, the random survival forest model achieves lower prediction error for predicting death due to bladder cancer than the componentwise likelihood-based boosting. This may indicate that the likelihood-based models misspecify the functional relationship between the covariates and the risk of cause 1. Both the componentwise likelihood-based boosting and the random survival forest show only slightly higher discrimination ability compared to the clinical covariate Fine–Gray model. This indicates that the expression array data provides only little additional information. The right panels show results for predicting death due to other causes. Here neither the models that use the clinical covariates nor the models that use both the clinical covariates and the expression array can outperform the null model in terms of prediction error.

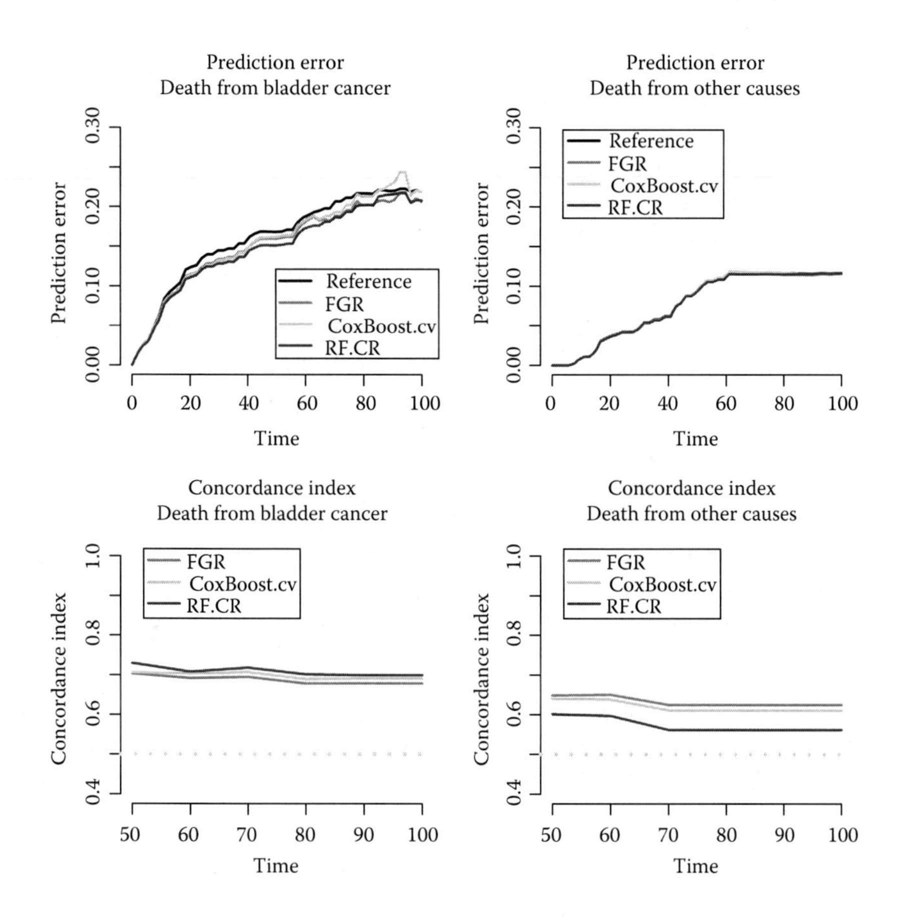

FIGURE 15.2
(See color insert.) Estimated Brier scores (upper panels) and time-truncated concordance index (lower panels) for risk prediction models from Fine–Gray regression with clinical covariates only (FGR), componentwise boosting (CoxBoost.cv), and random forests (RF.CR) for predicting progression and cancer-related death (left panels) and death from other causes (right panels). All estimates are obtained by averaging 100 bootstrap subsample cross-validation runs. In each run, training data are drawn without replacement and include 90% of all patients.

15.6 Concluding Remarks

When predicting risk in a setting with survival data, specific techniques are needed to deal with the time-to-event structure. We have shown how such techniques for risk prediction with high-dimensional molecular data can be derived from classical biostatistical approaches, for example, by regularized regression, or by adapting machine learning approaches, such as random forests.

Regardless of the specific techniques, it is important to carefully consider the event structure. We specifically illustrated risk prediction in a competing risks setting. There, the Fine–Gray model was seen to provide a summary interpretation. Alternatively, a composite endpoint could have been considered, for example, comprising progression or death from any cause. While this would have avoided the Fine–Gray modeling, it would have neither provided the biological interpretation of the cause-specific models nor the direct link to the cumulative incidence.

Generally, the endpoint should not be oversimplified when considering risk prediction in a survival setting. While simplification of the endpoint, for example, transforming it into a binary response and ignoring censoring, or ignoring a competing event type, might have seemed to be the only feasible approach some time ago, due to a lack of approaches for analysis tools, there are now several approaches available that can deal with complex endpoints. For example, the implementation of componentwise likelihood-based boosting can deal with competing risks settings in a straightforward way, or alternatively, random survival forest might be used. This also extends to the techniques used for performance evaluation. As indicated, there are many measures available, where several have been adapted for settings with complex endpoints, such as competing risks. Therefore, the endpoint can be analyzed in the form that is required by subject matter considerations, and performance measures can be chosen according to desired properties, such as providing a strictly proper scoring rule.

15.7 Appendix: Likelihood-Based Boosting

In the following, we briefly sketch the algorithm for componentwise likelihood-based boosting for fitting a Cox proportional hazards model in a time-to-event setting with a single event type, as proposed in [7]. For estimating the parameter vector β of the linear predictor $\eta = X'\beta$ of a Cox model (15.1), the algorithm starts with an estimate $\hat{\beta}^{(0)} = \left(\hat{\beta}_1^{(0)}, \ldots, \hat{\beta}_p^{(0)}\right)'$ and an offset $\hat{\eta}_i^{(0)} = 0, i = 1, \ldots, n$, subsequently performing updates in $m = 1, \ldots, M$, boosting steps. Each boosting step m has the following form:

1. Update the elements $j \in J_{mand}$ of $\hat{\beta}^{(m-1)}$ that correspond to mandatory covariates, such as established clinical predictors, by standard maximum partial likelihood estimation with offset $\hat{\eta}^{(m-1)}$, and subsequently update the offset by $\hat{\eta}_i^{(m-1)} = X_i'\hat{\beta}^{(m-1)}$.
2. Fit candidate models for each covariate $j \notin J_{mand}$, with linear predictor

$$\hat{\eta}_i^{(m-1)} + \gamma_j^{(m)} X_{ij},$$

by performing one Fisher scoring step with respect to the penalized partial log-likelihood $l_{pen}(\gamma_j) = l(\gamma_j) + \lambda\gamma_j^2$, where the partial log-likelihood $l(\gamma)$ incorporates the fixed offset $\hat{\eta}_i^{(m-1)}$, and λ is a penalty parameter that is chosen as indicated in Section 15.4.3.

3. Select the best candidate model j^* according to the penalized score-statistic

$$\frac{U_j^{(m)}(0)^2}{\left(I_j^{(m)} + \lambda\right)},$$

with score function $U_j^{(m)}(\gamma_0) = (\partial l / \partial \gamma)(\gamma_0)$ and Fisher information $I_j^{(m)}(\gamma_0) = (\partial^2 l / \partial^2 \gamma)(\gamma_0)$, for the updates

$$\hat{\beta}_j^{(m)} = \begin{cases} \hat{\beta}_j^{(m-1)} + \hat{\gamma}_j^{(m)} & \text{for } j = j^* \\ \hat{\beta}_j^{(m-1)} & \text{for } j \neq j^* \end{cases}$$

and $\hat{\eta}_i^{(m)} = X_i' \hat{\beta}^{(m)}$.

Selection according to the penalized score statistic ensures that the first boosting steps select the same covariate into the model that would also be the top candidate according to univariate testing, assuming covariates with equal variance.

References

1. O. Aalen and S. Johansen. An empirical transition matrix for non-homogenous Markov chains based on censored observations. *Scandinavian Journal of Statistics*, 5:141–150, 1978.
2. P.K. Andersen, Ø. Borgan, R.D. Gill, and N. Keiding. *Statistical Models Based on Counting Processes*. Springer, Berlin, Germany, 1993.
3. P.K. Andersen, J.P. Klein, and S. Rosthøj. Generalised linear models for correlated pseudo-observations, with applications to multistate models. *Biometrika*, 90(1):15–27, 2003.
4. J. Beyersmann, A. Allignol, and M. Schumacher. *Competing Risks and Multistate Models with R*. Springer, New York, 2012.
5. H. Binder, A. Allignol, M. Schumacher, and J. Beyersmann. Boosting for high-dimensional time-to-event data with competing risks. *Bioinformatics*, 25(7): 890–896, 2009.

6. H. Binder, A. Benner, L. Bullinger, and M. Schumacher. Tailoring sparse multivariable regression techniques for prognostic single-nucleotide polymorphism signatures. *Statistics in Medicine*, 32(10):1778–1791, 2013.
7. H. Binder and M. Schumacher. Allowing for mandatory covariates in boosting estimation of sparse high-dimensional survival models. *BMC Bioinformatics*, 9:14, 2008.
8. H. Binder, C. Porzelius, and M. Schumacher. An overview of techniques for linking high-dimensional molecular data to time-to-event endpoints by risk prediction models. *Biometrical Journal*, 53:170–189, 2011.
9. N. Binder, T.A. Gerds, and P.K. Andersen. Pseudo-observations for competing risks with covariate dependent censoring. *Lifetime Data Analysis*, 20(2): 303–315, 2014.
10. P. Blanche, J.-F. Dartigues, and H. Jacqmin-Gadda. Estimating and comparing time-dependent areas under receiver operating characteristic curves for censored event times with competing risks. *Statistics in Medicine*, 32(30):5381–5397 2013.
11. P. Blanche, J.-F. Dartigues, and H. Jacqmin-Gadda. Review and comparison of roc curve estimators for a time-dependent outcome with marker-dependent censoring. *Biometrical Journal*, 55(5):687–704, September 2013.
12. H.M. Bøvelstad, S. Nygård, H.L. Størvold et al. Predicting survival from microarray data—A comparative study. *Bioinformatics*, 23(16):2080–2087, 2007.
13. L. Breiman. Random forests. *Machine Learning*, 45(1):5–32, 2001. doi: 10.1023/A:1010933404324.
14. P. Bühlmann and B. Yu. Boosting with the l2 loss: Regression and classification. *Journal of the American Statistical Association*, 98:324–339, 2003.
15. T. Cai, J. Huang, and K. Tian. Regularized estimation for the accelerated failure time model. *Biometrics*, 65(2):394–404, 2009.
16. K.A. Doksum and M. Gasko. On a correspondence between models in binary regression and in survival analysis. *International Statistical Review*, 58:243–252, 1990.
17. L. Dyrskjøt, K. Zieger, F.X. Real et al. Gene expression signatures predict outcome in non-muscle-invasive bladder carcinoma: A multicenter validation study. *Clinical Cancer Research*, 13(12): 3545–3551, 2007.
18. B. Efron and R. Tibshirani. Improvements on cross-validation: The .632+ bootstrap method. *Journal of the American Statistical Association*, 92(438):548–560, 1997.
19. D. Engler and Y. Li. Survival analysis with high-dimensional covariates: An application in microarray studies. *Statistical Applications in Genetics and Molecular Biology*, 8(1):Article 14, January 2009.
20. L. Evers and C.M. Messow. Sparse kernel methods for high-dimensional survival data. *Bioinformatics*, 24(14):1632–1638, 2008.
21. J.P. Fine and R.J. Gray. A proportional hazards model for the sub-distribution of a competing risk. *Journal of the American Statistical Association*, 94(446):496–509, 1999.
22. Y. Freund and R.E. Schapire. Experiments with a new boosting algorithm. In *Machine Learning: Proceedings of Thirteenth International Conference*, pp. 148–156, San Francisco, CA, 1996. Morgan Kaufman.
23. J.H. Friedman, T. Hastie, and R. Tibshirani. Additive logistic regression: A statistical view of boosting. *The Annals of Statistics*, 28:337–407, 2000.

24. T.A. Gerds, T. Cai, and M. Schumacher. The performance of risk prediction models. *Biometrical Journal*, 50(4):457–479, 2008.
25. T.A. Gerds, M.W. Kattan, M. Schumacher, and C. Yu. Estimating a time-dependent concordance index for survival prediction models with covariate dependent censoring. *Statistics in Medicine*, 32(13):2173–2184, 2013.
26. T.A. Gerds and M. Schumacher. Efron-type measures of prediction error for survival analysis. *Biometrics*, 63(4):1283–1287, 2007.
27. T.A. Gerds, T.H. Scheike, and P.K. Andersen. Absolute risk regression for competing risks: Interpretation, link functions, and prediction. *Statistics in Medicine*, 31(29):3921–3930, 2012.
28. J.J. Goeman. L1 penalized estimation in the Cox proportional hazards model. *Biometrical Journal*, 52(1):70–84, 2010.
29. N. Grambauer, M. Schumacher, and J. Beyersmann. Proportional subdistribution hazards modeling offers a summary analysis, even if misspecified. *Statistics in Medicine*, 29(7–8):875–884, March 2010.
30. R.J. Gray. A class of k-sample tests for comparing the cumulative incidence of a competing risk. *Annals of Statistics*, 16(3):1141–1154, 1988.
31. F.E. Harrell, R.M. Califf, D.B. Pryor, K.L. Lee, and R.A. Rosati. Evaluating the yield of medical tests. *Journal of the American Medical Association*, 247: 2543–2546, 1982.
32. T. Hastie, J. Taylor, R. Tibshirani, and G. Walther. Forward stagewise regression and the monotone lasso. *Electronic Journal of Statistics*, 1:1–29, 2007.
33. T. Hastie, R. Tibshirani, and J. Friedman. *The Elements of Statistical Learning*, 2nd ed. Springer, New York, 2009.
34. P.J. Heagerty, T. Lumley, and M.S. Pepe. Time-dependent roc curves for censored survival data and a diagnostic marker. *Biometrics*, 56(2):337–344, 2000.
35. A.E. Hoerl and R.W. Kennard. Ridge regression: Biased estimation for nonorthogonal problems. *Technometrics*, 12(1):55–67, 1970.
36. T. Hothorn, B. Lausen, A. Benner, and M. Radspiel-Tröger. Bagging survival trees. *Statistics in Medicine*, 23(1):77–91, 2004.
37. H.C. van Houwelingen, T. Bruinsma, A.A.N. Hart, L.J. Veer, and L.F.A. Wessels. Cross-validated cox regression on microarray gene expression data. *Statistics in Medicine*, 25:3201–3216, 2006.
38. J. Huang, S. Ma, and H. Xie. Regularized estimation in the accelerated failure time model with high-dimensional covariates. *Biometrics*, 62(3):813–820, 2006.
39. H. Ishwaran, U.B. Kogalur, E.Z. Gorodeski, A.J. Minn, and M.S. Lauer. High-dimensional variable selection for survival data. *Journal of the American Statistical Association*, 105(489):205–217, 2010.
40. H. Ishwaran, U.B. Kogular, E.H. Blackstone, and M.S. Lauer. Random survival forests. *Annals of Applied Statistics*, 2(3):841–860, 2008.
41. N.P. Jewell. Correspondence between regression models for complex binary outcome and those for structured multivariate survival analysis. *U.C. Berkeley Division of Biostatistics Working Paper Series*, 195, 2005.
42. C. Kahl, B.E. Storer, B.M. Sandmaier, M. Mielcarek, M.B. Maris, K.G. Blume, D. Niederwieser et al. Relapse risk in patients with malignant diseases given allogeneic hematopoietic cell transplantation after nonmyeloablative conditioning. *Blood*, 110(7):2744–2748, 2007.
43. J.D. Kalbfleisch and R.L. Prentice. *The Statistical Analysis of Failure Time Data*, 2nd ed. Wiley, Hoboken, NJ, 2002.

44. J.P. Klein and M.L. Moeschberger. *Survival Analysis: Techniques for Censored and Truncated Data*. Springer, New York, 2003.
45. C. Leng and S. Ma. Path consistent model selection in additive risk model via lasso. *Statistics in Medicine*, 26(20):3753–3770, 2007.
46. S. Ma, J. Huang, M. Shi, Y. Li, and B.-C. Shia. Semiparametric prognosis models in genomic studies. *Briefings in Bioinformatics*, 11(4):385–393, 2010.
47. E. Marubini and M.G. Valsecchi. *Analysing Survival Data from Clinical Trials and Observational Studies*. Wiley, New York, 2004.
48. U.B. Mogensen and T.A. Gerds. A random forest approach to competing risks based on pseudo-values. *Statistics in Medicine*, 32(18):3102–3114, 2013.
49. C. Porzelius, M. Schumacher, and H. Binder. A general, prediction error-based criterion for selecting model complexity for high-dimensional survival models. *Statistics in Medicine*, 29(7–8):830–838, 2010.
50. C. Porzelius, M. Schumacher, and H. Binder. The benefit of data-based model complexity selection via prediction error curves in time-to-event data. *Computational Statistics*, 26(2):293–302, June 2011.
51. P. Saha and P.J. Heagerty. Time-dependent predictive accuracy in the presence of competing risks. *Biometrics*, 66(4):999–1011, 2010.
52. T.H. Scheike, M.J Zhang, and T.A. Gerds. Predicting cumulative incidence probability by direct binomial regression. *Biometrika*, 95(1):205–220, 2008.
53. R. Schoop, J. Beyersmann, M. Schumacher, and H. Binder. Quantifying the predictive accuracy of time-to-event models in the presence of competing risks. *Biometrical Journal*, 53(1):88–112, 2011.
54. M. Schumacher, H. Binder, and T.A. Gerds. Assessment of survival prediction models based on microarray data. *Bioinformatics*, 23(14):1768–1774, 2007.
55. R.M. Simon, J. Subramanian, M.-C. Li, and S. Menezes. Using cross-validation to evaluate predictive accuracy of survival risk classifiers based on high-dimensional data. *Briefings in Bioinformatics*, 12(3):203–214, 2011.
56. E.W. Steyerberg. *Clinical Prediction Models: A Practical Approach to Development, Validation, and Updating*. Springer, New York, 2009.
57. R. Tibshirani. Regression shrinkage and selection via the lasso. *Journal of the Royal Statistical Society Series B*, 58(1):267–288, 1996.
58. R. Tibshirani. The lasso method for variable selection in the Cox model. *Statistics in Medicine*, 16(4):385–395, 1997.
59. H. Uno, T. Cai, M.J. Pencina, R.B. D'Agostino, and L.J. Wei. On the C-statistics for evaluating overall adequacy of risk prediction procedures with censored survival data. *Statistics in Medicine*, 30:1105–1117, 2011.
60. V.V. Belle, K. Pelckmans, S.V. Huffel, and J.A.K. Suykens. Improved performance on high-dimensional survival data by application of Survival-SVM. *Bioinformatics*, 27:87–94, 2011.
61. S. Varma and R. Simon. Bias in error estimation when using cross-validation for model selection. *BMC Bioinformatics*, 7:91, 2006.
62. P.J.M. Verweij and H.C. van Houwelingen. Penalized likelihood in cox regression. *Statistics in Medicine*, 13:2427–2436, 1994.
63. S. Wang, B. Nan, J. Zhu, and D.G. Beer. Doubly penalized buckley–James method for survival data with high-dimensional covariates. *Biometrics*, 64(1):132–140, 2008.
64. D.M. Witten and R. Tibshirani. Survival analysis with high-dimensional covariates. *Statistical Methods in Medical Research*, 19(1):29–51, 2010.

65. M. Wolbers, M.T. Koller, J.C.M. Witteman, and T.A. Gerds. Concordance for prognostic models with competing risks. Technical Report 3, Department of Biostatistics, University of Copenhagen, Copenhagen, Denmark, 2013.
66. M. Zhu. Kernels and ensembles: Perspectives on statistical learning. *The American Statistician*, 62(2):97–109, 2008.

Section V

Randomized Trials with Biomarker Development and Validation

16

Adaptive Clinical Trial Designs with Biomarker Development and Validation

Boris Freidlin and Richard Simon

CONTENTS

16.1 Introduction

Human cancers are heterogeneous with respect to their molecular and genomic properties. Therefore, a given therapy may benefit only a subset of treated patients. This is particularly relevant for the new generation of cancer therapies that target specific molecular pathways. Recent developments in molecular medicine provide new tools for identifying biomarkers to select patients who benefit from a targeted agent.

Ideally, biomarkers to identify sensitive subpopulations should be developed and clinically validated during the early stages of drug development before the definitive phase III randomized clinical trial (RCT) is designed. In this case, enrichment design [1] that restricts eligibility to sensitive patients should be used. However, biomarker development often lags behind drug development. In the absence of a reliable biomarker, broad eligibility clinical trials are routinely used. Most of these trials use conventional design with the primary analysis based on comparison of all randomized patients. This may lead to missing effective agents due to the dilution of the treatment effect by the presence of the patients who do not benefit from the agent. Moreover, phase III RCTs require considerable investment of time and resources. Therefore, clinical trial designs that allow combining definitive evaluation of a new agent with development of the companion diagnostic test to identify sensitive patients can considerably speed up introduction of new cancer therapies [2].

In this chapter, we discuss designs that allow a statistically rigorous codevelopment of a new treatment and a companion biomarker to identify a sensitive subpopulation. First, we consider settings where a candidate biomarker score is available but no cutoff to distinguish sensitive versus nonsensitive subpopulation is predefined. For these settings, we describe the biomarker adaptive threshold design (BATD) [3] that combines a test for overall treatment effect in all randomized patients with the establishment and validation of the biomarker cut-point for identifying the sensitive subpopulation. Next we consider situations where no candidate biomarker to identify sensitive patients is available at the outset of the study. For these settings, the adaptive signature design (ASD) [4] that combines a prospective development and validation of a biomarker classifier to select sensitive patients with a properly powered test for overall effect is proposed. We then describe a cross-validated version of the ASD (CVASD) procedure [5] that allows one to optimize efficiency of both the signature development and validation components of the design.

16.2 Biomarker-Adaptive Threshold Design

Often, when a phase III trial to evaluate a new therapy is designed, a candidate biomarker score to identify the sensitive subpopulation is available but an appropriate cutoff value has not been properly established (or validated). Many biomarkers that are originally measured on a continuous or graded scale (such as proportion of cells in S-phase) are then used to categorize patients into several distinct categories for clinical management. In particular, molecularly targeted drugs often rely on assays to measure target expression (e.g., HER2 or EGFR) that are graded and then are converted to dichotomous (positive/negative) status based on a cutoff that has not been properly validated. For example, when EGFR expression is measured by immunohistochemistry using the DAKO kit, various cut-points have been used [6].

In this section, we describe a statistically rigorous phase III design for settings where the putative biomarker is measured on a continuous or graded scale. The design combines a test for overall treatment effect in all randomized patients with establishment and validation of a cut-point for a prespecified biomarker for identifying the sensitive subpopulation. The procedure provides prospective tests of the hypotheses that the new treatment is beneficial for the entire patient population or for a subset of patients that is defined by the biomarker.

In addition to a formal test for any treatment effect (overall or in subpopulation), the BATD procedure can be used to provide point and interval estimates of the optimal biomarker cutoff and a graph for estimating the probability that a patient with given biomarker value will benefit from the new therapy. These tools can be useful in selecting a biomarker defined subpopulation with improved risk–benefit ratio as well as in guiding treatment decisions for individual patients.

16.2.1 Design

Consider a RCT designed to assess whether a new therapy is better than the standard care. Patients are randomized between the new treatment (arm E) and the standard treatment (arm C). In this presentation, we assume time-to-event clinical outcome (e.g., overall survival [OS] or progression-free survival [PFS]) and use the proportional hazards model [7]; however, the overall algorithm behind the design can be used with any outcome using a likelihood ratio-type statistic. Under the assumption of uniform treatment effect in the entire study population, the proportional hazards model is

$$\log\left(\frac{h_E(t)}{h_C(t)}\right) = \gamma \tag{16.1}$$

where

t denotes time form randomization

$h_E(t)$ and $h_C(t)$ denote the hazard functions for experimental and control arms, respectively

γ denotes treatment effect

If one hypothesizes that the new therapy may only be beneficial in a *sensitive* subset of patients defined by a quantitative biomarker and the risk–benefit ratio is maximized in patients with biomarker above some unknown cutoff value, then for a patient with biomarker value v, a general representation of the model is

$$\log h(t) = \log h_0(t) + \mu\tau + \eta I\left(v > c_0\right) + \gamma\tau I\left(v > c_0\right) \tag{16.2}$$

where

μ is the main treatment effect
η is the main biomarker effect
γ is treatment by biomarker interaction
τ is the treatment group indicator ($\tau = 0$ for arm C and $\tau = 1$ for arm E)
c_0 denotes the unknown cutoff value
I is an indicator function that takes value 0 when $v \le c_0$ and 1 when $v > c_0$

Without loss of generality, it can be assumed that the biomarker (and c_0) takes values in interval [0, 1]. If the main treatment effect μ is assumed to be 0, one obtains a simplified *cut-point* model [8]:

$$\log\left(\frac{h_E(t)}{h_C(t)}\right) = \begin{cases} 0 & \text{for patients with biomarker values below } c_0 \\ \gamma & \text{for patients with biomarker values above } c_0 \end{cases} \tag{16.3}$$

Note that model (16.3) reduces to model (16.1) when $c_0 = 0$.

In the following presentation, we will use model (16.3) for developing likelihood-ratio-based testing procedures. The objective of the analysis is to determine whether the experimental arm is better than the control arm for all randomized patients or for a subset of patients defined by values of the biomarker greater than some value c_0. Two alternative procedures are described.

A simple approach (procedure A) can be constructed as follows. First, test for treatment effect in all patients at a reduced significance level α_1. If the test is significant then, for the purpose of formal evaluation, the procedure rejects the null hypothesis of no treatment effect in the entire study population. Otherwise, the procedure uses an algorithm to test for treatment effect in a biomarker-defined subset of patients, at significance level $\alpha_2 = \alpha - \alpha_1$. The specific algorithm will be described later. This procedure controls the probability of making any false-positive claim at the prespecified level α. To preserve the ability of the procedure to detect an overall effect without a major increase in sample size, we often recommend setting α_1 to 80% of α and α_2 to 20% of α. For example, setting a $\alpha_1 = 0.04$ and $\alpha_2 = 0.01$ corresponds to procedure-wise α level of 0.05.

The advantage of procedure A is its simplicity and that it explicitly separates the test of treatment effect in the broad population from the subset selection. Thus, at the end of the study, one of the three distinct outcomes is established (1) treatment benefit in broad population is shown, (2) treatment effect in a biomarker-defined subset of patients is shown, or (3) no treatment effect is detected. However, the procedure takes a conservative approach in adjusting for multiplicity of combining the overall and subset tests.

A more efficient approach to combining the overall and subset tests can be constructed by accounting for the correlation structure of the test statistics (procedure B) as follows: For each candidate biomarker cutoff value of c in the interval [0, 1], fit model (16.3) on the subset of patients with biomarker values above c. Then, the log-likelihood ratio statistic $S(c)$ for testing $\gamma=0$ is calculated. (Note that for cutoff value of 0 the likelihood ratio statistic is the overall effect statistic $S=S(0)$.) A natural approach to converting a series of statistics calculated over the range of possible cutoff values into a single test is to take the maximum [9]. To ensure that the resulting procedure has reasonable power when the new treatment is effective for the entire population, we weigh up the contribution of the overall test S. This is achieved by adding a positive constant R to statistic S before taking the maximum; the resulting statistic is denoted $T=\max\left(\left(S(0)+R\right),\max\limits_{0<c<1}\{S(c)\}\right)$. Note that adding a constant to S could be seen as a generalization of the approach taken in procedure A where a higher portion of procedure-wise error rate is allocated to the overall effect test. In our simulation study, several values of R were investigated. The value $R=2.2$ was shown to provide a good balance between the ability of the procedure to detect an overall effect and its ability to detect a subset effect. In the second stage of procedure A, $T_A=\max\limits_{0.5<c<1}\{S(c)\}$ is used to test the null hypothesis that the treatments are equivalent for the subset of patients with biomarker values above any specified cut-point.

Statistics T and T_A use an optimized cutoff value. Because of the well-known multiple testing problem, the standard asymptotic theory does not apply [8,9]. To adjust for the multiple testing inherent in the construction of the statistics, a resampling-based approach is used [10]. First, statistic T is evaluated on the observed data. Then, K permuted datasets are constructed by randomly permuting treatment labels. For each permuted dataset, the corresponding test statistic T^* is calculated. The permutation p-value is given by

$$\frac{1+\text{number of permutations where } T^*\geq T}{1+\text{number of permutations}}.$$

If procedure B or the second part of procedure A rejects the null hypothesis of no treatment effect, the next step is to identify the biomarker threshold c_0 above which the new treatment is more effective than the control. A point estimator $\hat{c}_0$, for the cutoff value c_0 is obtained as

$$\hat{c}_0=\underset{c_0}{\operatorname{argmax}}\, l(c_0)$$

where $l(c_0)$ is the partial log likelihood function based on model (16.2):

$$l(c_0)=\max_{\mu\eta\gamma} l(\mu,\eta,\gamma,c_0) \text{ for } c_0\in[0,1].$$

In addition, one can use a graphical representation of the distribution function of the estimate of c_0 as a convenient tool for communicating the study result to patients and clinicians. An estimate $\hat{F}_{\hat{c}0}$ of the distribution function $F_{\hat{c}0}$ of $\hat{c}_0$ is estimated as follows. B random bootstrap samples from the observed data are drawn. For each bootstrap sample, an estimate $\hat{c}_0^*$ is obtained, $\hat{F}_{\hat{c}0}$ is estimated by the empirical distribution of $\hat{c}_0^*$. For a given biomarker value, function $\hat{F}_{\hat{c}0}$ gives the estimated probability that the true cutoff level c_0 is below that value. When there is no overall treatment effect, this function is interpreted as the probability that a patient with given biomarker value will benefit from the new therapy. (It can be used as a clinical management tool for guiding individual patient decisions.) Percentiles of the empirical distribution function provide a confidence interval for c_0. Confidence intervals for $\hat{F}_{\hat{c}0}$ are obtained by double bootstrap: first B_1 random first-level bootstraps are drawn from the observed data. For each first-level bootstrap sample, an estimate of the distribution function $\hat{F}^*_{\hat{c}0}$ is obtained using B_2 second-level bootstraps. Percentiles of the empirical distribution of $\hat{F}^*_{\hat{c}0}$ provide a confidence interval for $\hat{F}_{\hat{c}0}$.

It is important to prospectively incorporate the biomarker-based procedures into the study design and describe them in the study protocol. In particular, the procedures require careful sample size planning: an approach to sample size calculation for BATD procedures is described in Jiang et al. [3].

16.2.2 Evaluation of the BATD Procedures

In this section, we use simulations to illustrate the performance of procedures A and B relative to a standard broad eligibility phase III design (which is based on testing overall effect in the entire study population). The simulations correspond to clinical trials with 200 patients randomized between experimental and control arms. Outcome data were generated from model (16.3) with an exponential model ($h_E(t) = h_C(t) = 1$). Biomarker values were generated from a uniform distribution on the interval (0, 1). Administrative censoring resulting from staggered entry ranged between 10% and 20%. In implementing the procedures, we used a grid of candidate biomarker cutoff values of (0, 0.1, 0.2, 0.3, 0.4, 0.5, 0.6, 0.7, 0.8, and 0.9). Procedure A used $\alpha_1 = 0.04$ and $\alpha_2 = 0.01$. Constant $R = 2.2$ was used in procedure B.

Procedures were evaluated under a range of settings. In the first set of simulations, all patients benefit from new therapy (corresponding to model [16.1]). In the second set of simulations data were generated using model (16.3) where only patients with biomarker values above the true cut-point benefit from the new treatment. We performed simulations with cut-point values of $c_0 = 0.25$, 0.5, 0.75, and 0.9. In order to evaluate the performance of the proposed procedures under a departure from model (16.3), we considered two additional situations. In one, the log hazard ratio of the experimental over the standard arm increased linearly over the entire range of biomarker values (*linear trend*). In the other (*delayed linear trend*), there is no benefit (log hazard ratio equals 0) for patients with biomarker value below 0.5 and a linear increase in log hazard ratio for patients with biomarker values above 0.5.

Each of the seven simulation settings are presented in a separate panel in Table 16.1. Within each panel rows represent different magnitudes of the treatment effect. We tabulated empirical power of the test for overall treatment effect (column 4) and empirical powers for procedures A and B (columns 5 and 6, respectively). The tests were conducted at a two-sided 0.05 significance level.

TABLE 16.1

Empirical Power: Procedures A and B versus Overall Test

		Effect Size: Reduction in Hazard (Hazard Ratio)	Empirical Power[a]		
Sim #	Model		Overall Test	Procedure A	Procedure B
1	Everybody benefits from new therapy	20% (0.8)	0.330	0.304	0.313
		33% (0.67)	0.775	0.751	0.732
		43% (0.57)	0.965	0.957	0.943
2	Only patients with biomarker values above 0.25 benefit from new therapy	43% (0.57)	0.819	0.802	0.837
		60% (0.4)	0.996	0.997	0.998
3	Only patients with biomarker values above 0.5 benefit from new therapy	43% (0.57)	0.505	0.562	0.607
		60% (0.4)	0.888	0.932	0.952
4	Only patients with biomarker values above 0.75 benefit from new therapy	43% (0.57)	0.196	0.280	0.311
		60% (0.4)	0.429	0.604	0.641
		69% (0.31)	0.600	0.806	0.846
5	Only patients with biomarker values above 0.9 benefit from new therapy	60% (0.4)	0.105	0.238	0.274
		69% (0.31)	0.162	0.401	0.412
		79% (0.21)	0.238	0.632	0.624
6	Linear increase in hazard ratio	43% (0.57)[b]	0.497	0.504	0.542
		60% (0.4)[b]	0.887	0.892	0.909
		69% (0.31)[b]	0.974	0.981	0.985
7	Linear increase in hazard ratio for patients with biomarker values above 0.5	43% (0.57)[c]	0.166	0.212	0.262
		60% (0.4)[c]	0.386	0.514	0.541
		69% (0.31)[c]	0.559	0.744	0.741

[a] Overall test, procedures A and B performed at a two-sided 0.05 significance level.
[b] Maximum effect, effect increases linearly in biomarker from 0 to the maximum.
[c] Maximum effect, effect increases linearly in biomarker from 0.5 to the maximum.

Panel 1 considers the situation where the new therapy is beneficial for all patients. Naturally, the overall effect test has the highest power under this model. However, the proposed procedures have similar power, with only marginal loss relative to the overall test. Panels 2–5 consider situations in which only a proportion of patients benefits from the new therapy. The standard phase III design, relying on the test for overall effect, generally results in a considerable loss of power. The ability of the standard design to detect treatment effect decreases as the proportion of the sensitive patients in the population decreases. For example, for a 43% reduction in hazard the power is reduced from 97% when all patients benefit (panel 1, third line) to less than 20% when only 25% of patients benefit (those with biomarker values greater than 0.75) (panel 4, first line). The proposed procedures provide improved power under the subset effect scenarios 2 through 5. In many instances, the improvement is substantial.

Under a linear trend model (panel 6), the proposed procedures have slightly better power than the standard design. Under the delayed trend model, power advantage of procedure B is considerable (panel 7).

Procedures A and B provide good power for detecting a subset effect while preserving the ability to detect overall treatment effect when it is present. In general, procedure B has a higher power than procedure A across the settings considered.

16.2.3 Example: Prostate Cancer Data

We now use the proposed procedures to analyze data from the second Veterans Administration Cooperative Urologic Research Group clinical trial [11,12]. This double-blind clinical trial randomized 506 prostate cancer patients to one of four arms: placebo, 0.2 mg of diethylstilbestrol (DES), 1.0 or 5.0 mg DES. Similar to Byar and Corle [11], in our analysis the two lower doses (placebo and the 0.2 mg DES) are combined into a single arm (designated arm C) and the two higher doses (1.0 and 5.0 mg DES) are combined into a single arm (designated arm E). Arms E and C are compared with respect to OS.

We investigated whether serum prostatic acid phosphatase (AP) or the combined index of tumor stage (SG) can be used to identify a subset of patients for whom DES is beneficial. The variable AP measures the serum prostatic AP in King-Armstrong units; the numbers are continuous from 1 to 5960 with a median value of 7. SG records the combined index of tumor stage and histological grade; it takes integer values ranging from 5 to 15 with a median of 10. The results are presented in Table 16.2.

A standard clinical trial design based on testing overall treatment effect (in all randomized patients) fails to detect a significant benefit for DES at 0.05 significance level (p-value 0.084); see Table 16.2. In applying procedure A to AP, one first performs the overall test at a 0.04 significance level. Since it fails to reach the required significance, one then proceeds to testing for subset effect at 0.01 level. From Table 16.2, the subset test p-value is 0.019.

TABLE 16.2

Prostate Cancer Study Results

Variable	# Patients with Measured Covariate	*p*-Value			Estimate and Confidence Interval	
		Overall Test	Procedure A, Stage 2	Procedure B[a]	Estimated Cutoff	95% CI
AP	505	0.084	0.019	0.041	36	(9, 170)
SG	494	0.110	0.025	0.050	11	(10, 13)

[a] Procedure B used $R=2.2$.

Thus, procedure A fails to reject the null hypothesis of no effect (at overall 0.05 level). Procedure B applied to AP gives *p*-value 0.041 indicating that treatment is effective in a subset of population with high stage-grade values. The estimated cutoff value is 36 with 95% confidence interval [9, 170] (Table 16.2). The implications for a patient with a given value of AP are summarized by the estimated probability of benefit (Figure 16.1). For example, a patient with AP value of 100 is estimated to have over 90% probability of benefit, while a patient with AP value of 20 has only about 10% chance of benefit.

Similarly, for SG, the procedure A fails to reject the null hypothesis (overall test *p*-value 0.1, subset effect test *p*-value 0.025). Procedure B indicates that DES is beneficial in a subset of patients with high SG values (*p*-value 0.05). The cutoff is estimated to be 11 (95% confidence interval is [10,13]; Table 16.2), that is, patients with SG values above 11 benefit from the treatment.

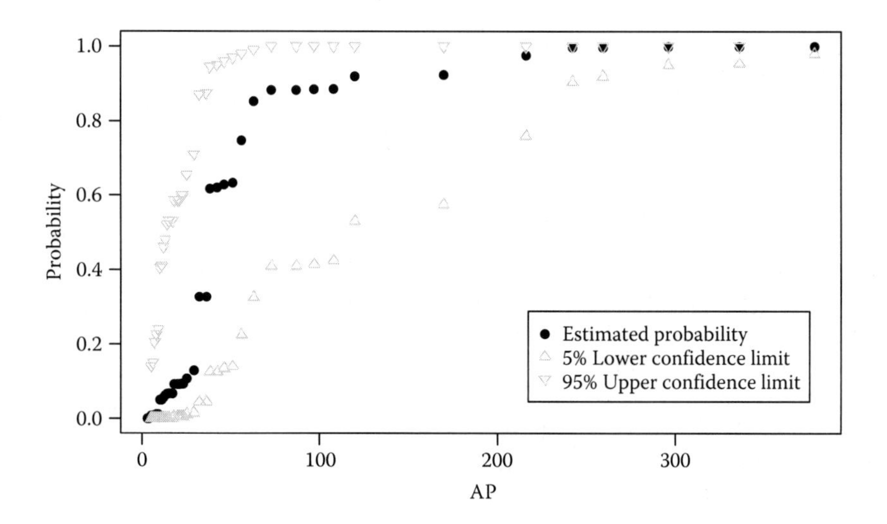

FIGURE 16.1
Estimated probability that a prostate cancer patient with a given value of serum prostatic AP will benefit from treatment with DES.

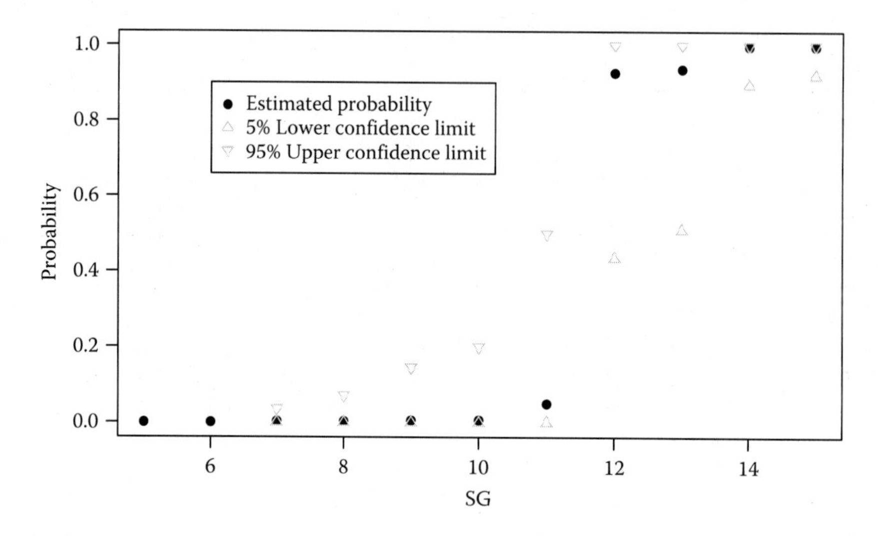

FIGURE 16.2
Estimated probability that a prostate cancer patient with a given value on a combined index of tumor stage and histological grade (SG) will benefit from treatment with DES.

The implications for a patient with a given value of SG are summarized in Figure 16.2. For example, a patient with SG value of 12 is estimated to have over 90% probability of benefit while a patient with SG value of 10 has less than 5% probability of benefit.

16.3 Adaptive Signature Designs

We now focus on settings where a prespecified biomarker or classifier to identify sensitive patients is not available. For this setting, ASD was developed [4]. The design combines (1) prospective development and validation of a pharmacogenomic diagnostic test (signature) to select sensitive patients and (2) a properly powered test for overall effect. The two components are prospectively incorporated into a single-phase III RCT with the overall false-positive error rate controlled at a prespecified level. Although the ASD was originally developed for gene expression profile classifiers, it is much more widely applicable [13,14]. For example, Sher et al. [15] describe use of the design for planning clinical trials in advanced hormone-resistant prostate cancer with four candidate biomarkers.

In the original ASD procedure, the signature development and validation steps are carried out on the two mutually exclusive subgroups of patients in the clinical trial (e.g., half of the study population is used to develop a signature and another half to validate it). While conceptually simple, this approach limits the power as only half of the patients are used in each step. (This is especially problematic in settings with high-dimensional data.) To improve ASD efficiency, a version of the design in which signature development and validation are embedded in a complete CVASD has been described [5]. The CVASD procedure allows us to use virtually the entire study population in both signature development and validation steps.

This section describes the ASD and CVSD procedures. We then present a simulation study that compares the designs to each other and to the traditional phase III RCT design that tests treatment in overall population. We also examine approaches to estimating treatment effect in the identified sensitive subpopulation.

16.3.1 Adaptive Signature Design

Consider an RCT that randomly assigns patients to the new treatment (arm E) or the standard treatment (arm C). In defining the design for the high-dimensional modeling setting, we make the following modeling assumptions: among H evaluated markers there is a subset of L predictive (*sensitivity*) markers. The identities of the predictive markers are unknown, but responsiveness to treatment is influenced by them through the following model. We consider a binary response endpoint but the design can be easily generalized to a proportional hazards model for time-to-event data. For a given patient, let p denote the probability of response, t denote the treatment indicator ($t=0$ for arm C and $t=1$ for arm E), and $x_1,\ldots, x_L$ denote the levels of the L unknown predictive markers. Then,

$$\log\left(\frac{p}{1-p}\right) = \mu + \lambda t + \xi_1 x_1 + \cdots + \xi_L x_L + \gamma_1 t x_1 + \cdots + \gamma_L t x_L \tag{16.4}$$

where

λ is treatment main effect of treatment

ξ_i is main effect for ith sensitivity marker

γ_i is treatment–marker interaction effect that reflects the degree by which the difference in treatment arms is influenced by the ith sensitivity marker level

To simplify the presentation, main effects and the treatment–marker interactions for the nonpredictive markers are assumed to be 0.

If the interaction parameters are positive, patients with higher levels of those markers have a higher probability of response on arm E compared to arm C.

Similar to the traditional RCT design, the ASD is based on randomizing a total of N patients between the two treatment arms and provides control of the overall type I error at level α. The final analysis begins with an overall comparison between arms E and C using data from all N patients. If the comparison is significant at a prespecified significance level α_1 ($\alpha_1 < \alpha$), then the new treatment is considered beneficial in the entire population. Otherwise, the design proceeds to the signature development/validation stage. The study patients are divided into two cohorts: (1) the signature validation cohort that contains M patients, and (2) the classifier development (or training) cohort that contains the remaining $N - M$ patients. First, using the development cohort patients only, a classifier is developed to identify patients that have better outcomes on the new therapy than the standard therapy. The classifier is then applied to the validation cohort and classifier positive *sensitive* patients are identified.

For validation, outcomes for patients in the sensitive subset of the validation cohort who received the new therapy are compared to the outcomes for patients in the sensitive subset of the validation cohort who received the standard therapy. A statistical significance test is performed at significance level $\alpha_2 = \alpha - \alpha_1$ to ensure that overall type I error of the design is no greater than $\alpha = \alpha_1 + \alpha_2$.

The allocation of the experiment-wise significance level α between the overall and subset tests in a particular implementation of the design should be based on the context of the clinical trial and the credentials of the candidate markers available for developing a predictive classifier. For example, an 80%–20% allocation setting $\alpha_1 = 0.04$ and $\alpha_2 = 0.01$ protects the study-wise α-level of 0.05 for settings where the classifier development process is viewed as a fall-back strategy, the main focus is on the overall analysis and there is little interest in expanding the size of the clinical trial to accommodate classifier development and validation. When, however, the trial is to be sized for adequate power for both overall analysis and for classifier development and validation, an increase in sample size will be required and it may be efficient to allocate 80% of the alpha to the subset analysis (i.e., $\alpha_1 = 0.01$ and $\alpha_2 = 0.04$) as in [15] because the power for the subset analysis primarily determines the sample size.

Many types of algorithms for developing a predictive classifier on the training cohort are possible. It should be noted, however, that a predictive classifier is not the same as a prognostic classifier. A predictive classifier is a binary classifier that indicates whether one treatment is likely to be better than the other, not whether the patient will respond to a given treatment. Here we describe the approach originally used in [4] based on machine learning voting method [16].

Step 1: Using data from the development cohort patients, for each marker j fit the single marker logistic model $\log(p) = \mu + \lambda_j t + \beta_j t x_j$. Note the markers that have treatment–marker interaction $\hat{\beta}_j$ significant at a predetermined level η.

Step 2: Classify the validation cohort patients as sensitive or nonsensitive to the new treatment based on the markers with significant interactions in step 1. Validation cohort patient is designated sensitive if the predicted new versus control arm odds ratio exceeds a specified threshold (R) for at least G of the significant markers j (i.e., $e^{\hat{\lambda}_j+\hat{\beta}_j x_j} > R$).

A list Θ of plausible sets of the three tuning parameters (η, R, and G) should be identified prospectively based on the range of feasible models. Freidlin and Simon [4] described selection of tuning parameter set from the list.

16.3.2 Cross-Validated Adaptive Signature Design (CVASD)

The classifier development and validation stages of the ASD procedure are carried out on two nonoverlapping subpopulations; therefore, the nominal significance level of the test of treatment effect in the adaptively determined sensitive subset is preserved at the nominal α_2 level. While this makes ASD conceptually simple, it also results in loss of efficiency since only a portion of the trial patients contribute to each stage. The CVASD allows a more efficient use of patient data by employing a cross-validation approach for the signature development and subset effect testing. A K-fold cross-validation for an N-patient trial proceeds as follows: First, the trial population is split into an M-patient validation cohort and an (N – M)-patient development cohort (where $M = N/K$). Let D_k denote the set of patients in the kth development cohort, and V_k the set of patients in the corresponding validation cohort. For each D_k ($k = 1,\ldots, K$), a predictive classifier is developed. The classifier is applied to identify a sensitive patient subset S_k of V_k. This procedure is repeated K times over all M-patient nonoverlapping validation cohorts V_k (and the corresponding D_k). Each study patient appears in exactly one of the validation cohorts.

At the end of the cross-validation procedure, each of the study patients is classified as either sensitive or not. The sensitive patient subset of the entire study population is identified as $S = \bigcup_{k=1}^{K} S_k$. The outcomes for the sensitive patients who received the experimental therapy are compared to the outcomes for the sensitive patients who received the standard therapy using an appropriate statistic T. Since this subset of sensitive patients is obtained by cross-validation, the standard asymptotic theory for distribution of T does not apply. Similar to the BATD procedures A and B (described in Section 16.2) a valid p-value is obtained by permutation method. In practice the permutation distribution is usually approximated by a resampling-based approach. First, statistic T is evaluated on the observed data. Then, a permuted dataset is constructed by randomly permuting treatment labels. The entire cross-validation procedure is repeated for the permuted data set and the corresponding test statistic T^* is computed. This procedure is repeated for B permuted datasets. The permutation p-value is given by

$$\frac{1 + \text{Number of permutations where } T^* \geq T}{1 + B}.$$

In order to obtain a valid p-value, all steps of the signature development algorithm (including selection of tuning parameters) must be incorporated into each loop of the cross-validation procedure for each permuted dataset [10]. The CVASD implements this in the following way for the machine learning classifier algorithm described in the previous section. A list Θ of plausible tuning parameter sets (η, R, G) is prespecified; then, on each ($N - M$)-patient development cohort D_k, a nested inner-loop of K-fold cross-validation is applied to obtain a set of sensitive patients corresponding to each of the parameter sets. The tuning parameter set corresponding to the sensitive subset with smallest p-value (for the difference between arms) is selected for use in the corresponding development cohort. Finally, to ensure strict validity and reproducibility of the procedure, patient allocation to the cross-validation cohorts D_k and V_k ($k = 1, \ldots, K$) should be prospectively defined.

16.3.3 Evaluation of ASD and CVASD

A simulation study is presented to illustrate the performance of ASD and CVASD with $K = 10$ (tenfold cross-validation). The results are given for a 10,000-gene array with $L = 10$ predictive genes (it was shown [4] that the design performance is similar over a range of values of L). Gene main effects, ξ_i, were assumed to be 0. Treatment–expression interaction levels were kept constant across predictive genes ($\gamma = \gamma_1 = \gamma_2 = \cdots = \gamma_L$). An intercept ($\mu$) value corresponding to control arm response rate of 25% was used (previous simulation suggested similar results for other intercept values [4]). The simulations were based on 1000 replications and $B = 99$ (see [5] for more details).

The simulations are reported in Tables 16.3 through 16.5 and represent a clinical trial in which $N = 400$ patients were randomized between the experimental and control arms. Both CVASD and ASD procedures use 80%–20% alpha-level split with an overall 0.05 (two-sided) significance level (corresponding to $\alpha_1 = 0.04$ and $\alpha_2 = 0.01$). We tabulated empirical powers of the overall arm comparison at 0.05 and 0.04 significance levels and comparison in the selected sensitive subset at 0.01 two-sided significance levels. In addition, the overall empirical power of the adaptive designs is calculated as the percentage of replications with either positive overall 0.04 level test or positive 0.01 level sensitive subset test. Since ASD and CVASD simulations were run independently, we report empirical power for the overall tests for each procedure separately (note that the small discrepancies between the power of the overall tests for the two procedures reflect the random variation in the simulation results).

TABLE 16.3

Empirical Power: ASD and CVASD as a Function of the Subset Treatment Effect

Test	ASD	CVASD (10-Fold Cross-Validation)
90% response in sensitive patients on the experimental arm and 25% in all other patients		
Overall 0.05 level test	0.301	0.291
Overall 0.04 level test	0.261	0.256
Sensitive subset 0.01 level test	0.495	0.880
Overall ASD	0.605	0.909
80% response in sensitive patients on the experimental arm and 25% in all other patients		
Overall 0.05 level test	0.232	0.240
Overall 0.04 level test	0.203	0.209
Sensitive subset 0.01 level test	0.202	0.661
Overall ASD	0.348	0.714
70% response in sensitive patients on the experimental arm and 25% in all other patients		
Overall 0.05 level test	0.177	0.183
Overall 0.04 level test	0.147	0.155
Sensitive subset 0.01 level test	0.066	0.371
Overall ASD	0.191	0.450
60% response in sensitive patients on the experimental arm and 25% in all other patients		
Overall 0.05 level test	0.121	0.129
Overall 0.04 level test	0.105	0.107
Sensitive subset 0.01 level test	0.015	0.135
Overall ASD	0.115	0.229

Note: 10% of patients sensitive.

First we consider a situation where the benefit of the new drug is restricted to a small fraction of patients: 10% of the eligible patient population that over-expresses the predictive genes. Table 16.3 presents results for a range of treatment effects. The first panel corresponds to a very strong subset effect: 90% response rate in sensitive patients on the experimental arm and a 25% response rate in all other patients (nonsensitive patients on the experimental arm and all control arm patients). In this case, the traditional broad eligibility design that relies on an overall 0.05 level test has a 30% power to detect difference between the arms. This can be contrasted with the performance of the signature designs: for both ASD and CVASD, the overall difference was declared with 26% probability (using a 0.04 level overall test). In ASD, the sensitive subset test was significant (at 0.01 level) in 50% of cases, resulting in 61% overall power for the design (a 61% probability of either detecting a significant overall effect or a significant subset effect). For CVASD, the sensitive subset test was significant (at 0.01 level) in 88% of cases, resulting in 91% overall power. As the magnitude of the treatment effect in the subset becomes smaller (Table 16.3, panels 2–4), ASD's ability to detect the subset effect is reduced; on the other hand, CVASD continues to demonstrate a robust ability to detect subset effect

TABLE 16.4

Empirical Power: ASD and CVASD as a Function of Fraction of Sensitive Patients

Test	ASD	CVASD (10-Fold Cross-Validation)
70% response in sensitive patients on the experimental arm and 25% in all other patients		
20% of patients are sensitive		
Overall 0.05 level test	0.518	0.503
Overall 0.04 level test	0.478	0.471
Sensitive subset 0.01 level test	0.192	0.588
Overall ASD	0.543	0.731
30% of patients are sensitive		
Overall 0.05 level test	0.846	0.838
Overall 0.04 level test	0.822	0.808
Sensitive subset 0.01 level test	0.295	0.723
Overall ASD	0.836	0.918
40% of patients are sensitive		
Overall 0.05 level test	0.969	0.961
Overall 0.04 level test	0.962	0.955
Sensitive subset 0.01 level test	0.412	0.812
Overall ASD	0.963	0.972
60% response in sensitive patients on the experimental arm and 25% in all other patients		
20% of patients are sensitive		
Overall 0.05 level test	0.359	0.349
Overall 0.04 level test	0.323	0.313
Sensitive subset 0.01 level test	0.051	0.196
Overall ASD	0.342	0.421
30% of patients are sensitive		
Overall 0.05 level test	0.620	0.622
Overall 0.04 level test	0.584	0.582
Sensitive subset 0.01 level test	0.047	0.254
Overall ASD	0.589	0.641
40% of patients are sensitive		
Overall 0.05 level test	0.861	0.856
Overall 0.04 level test	0.841	0.829
Sensitive subset 0.01 level test	0.089	0.274
Overall ASD	0.842	0.843

across the range of treatment effects. For example, when the response rate in sensitive patients on the experiment arm is 70%, the sensitive subset test was significant in 37% of cases in CVASD versus 7% in ASD (45% versus 19% overall power). For smaller treatment effects (panels 3 and 4), the power advantage for the adaptive designs versus the traditional broad eligibility design (which relies on overall effect test) is limited to the CVASD procedure.

TABLE 16.5

Empirical Power: No Subset Effect

Test	ASD	CVASD (10-Fold Cross-Validation)
No subset effect: 35% response in all patients on the experimental arm 25% response rate in all patients on the control arm		
Overall 0.05 level test	0.572	0.594
Overall 0.04 level test	0.534	0.554
Sensitive subset 0.01 level test	0.009	0[a]
Overall ASD	0.534	0.554
No treatment effect 25% response in all patients		
Overall 0.05 level test	0.050	0.056
Overall 0.04 level test	0.038	0.048
Sensitive subset 0.01 level test	0.001	0[a]
Overall ASD	0.038	0.048

[a] When no sensitive patients are identified, the test statistic is given the lowest possible value.

Table 16.4 illustrates the performance of the ASD with increasing fraction of the sensitive patients (strong subset effect in panels 1–3 and moderate subset effect in panes 4–6). The difference in overall power between ASD, CVASD, and the traditional design becomes smaller as the fraction of sensitive patients increases (when sensitive fraction is 40% or higher, the overall power is similar). For example, when 40% of the study patients are sensitive overall powers of the ASD, CVASD, and the traditional design are 84%, 84%, and 86%, respectively (panel 6). In terms of ability to identify the subset effect, CVASD provides an improved power (relative to ASD) to detect the sensitive subpopulation.

When the effect of the new treatment is homogeneous across the patient population (i.e., all patients benefit equally), the adaptive procedures preserve the power to detect the overall effect while correctly indicating the absence of sensitive subpopulation (Table 16.5, panel 1). Under the null hypothesis (when there is no overall or subset effect), both ASD and CVASD preserve the overall type I error rate (Table 16.5, panel 2).

The simulation results demonstrate that the cross-validation approach can considerably enhance the ASD performance. Cross-validation permits maximization of the portion of study patients contributing to the development of the diagnostic classifier. Cross-validation also maximizes the size of the sensitive patient subset used to test (validate) the classifier, and this is important in settings where the fraction of the sensitive patients is small.

16.3.4 Estimation of the Treatment Effect in the Sensitive Population

An important issue with adaptive designs is interpretation of a positive study that concludes that the treatment benefit is limited to a subgroup of patients.

In this case, the design needs to provide (1) an explicitly defined diagnostic classifier to identify the sensitive subpopulation of future patients and (2) an estimate of the treatment effect in that sensitive subpopulation. Consider a study that followed CVASD and concluded a significant treatment effect in a subpopulation but not for the overall population. To obtain the final classifier to identify future patients who benefit from the new drug, we recommend applying the signature development algorithm to the entire study population. A relevant measure of the treatment effect is then the predicted treatment effect in the future patients that are classified as sensitive by the final signature. Two possible estimators for the predicted effect could be considered: (1) the treatment effect observed in patients identified as sensitive by applying the final signature to the entire study population (since this estimator is obtained by applying the signature to the patients that were used in the signature development we refer to this as the resubstitution estimator) and (2) the treatment effect observed in patients identified as sensitive by K-fold cross-validation using the tuning parameters selected from the entire study population (as in the resubstitution estimator given earlier), we refer to this as CV estimator. The performance of the two estimators is illustrated in Table 16.6 for two settings with 10% fraction of sensitive patients. The table presents resubstitution and the 10-fold CV treatment effect estimates for a simulated 400-patient trial. The treatment effect observed by applying the final signature to an independent set of 1000 patients is used as a reference value for the true predicted effect (*predicted rates* column in Table 16.6). The results were then averaged over 1000 simulations. As expected, the resubstitution estimate tends to overestimate the predicted effect since it uses the same data to develop the signature and estimate the treatment effect. On the other hand, the 10-fold CV estimate tends to underestimate the predicted effect. Therefore, we recommend using 10-fold CV method to obtain a conservative estimate of the treatment effect in the signature-defined subpopulation of the future patients.

TABLE 16.6

Resubstitution and CV Estimates of the Predicted Treatment Effect in the Sensitive Subpopulation

	Predicted Rates	Resubstitution Rates	CV Rates
90% in sensitive patients, 25% response in all other patients			
Experimental arm	90%	91%	87%
Control arm	25%	23%	27%
Difference	65%	68%	60%
70% in sensitive patients, 25% response in all other patients			
Experimental arm	74%	88%	65%
Control arm	25%	19%	28%
Difference	49%	69%	37%

Note: 10% patients sensitive, 1000 replications.

16.4 Conclusion

When a predictive classifier to identify sensitive subpopulation for a new targeted therapy is not available at the time of definitive testing, the BATD and ASD procedures provide a statistically rigorous approach for integrating in a pivotal trial: (1) evaluation of the new treatment and (2) development of a companion diagnostic to select patients who are likely to benefit. For the ASD procedure, use of cross-validation improves performance by allowing a more efficient use of the available data. These methods are very powerful for enabling the clinical trial to adaptively determine the population who benefit from the test regimen. This is very important for patients and for controlling medical expenditures. Most regimens currently in use in oncology benefit only a minority of the patients to whom they are administered. These methods do not modify eligibility criteria or randomization weights based on interim data and thus avoid some of the complexity and questions of validity associated with other adaptive methods. The cross-validated ASD has been extended by Matsui et al. [17] (see also Chapter 17).

References

1. Simon R, Maitournam A. Evaluating the efficiency of targeted designs for randomized clinical trials. *Clinical Cancer Research* 2004;10:6759–6763.
2. Simon R, Wang SJ. Use of genomic signatures in therapeutics development in oncology and other diseases. *The Pharmacogenomics Journal* 2006;6:166–173.
3. Jiang W, Freidlin B, Simon R. Biomarker-adaptive threshold design: A procedure for evaluating treatment with possible biomarker-defined subset effect. *Journal of the National Cancer Institute* 2007;99:1036–1043.
4. Freidlin B, Simon R. Adaptive signature design: An adaptive clinical trial design for generating and prospectively testing a gene expression signature for sensitive patients. *Clinical Cancer Research* 2005;11:7872–7878.
5. Freidlin B, Jiang W, Simon R. The cross-validated adaptive signature design. *Clinical Cancer Research* 2010;16:691–698.
6. Dziadziuszko R, Hirsch FR, Varella-Garcia M, Bunn PA Jr. Selecting lung cancer patients for treatment with epidermal growth factor receptor tyrosine kinase inhibitors by immunohistochemistry and fluorescence in situ hybridization—Why, when, and how? *Clinical Cancer Research* 2006;12:4409s–4415s.
7. Cox DR. Regression models and life tables (with discussion). *Journal of the Royal Statistical Society Series B* 1972;34:187–220.
8. Altman DG, Lausen B, Sauerbrei W, Schumacher M. Dangers of using "optimal" cutpoints in the evaluation of prognostic factors. *Journal of the National Cancer Institute* 1994;86:829–835.
9. Miller R, Siegmund D. Maximally selected chi-square statistics. *Biometrics* 1982;38:1011–1016.

10. Simon RM, Korn EL, McShane LM, Radmacher MD, Wright GW, Zhao Y. *Design and Analysis of DNA Microarray Investigations*. New York: Springer; 2004.
11. Byar DP, Corle DK. Selecting optimal treatment in clinical trials using covariate information. *Journal of Chronic Diseases* 1977;30:445–459.
12. Andrews DF, Herzberg AM. *Data*, Chapter 46, pp. 261–274. New York: Springer; 1985.
13. Simon R. *Genomic Clinical Trials and Predictive Medicine*. Cambridge, U.K.: Cambridge University Press; 2012.
14. Simon R. Clinical trials for predictive medicine. *Statistics in Medicine* 2012;31:3031–3040.
15. Sher HI, Nasso SF, Rubin E, Simon R. Adaptive clinical trial designs for simultaneous testing of matched diagnostics and therapeutics. *Clinical Cancer Research* 2011;17:6634–6640.
16. Breiman L. Bagging predictors. *Machine Learning* 1996;24:123–140.
17. Matsui S, Simon R, Qu P, Shaughnessy JD, Barlogie B, Crowley J. Developing and validating continuous genomic signatures in randomized clinical trials for predictive medicine. *Clinical Cancer Research* 2012;18:6065–6073.

17

Development and Validation of Continuous Genomic Signatures in Randomized Clinical Trials

Shigeyuki Matsui

CONTENTS

17.1 Introduction

The biology of many human diseases is very complex and highly heterogeneous. In recent years, with rapid advances in genomics and biotechnology, the molecular characteristics of diseases, such as cancer, have been gradually revealed. Accordingly, the development of therapeutics embarks on a new era, arising a new paradigm to develop molecularly targeted treatments and companion predictive molecular markers to identify responsive patients simultaneously toward personalized or predictive medicine.

In clinical development, the predictive marker should be developed in advance of a pivotal phase III trial (e.g., Chapter 2 of this volume). However, this is generally difficult because of the complexity of disease biology and the inherent difficulty in developing reliable predictive markers for clinical endpoints, such as survival or disease-free survival, using early phase II data. One approach to address this issue, where a reliable predictive marker is unavailable at the initiation of a phase III trial, is to design and analyze the phase III trial in such a way that both developing a genomic signature and testing treatment efficacy based on the developed signature are possible and performed validly. The adaptive signature design (Freidlin and Simon 2005) and the cross-validated adaptive signature design (Freidlin et al. 2010) have been proposed for this purpose (see also Chapter 16).

A genomic signature is usually developed as a composite score integrating the status or values of multiple component genomic features. Such signatures are continuously valued in nature and represent varying treatment effects across patients (Hoering et al. 2008; Janes et al. 2011; see also Chapter 9), reflecting the complexity of disease biology. For developing a diagnostic test, one conventional framework is to define responsive and non–responsive patients by invoking a thresholding of the continuous score (i.e., patients whose scores are higher or smaller than a threshold are defined as responsive patients) as done in the adaptive signature designs. However, in this framework, information regarding varying treatment effects among responsive patients would be lost. This can be a concern for plausible situations where treatment selection is affected by many factors, including adverse effects, cost of treatment, and patient's preference, and thus, the size of treatment effect that leads to a patient's selecting the treatment can differ among patients. This suggests the need for another framework that presents the treatment effect as a function of the continuous genomic signature as a more relevant diagnostic tool for personalized or predictive medicine.

In this chapter, we consider this framework and present a methodology for developing and validating continuous genomic signatures in phase III randomized trials proposed by Matsui et al. (2012). In this framework, the underlying profile of the variation of treatment effects is estimated as a function of continuous genomic signatures. On the basis of an estimate of this function, we can provide a cross-validation-based test of treatment efficacy for the patient population. Furthermore, our framework allows prediction of patient-level survival curves for each treatment for any subset of patients with various degrees of responsiveness to treatments and various degrees of baseline risks, represented by the predictive and prognostic signatures, respectively. Such prediction curves can serve as a basic diagnostic tool for selecting appropriate treatments for future patients.

17.2 Framework for Developing and Validating Continuous Genomic Signatures

We consider a randomized trial to compare an experimental (E) and control treatment (C). We suppose that pretreatment genomic data for signature development is available for a total of n patients. Specifically, we suppose that pretreatment expression levels for a total of G genes are measured using microarrays for each patient. Other types of genomic data, such as single nucleotide polymorphism genotyping, copy number profiling, and proteomic profiling data, can be used similarly.

Matsui et al. (2012) have proposed a framework for developing and validating continuous genomic signatures in randomized trials with genomic data. This framework consists of the following four components:

1. Development of a continuous signature score
2. Estimation of the treatment effects as a function of the developed score
3. Test of the strong null hypothesis that the treatment has no effect on any patients
4. Prediction of patient-level survival curves for future patients

Figure 17.1 outlines the framework. The statistical models and procedures used in all the components must be prespecified. The last component is a step for developing a basic diagnostic tool to aid selecting appropriate treatments for individual future patients. This is different from the purpose of assessing treatment efficacy for a patient population in the second and third components.

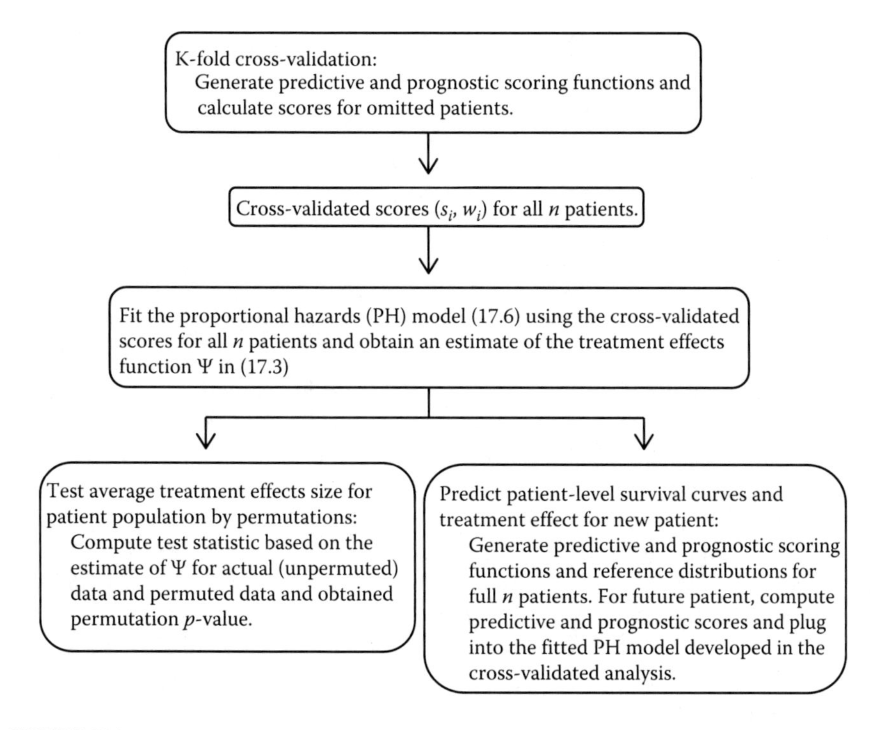

FIGURE 17.1
Outline of the proposed methodology. (From Matsui, S. et al., *Clin. Cancer Res.*, 18, 6065, 2012.)

Let P denote the set of all patients with size n in the randomized trial. We observe the dataset $D = \{(y, z, \boldsymbol{x})\}$ for P, consisting of a survival outcome y, a treatment indictor z, and a covariate vector $\boldsymbol{x}$ for P. The survival outcome y involves a pair of survival time and censoring indicator for each patient. The covariate vector $\boldsymbol{x}$ involves the baseline genomic data and baseline clinical characteristics.

We define an algorithm A for developing a predictive (continuous) signature score. For example, when applying the algorithm A to the dataset D as a training set, we obtain a predictive signature score function and express it as $U(\boldsymbol{x}^*; A, D)$ for a given value of the covariate vector, $\boldsymbol{x}^*$. Without loss of generality, we suppose that the signature score is developed such that, for a patient with a low value of the score, the survival probability when receiving E is predicted to be higher than that when receiving C; as such, this patient is predicted to be responsive to E. The algorithm A can be of any type, for example, Cox's proportional hazard regression, tree-based methods, and so on (e.g., Kalbfleisch and Prentice 2002; Zhang and Singer 2010; van Houwelingen and Putter 2012). For high-dimensional microarray data, the algorithm A may involve feature selection algorithms, for example, multiple univariate tests for detecting treatment by gene interactions on survival outcomes. A wide variety of prediction algorithms have been proposed for survival outcomes in high dimension (van Wieringen et al. 2009; Witten and Tibshirani 2010; Binder et al. 2011; see also Chapter 15).

17.2.1 Development of Genomic Signature Score

We consider a framework of prediction analysis and apply complete K-fold cross-validation as in the cross-validated adaptive signature design, because it is more efficient than the split-sample approach (Freidlin et al. 2010; see also Chapter 16). In the K-fold cross-validation, the trial population, P, is split into K roughly equal-sized parts, $P_1, \ldots, P_K$. The patient allocation must be prospectively defined. The kth training set consists of the full set of patients except for the kth subset, that is, the complement of P_k in P, $P_{-k} = P - P_k$. Similarly, let D_{-k} denote the kth training dataset from P_{-k}, that is, the full dataset D minus data for patients in P_k ($k = 1, \ldots, K$). We apply the defined algorithm A to the training dataset D_{-k} to obtain a prediction score function $U_{-k}(\bullet; A, D_{-k})$. Note that the complete cross-validation requires that the algorithm A involves all aspects of the signature development, including feature selection, and is reperformed in each fold of the cross-validation (Ambroise and McLachlan 2002; Simon et al. 2003). When feature selection and/or prediction models to develop the signature are optimized based on cross-validated predictive accuracy, the optimization process should be included in the K-fold cross-validation with application of a nested inner loop of K-fold cross-validation (Dudoit and Fridlyand 2003; Varma and Simon 2006).

After developing the signature scoring function, $U_{-k}(\bullet; A, D_{-k})$, using the kth training set, we apply it to compute predicted scores for all patients in the test set, P_k, that is, $U_{-k}(\boldsymbol{x}_k; A, D_{-k})$. We then normalize the predicted scores based on a quantile (or percentile) value based on the distribution of the score, $U_{-k}(\boldsymbol{x}_{-k}; A, D_{-k})$, in the training set. Specifically, using an empirical cumulative density distribution $F_{-k}(u)$ of $U_{-k}(\boldsymbol{x}_{-k}; A, D_{-k})$, we obtain the normalized score for the test set as $S_{-k}(\boldsymbol{x}_k) = F_{-k}\{U_{-k}(\boldsymbol{x}_k; A, D_{-k})\}$ $(k = 1, \ldots, K)$.

After completion of the *K*-fold cross-validation, we have the predicted (quantile) scores $\{S_{-k}(\boldsymbol{x}_k)\}$ $(k = 1, \ldots, K)$ for all n patients. For ease of notation, we denote the score for patient i as $S_i \in (0, 1)$ $(i = 1, \ldots, n)$. Note that, because S_i is a quantile measure, it is essentially continuously valued. Again, for patients with lower values of S_i, the survival probabilities when receiving E are predicted to be higher than those when receiving C. We then use the predicted score S_i from the cross-validation for modeling treatment responsiveness using the entire patients as described in the following text. This analysis corresponds to the *prevalidation* analysis (Tibshirani and Efron 2002; Höfling and Tibshirani 2008), where the score S_i can be regarded as a prevalidated score.

17.2.2 Estimation of the Treatment Effects Function

We estimate the treatment effects as a function of S_i, $\Psi(s)$ say. As a basic measure of treatment effects, we consider a logarithm of the hazard ratio between the two treatment arms under the proportional hazards assumption that the hazard ratio is constant over time. Specifically, for a patient with the score value $S = s$,

$$\begin{aligned}\Psi(s) = &(\text{The log hazard for a patient with } S = s \text{ when receiving } E) \\ &- (\text{The log hazard for a patient with } S = s \text{ when receiving } C) \qquad (17.1)\end{aligned}$$

represents the treatment effect for that patient. We assume the multivariate Cox proportional hazards model,

$$h_i(t \mid r_i, s_i) = h_0(t)\exp\{\beta_1 r_i + f_2(s_i) + r_i f_3(s_i)\}, \qquad (17.2)$$

where

r_i is the treatment assignment indicator such that $r_i = 1$ if patient i is assigned to treatment E and $r_i = 0$ otherwise

Here the functions f_2 and f_3 capture the main effects of S and the interactions between S and r, respectively.

These effects can be nonlinear, but should be monotonic in S, because the score S has been developed such that its lower value represents greater responsiveness to E. One simple specification to have monotonic effects for S is to use the fractional polynomials (FPs) (Royston and Altman 1994). For example, one term FP functions (FP1), expressed as $f_3(s) = \beta_3 s^a$ $(a \in \{-2, -1,$

−0.5, 0, 0.5, 1, 2, 3} with $a=0$ identical to log(s), the natural logarithm of s, are always monotonic. See Royston and Sauerbrei (2004) for modeling interactions between treatment and continuous covariates using FPs in clinical trials. Other types of monotonic specification include monotone smoothing functions (Kelly and Rice 1990; Leitenstorfer and Tutz 2007). The model (17.2) is fitted by maximum (partial) likelihood.

Under the model (17.2), the treatment effects function Ψ will be expressed as

$$\Psi(s_i) = \beta_1 + f_3(s_i). \tag{17.3}$$

Under the specification of monotonic effects for the interaction f_3, the estimated function, $\hat{\Psi}$, will also be monotone. In particular, if the developed signature score S is truly effective in predicting the effect of E, a nondecreasing shape of $\hat{\Psi}$ is expected for increasing S, such that lower values of s are linked to larger negative values of $\Psi(s)$, that is, greater responsiveness to E. If the shape of $\hat{\Psi}(s)$ is decreasing for increasing s, contrary to the intended increasing shape of $\hat{\Psi}(s)$, it indicates that no statistical evidence is obtained from the use of the genomic signature in assessing treatment efficacy. For this case, we remove the terms including the genomic signature from the model and refit the reduced model with only the main effect of r_i. Under the reduced model, we have $\Psi(s_i) = \beta_1$.

17.2.3 Test of Treatment Effects

We can perform a test of treatment efficacy for a patient population based on the estimated treatment effects function $\hat{\Psi}$. Because our models incorporate varying treatment effects on individual patients, it is natural to consider the strong null hypothesis, H_0, that the treatment has no effect on any patients. Under H_0, the null distribution of $\hat{\Psi}$ and p-values can be obtained by a permutation method that randomly permutes treatment labels. For permutation datasets, the entire cross-validation procedure, including the signature development and the estimation of Ψ, is repeated to obtain a null distribution of $\hat{\Psi}$. As the test statistic, we can use an average absolute effect size over the entire patient population,

$$T = \int_0^1 \left|\hat{\Psi}(s)\right| ds, \tag{17.4}$$

which represents a summation of absolute effect sizes, or equivalently, an average absolute effect size over the entire patient population. It corresponds to a two-sided alternative hypothesis to detect treatment effects in both directions where the treatment $E(C)$ is superior to $C(E)$. Another approach is, like in the second stage of the cross-validated adaptive signature designs, to test treatment effects for a subset of patients with $\widehat{\Psi}(s) < 0$, who are predicted to be responsive to *E*. Let *I* be $\{s : \widehat{\Psi}(s) < 0\}$, which represents a group of responsive patients to *E*, and *L* be the size or length of *I*, which represents the size of the group of responsive patients. Alternatively, one can define the responsive subset to be $\{s : \widehat{\Psi}(s) < c\}$, where *c* represents a minimum size of clinically meaningful effects. Then, as the counterpart of *T*, we can consider a one-sided test statistic,

$$T_R = \frac{1}{L} \int_{s \in I} \widehat{\Psi}(s) ds, \tag{17.5}$$

which represents an average treatment effect over the responsive patients.

In calculating *p*-values of the two-sided statistic *T* using the permutation method, we count the number of permutations when the values of *T* are equal or larger than the observed value of *T*. For the one-sided statistic T_R, we count the number of permutations when the values of T_R are equal or less than the observed value of T_R.

17.2.4 Prediction of Patient-Level Survival Curves

Although the estimation of the treatment effects function, $\Psi(s)$, provides direct information regarding the sizes of treatment effects for individual patients in terms of the (logarithm of) hazard ratio, information regarding the survival curves when individual patients receive either one of the two treatments would be more relevant. The patient-level survival curves can be predicted on the basis of the estimates of the baseline hazard function and regression coefficients by fitting the multivariate Cox proportional hazards model (17.2). However, this model, which can work well for estimating the treatment effects function ψ, may not be so accurate in predicting the patient-level survival curves, because it does not incorporate information about risk or prognostic factors. We therefore consider the extension of the model (17.2),

$$h_i(t \mid r_i, s_i) = h_0(t)\exp\{\beta_1 r_i + f_2(s_i) + r_i f_3(s_i) + f_4(w_i)\}, \tag{17.6}$$

where

the function f_4 represents an effect of a prognostic index w_i

Under the model (17.6), we have the same form of the treatment effects function (17.3) with that under the model (17.2), but the effects β_1 and f_3 are now interpreted with the use of the prognostic index w (or after adjustment for the prognostic term f_4).

The prognostic index, w, can be established based on clinical prognostic factors. However, recent prognostic studies have demonstrated improvement of the accuracy of prognostic prediction by incorporating genomic signatures

(Rosenwald et al. 2002; Paik et al. 2004; Shaughnessy et al. 2007). Because large-scale phase III trials with pretreatment genomic data also provide a precious chance for developing reliable prognostic signatures, in addition to reliable predictive signatures, codevelopment of them would be warranted. Our methodology can be easily extended in this direction. Within the K-fold cross-validation, we develop a prognostic signature score, independently of developing the predictive signature score, S, through correlating genomic data with survival outcomes without reference to treatment assignment. At each step of the K-fold cross-validation, we can fit a multivariate Cox model with the developed genomic signature score and clinical prognostic factors as covariates to obtain a composite prognostic signature. A quantile score can also be developed for the prognostic signature. Then, the developed (quantile) prognostic score is used for w in the model (17.6).

Based on the estimates under the model (17.6), for patient i with (s_i, w_i), we predict a patient-level survival curve or survival rate at a given time point for each treatment. We then compare the predicted survival curve when receiving E and that when receiving C to assess the benefit of receiving E for that patient.

Finally, we regard the entire n patients in the clinical trial as a training set and apply the entire procedure. That is, we develop predictive and prognostic scoring functions and compute scores for all n patients. When feature selection and/or prediction models are optimized in the prior K-fold cross-validation, we invoke a new session of K-fold cross-validation for n patients to determine optimal values of the tuning parameters using the same optimization procedure, and then compute scores at these values for n patients. The empirical distributions of those scores serve as reference distributions. For any new patient, the scoring functions are used to compute predictive and prognostic scores, which are then normalized using the reference distributions. For the new patient, we then assess the expected treatment effect by plugging these values into the estimated treatment effects function, $\widehat{\Psi}$, obtained in the cross-validated prediction analysis. From (17.6), one can also compute the predicted survival curves for the new patient under each treatment based on the cross-validated prediction analysis.

17.3 Multiple Myeloma Example

A large-scale randomized phase III trial was conducted to assess whether the addition of thalidomide, which has activity against advanced and refractory multiple myeloma, improves survival in the up-front management of patients with multiple myeloma undergoing melphalan-based tandem transplantation (Barlogie et al. 2006, 2010). A unique feature of this phase III trial, pretreatment RNA from highly purified plasma cells was applied to

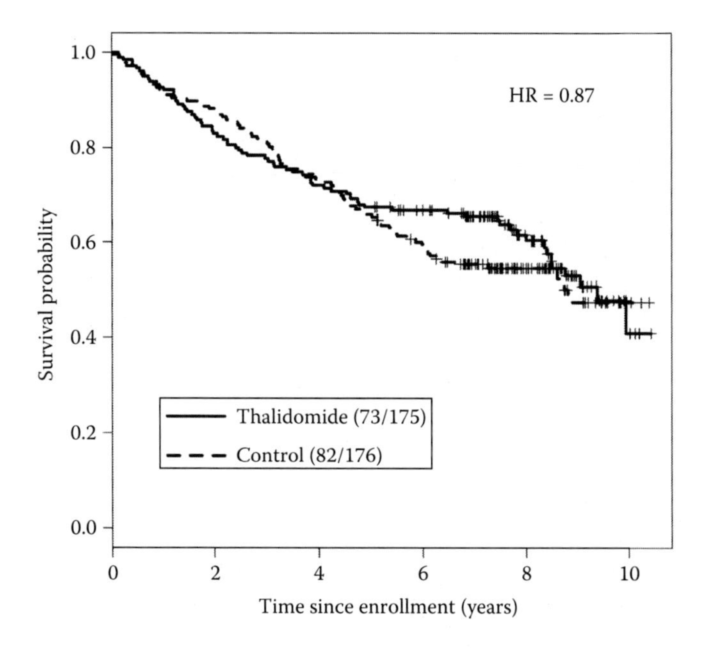

FIGURE 17.2
Survival curves for all 351 patients with genomic data in the randomized trial for multiple myeloma. (From Matsui, S. et al., *Clin. Cancer Res.*, 18, 6065, 2012.)

Affymetrix U133 Plus 2.0 microarrays for 351 patients, out of 668 randomized patients. In what follows, we provide an application of the predictive analysis described in Section 17.2 to overall survival (OS) at a median follow-up of 72 months (Barlogie et al. 2010) for 351 patients using the microarray gene expression data given by Matsui et al. (2012).

Figure 17.2 shows an OS curve for 351 patients by treatment arm (175 with thalidomide and 176 with no thalidomide [control]). For each of 54,675 gene features on the microarray, we standardized gene expression levels after normalization to have mean zero and standard deviation one across all 351 patients. We first developed the predictive signature score, S, and the prognostic signature score, W, using a fivefold cross-validation. For the training set, we screened predictive genes using a two-sided score test for no interaction between gene feature g and treatment, $\psi_g = 0$, in a gene-level Cox model with the patient i's hazard function, $h_{g,i}(t) = h_{g,0}(t)\exp(\tau_g r_i + \gamma_g x_{gi} + \psi_g r_i x_{gi})$, where x_{gi} is the expression level of the gene feature ($g = 1,\ldots, 54{,}675$). In this test, we used a significance level of 0.001 (Simon et al. 2004). For selected genes features, we developed a compound covariates predictor, $U_i = \sum_{g\in\Omega} z_g x_{gi}$, where Ω is the set of selected gene features and z_g is a standardized score test statistic of the interaction test for gene feature g (Tukey 1993; Matsui 2006; Emura et al. 2012). Similarly, but independently, we screened prognostic gene features using a two-sided univariate score (log-rank) test for no association of the gene feature and OS at a significance level of 0.001, and developed a compound covariates predictor based on the standardized statistics from the prognostic tests for selected gene features. We then obtained the predicted (quantile) signature scores S and W for the test set. After the completion of the fivefold cross-validation, we had obtained the predicted values of these scores for all 351 patients.

We fit the multivariate Cox proportional hazards model with both S and W in (17.6) for the entire patient cohort. We specified linear terms for the main effects of S and W, such that $f_2(s_i) = \beta_2 s_i$ and $f_4(w_i) = \beta_4 w_i$, but the FPs with one term (FP1) for the interaction of R and S, $f_3(s_i)$. The results were similar for the FPs with two terms (FP2) (Royston and Altman 1994). The estimated treatment effects function, $\hat{\Psi}(s)$, is provided in Figure 17.3. $\hat{\Psi}(s) < 0$ represents thalidomide's effects that prolong OS. The estimates $\hat{\Psi}(s)$ for $0 \le s \le 1$ represent the underlying smooth function regarding varying treatment effects for the whole range of the score S (i.e., the entire patient population). For approximately the half of patients with lower values of S, thalidomide is expected to prolong OS by varying degrees. On the other hand, for the rest of the patients with larger values of S, it could have small adverse effects on OS.

We performed a test of treatment efficacy for the subset of the patient population predicted to benefit from thalidomide based on $\hat{\Psi}(s)$. Because the interest in this randomized trial was to assess improvement in survival by adding thalidomide for patients with high-dose therapies, compared with the control arm with no thalidomide, it is reasonable to test treatment efficacy for a subset of patients who are considered to be responsive to thalidomide using the one-sided test statistic (17.5). The observed value of the test statistic was −0.47 in log hazard ratio (0.62 in hazard ratio). The p-value obtained

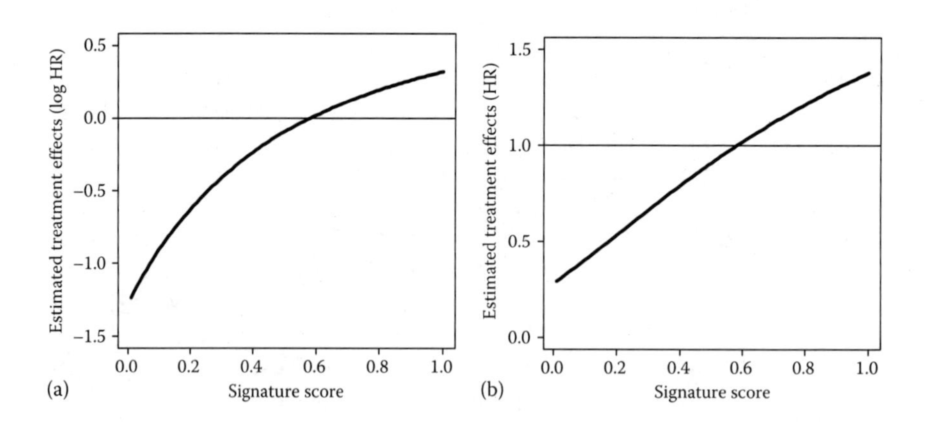

FIGURE 17.3
The estimated treatment effects functions for the predicted signature score, S, in terms of logarithm of hazard ratio, that is, $\hat{\Psi}$ (a) and hazard ratio, that is, $\exp(\hat{\Psi})$ (b). Here, $\hat{\Psi}(s) = 0.79 - 2.02(s+1)^{-2}$ derived from the fitted linear predictor, $0.79r - 0.69s - 2.02\{r(s+1)\}^{-2} + 1.72w$ for the model (17.6). (From Matsui, S. et al., *Clin. Cancer Res.*, 18, 6065, 2012.)

from 2000 permutations was 0.019, which is significant if our test is employed for a significance level 2% at the second stage of cross-validated adaptive signature designs (Freidlin et al. 2010). For reference, the permutation-based p-value for the observed two-sided test statistic (17.4), 0.35, was 0.038.

Based on the estimates obtained from fitting the model (17.6), we predicted patient-level survival rates for patients with $S=0.1$, 0.5, or 0.9 and $W=0.1$, 0.5, or 0.9. Again, lower values of S represent larger effects of prolonging OS by receiving thalidomide. Lower values of W represent higher survival rates (better prognosis). Figure 17.4 shows the predicted survival curves when receiving either of the two treatments (thalidomide and no thalidomide) for four combinations with $(S, W)=(0.1, 0.1)$, (0.1, 0.9), (0.5, 0.1), and (0.5, 0.9). Table 17.1 summarizes the predicted 5-year survival rates with thalidomide and no thalidomide and their difference for the all

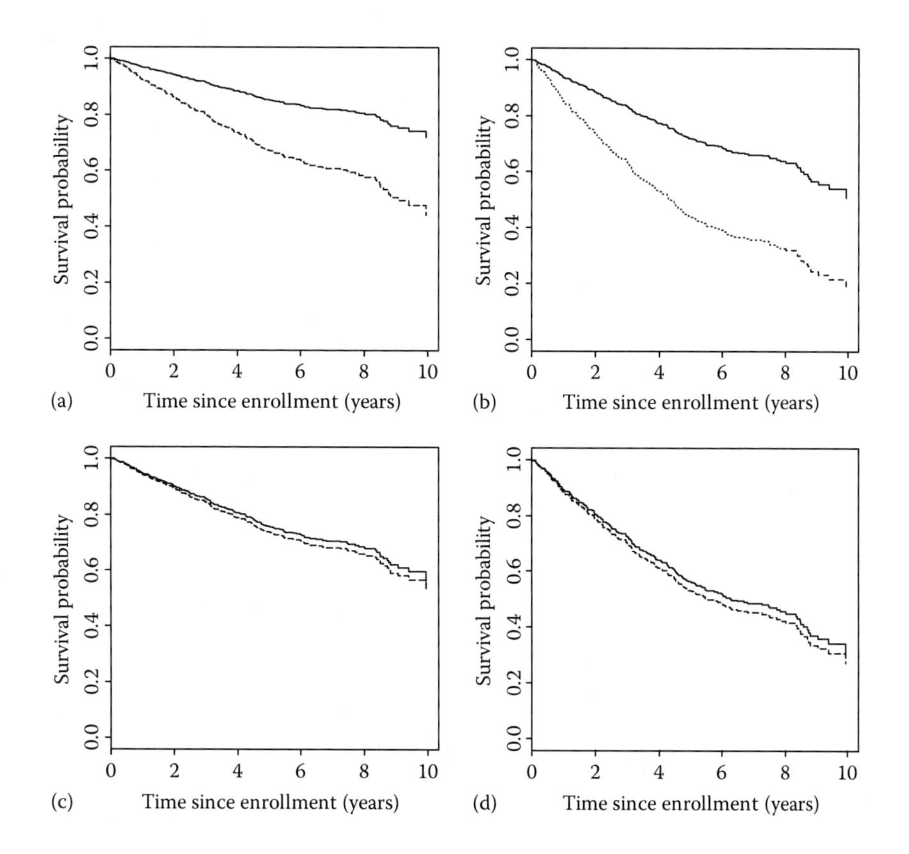

FIGURE 17.4
The predicted survival curves when receiving thalidomide (solid curves) and no thalidomide (dashed curves) for four patients with different values of the predictive score (S) and the prognostic score (W); $(s, w) = (0.1, 0.1)$, (0.1, 0.9), (0.5, 0.1), and (0.5, 0.9) (a–d). $s = 0.1$ (0.5) represents a high (small) responsiveness to thalidomide, while $w = 0.1$ (0.9) represents a good (poor) prognosis. (From Matsui, S. et al., *Clin. Cancer Res.*, 18, 6065, 2012.)

TABLE 17.1

Predicted 5-Year Survival Rates for Each Treatment

s	w	Survival Rate with Thalidomide (%)	Survival Rate with No Thalidomide (%)	Difference (%)
0.1	0.1	85.3	67.4	17.9
	0.5	79.5	56.6	22.9
	0.9	71.9	44.1	27.8
0.5	0.1	75.8	73.8	2.1
	0.5	67.1	64.5	2.6
	0.9	56.4	53.2	3.1
0.9	0.1	73.7	79.1	−5.4
	0.5	64.5	71.4	−6.9
	0.9	53.2	61.5	−8.3

combinations. Generally, even for the same level of the predictive score, S, the effect size of thalidomide was larger (larger absolute difference in the predicted survival rate under each treatment) for patients with poor prognosis (larger W). For example, for patients with $S = 0.1$, the difference in the predicted survival rate was 17.9% for $W = 0.1$, while it was 27.8% for $W = 0.9$ (see also Figure 17.4a and b).

Finally, we applied the procedures for selecting genes and developing signature scoring functions to the entire 351 patients; 81 and 662 genes with no overlap were selected using the significance level of 0.001 for developing the predictive and prognostic signature scoring functions, respectively. The empirical distributions of those scores will serve as reference distributions for predicting patient-level survival curves under each treatment for any new patient on the basis of the fitted model of (17.6) obtained in the cross-validated prediction analysis.

For treatment selection, it would be reasonable to withhold thalidomide for approximately the half of patients with $\widehat{\Psi}(s) > 0$, because no improvement in survival is expected by receiving thalidomide. For the rest of patients, the decision of whether to use thalidomide would take into consideration the estimated sizes of thalidomide's effects for individual patients as well as other factors such as safety issues, including severe peripheral neuropathy and deep-vein thrombosis (Barlogie et al. 2006).

17.4 Discussion

In this chapter, we have considered a framework for developing and validating continuous genomic signatures in phase III randomized trials.

We estimate treatment effects quantitatively over the entire patient population, rather than qualitatively classifying patients as in or not in a responsive subset.

We have provided an implementation of this framework with a combination of relatively simple, but effective statistical procedures, such as the FPs and the compound covariate predictors, for developing genomic signatures. Further research on the application of more complex procedures for each step of the framework or unified analytical approaches for the whole steps of the framework is worthwhile.

Our framework may be used as the second stage of the cross-validated adaptive signature design or a fallback option in all-comers or randomize-all designs (see Chapter 10). Another direction is to test the hypothesis of no heterogeneity in treatment effect using a test statistic, such as those for testing the interaction term in the multivariate Cox model in (17.2) or (17.6), and evaluating its distribution under permutations of the genomic covariate vectors (see Chapter 11 for a similar permutation approach). This test can serve as a preliminary interaction test in the treatment by biomarker designs (see Section 10.2.3). Incorporation of our framework in various all-comers designs, as well as sample size determination, is a subject for future research.

The one-sided test (17.5) is similar to the test of the average treatment effect for a subset of responsive patients proposed in the cross-validated adaptive signature design. These one-sided tests would be relevant typically when developing a new molecularly targeted agent, or more generally, when assessing improvement in survival by prescribing the experimental treatment, as in the multiple myeloma example. On the other hand, the two-sided test (17.4) for the entire patient population could be relevant when comparing two competitive treatments (or treatment regimens) to establish standard therapy. In such settings, the overall treatment effect for the entire population can be small (and thus not detected) due to combining reversed effects from distinct subsets of responsive patients to either one of the two treatments. The two-sided test would be particularly effective for such situations.

For licensing studies sponsored by pharmaceutical companies, although our framework can allow detecting treatment effects for a subset of responsive patients, uncertainty in identifying the responsive subset based on $\widehat{\Psi}(s)$ (due to possible model misspecification and random variation) may limit confidence in labeling of the new treatment for the identified patient subset (i.e., $\widehat{\Psi}(s) < 0$). Our framework, however, can provide useful information for designing a second confirmatory trial, possibly with a targeted or enrichment design with small sample sizes, especially when there is no overall treatment effect for the entire population.

Our framework can also be useful even if the overall average treatment effect is significant. In order to avoid overtreatment of the population, it is useful to identify patient subsets who receive large, small, or no benefits from the treatment and to predict patient-level survival curves to aid selecting treatment for individual patients. Provided that some conditions are met (Simon et al. 2009; see also Chapters 1 and 8), the framework could also be applied to genomic data from past randomized trials to analyze the heterogeneity in treatment effects over the study population and to develop diagnostic tools for established treatments.

Confidence intervals for the treatment effects function and patient-level survival curves are particularly important both in assessing the heterogeneity of treatment effects across patients and in developing diagnostic tools for individual patients. Construction of these intervals via resampling methods is another subject for future research.

Finally, for utilizing our framework, it is essential to plan for collection of genomic data in designing randomized clinical trials. The rapid development of high-throughput technologies, which has reduced the cost of microarrays and exome sequencing, and infrastructure development for genomic analysis in the context of clinical studies have allowed collection of large-scale genomic data in randomized trials, such as the illustrative example of the multiple myeloma trial. We hope the new framework for developing and validating continuous genomic signatures in randomized trials could contribute to accelerating modern clinical studies toward predictive medicine.

References

Ambroise, C. and McLachlan, G.J. (2002). Selection bias in gene extraction on the basis of microarray gene-expression data. *Proc Natl Acad Sci USA*, 99, 6562–6566.

Barlogie, B., Anaissie, E., van Rhee, F. et al. (2010). Reiterative survival analyses of total therapy 2 for multiple myeloma elucidate follow-up time dependency of prognostic variables and treatment arms. *J Clin Oncol*, 28, 3023–3027.

Barlogie, B., Tricot, G., Anaissie, E. et al. (2006). Thalidomide and hematopoietic-cell transplantation for multiple myeloma. *N Engl J Med*, 354, 1021–1030.

Binder, H., Porzelius, C., and Schumacher, M. (2011). An overview of techniques for linking high-dimensional molecular data to time-to-event endpoints by risk prediction models. *Biometrical J*, 53, 170–189.

Dudoit, S. and Fridlyand, J. (2003). Classification in microarray experiments. In Speed, T.P. ed. *Statistical Analysis of Gene Expression Microarray Data*. Boca Raton, FL: Chapman & Hall/CRC, pp. 93–158.

Emura, T., Chen, Y.H., and Chen, H.Y. 2012. Survival prediction based on compound covariate under Cox proportional hazard models. *PLOS ONE* 7:e47627.

Freidlin, B., Jiang, W., and Simon, R. (2010). The cross-validated adaptive signature design. *Clin Cancer Res*, 16, 691–698.

Freidlin, B. and Simon, R. (2005). Adaptive signature design: An adaptive clinical trial design for generating and prospectively testing a gene expression signature for sensitive patients. *Clin Cancer Res*, 11, 7872–7878.

Hoering, A., Leblanc, M., and Crowley, J.J. (2008). Randomized phase III clinical trial designs for targeted agents. *Clin Cancer Res*, 14, 4358–4367.

Höfling, H. and Tibshirani, R. (2008). A study of pre-validation. *Ann Appl Stat*, 2, 435–776.

Janes, H., Pepe, M.S., Bossuyt, P.M., and Barlow, W.E. (2011). Measuring the performance of markers for guiding treatment decisions. *Ann Intern Med*, 154, 253–259.

Kalbfleisch, J.D. and Prentice, R.L. (2002). *The Statistical Analysis of Failure Time Data*, 2nd ed. Hoboken, NJ: John Wiley & Sons.

Kelly, C. and Rice, J. (1990). Monotone smoothing with application to dose-response curves and the assessment of synergism. *Biometrics*, 46, 1071–1085.

Leitenstorfer, F. and Tutz, G. (2007). Generalized monotonic regression based on B-splines with an application to air population data. *Biostatistics*, 8, 654–673.

Matsui, S. (2006). Predicting survival outcomes using subsets of significant genes in prognostic marker studies with microarrays. *BMC Bioinformatics*, 7, 156.

Matsui, S., Simon, R., Qu, P., Shaughnessy, J.D. Jr., Barlogie, B., and Crowley, J. (2012). Developing and validating continuous genomic signatures in randomized clinical trials for predictive medicine. *Clin Cancer Res*, 18, 6065–6073.

Paik, S., Shak, S., Tang, G. et al. (2004). A multigene assay to predict recurrence of tamoxifen-treated, node-negative breast cancer. *N Engl J Med*, 351, 2817–2826.

Rosenwald, A., Wright, G., Chan, W.C. et al. (2002). The use of molecular profiling to predict survival after chemotherapy for diffuse large-B-cell lymphoma. *N Engl J Med*, 346, 1937–1947.

Royston, P. and Altman, D.G. (1994). Regression using fractional polynomials of continuous covariates: Parsimonious parametric modelling (with discussion). *Appl Stat*, 43, 429–467.

Royston, P. and Sauerbrei, W. (2004). A new approach to modelling interactions between treatment and continuous covariates in clinical trials by using fractional polynomials. *Stat Med*, 23, 2509–2525.

Shaughnessy, J.D. Jr., Zhan, F., Burington, B.E. et al. (2007). A validated gene expression model of high-risk multiple myeloma is defined by deregulated expression of genes mapping to chromosome 1. *Blood*, 109, 2276–2284.

Simon, R., Radmacher, M.D., Dobbin, K., and McShane, L.M. (2003). Pitfalls in the use of DNA microarray data for diagnostic and prognostic classification. *J Natl Cancer Inst*, 95, 14–18.

Simon, R.M., Korn, E.L., McShane, L.M., Radmacher, M.D., Wright, G.W., and Zhao, Y. (2004). *Design and Analysis of DNA Microarray Investigations*. New York: Springer.

Simon, R.M., Paik, S., and Hayes, D.F. (2009). Use of archived specimens in evaluation of prognostic and predictive biomarkers. *J Natl Cancer Inst*, 101, 1446–1452.

Tibshirani, R.J. and Efron, B. (2002). Pre-validation and inference in microarrays. *Stat Appl Genet Mol Biol*, 1, 1–18. MR2011184.

Tukey, J.W. (1993). Tightening the clinical trial. *Control Clin Trials*, 14, 266–285.

van Houwelingen, H.C. and Putter, H. (2012). *Dynamic Prediction in Clinical Survival Analysis*. Boca Raton, FL: CRC Press.

van Wieringen, W.N., Kun, D., Hampel, R., and Boulesteix, A.-L. (2009). Survival prediction using gene expression data: A review and comparison. *Comput Stat Data Anal*, 53, 1590–1603.

Varma, S. and Simon, R. (2006). Bias in error estimation when using cross-validation for model selection. *BMC Bioinformatics*, 7, 91.

Witten, D.M. and Tibshirani, R. (2010). Survival analysis with high-dimensional covariates. *Stat Methods Med Res*, 19, 29–51.

Zhang, H. and Singer, B.H. (2010). *Recursive Partitioning and Applications*, 2nd ed. New York: Springer.

Section VI

Evaluation of Surrogate Biomarkers

18

Biomarker-Based Surrogate Endpoints

Marc Buyse, Tomasz Burzykowski, Geert Molenberghs, and Ariel Alonso

CONTENTS

18.1 Introduction

The development of new drugs is facing unprecedented challenges today. More molecules than ever are potentially available for clinical testing, and advances in molecular biology make it possible to target patient subsets likely to respond. However, drug development remains a slow, costly, and inefficient process. A very important factor influencing the duration and complexity of this process is the choice of endpoint(s) used to assess drug efficacy. Often, the most clinically relevant endpoint is difficult to use in a trial. This happens if the measurement of this clinical endpoint (1) is costly or difficult to measure (e.g., quality-of-life assessments involve complex multidimensional instruments); (2) requires a large sample size because of low incidence of the event of interest (e.g., cytotoxic drugs may have rare but serious side effects, such as leukemias induced by topoisomerase inhibitors); or (3) requires a long follow-up time (e.g., survival in early stage cancers). A potential strategy in all these cases is to look for surrogate endpoints that can be measured more cheaply, more conveniently, more frequently, or earlier than the true clinical endpoint of interest. In the ideal case, these surrogate endpoints are based on biomarkers that are easily and repeatedly measured to assess the evolution of the disease of interest over time, and any treatment effect on this evolution.

Surrogate endpoints have been used in medical research for a long time (CAST, 1989; Fleming and DeMets, 1996). Despite the potential advantages of surrogates, their use has been surrounded by controversy. An unfortunate precedent set the stage for heightened skepticism about surrogates in general: the US Food and Drug Administration (FDA) approved three antiarrhythmic drugs (encainide, flecainide, and moricizine) based on their major effects on the suppression of arrhythmias. It was believed that, because arrhythmias are associated with an almost fourfold increase in the rate of cardiac-complication-related death, drugs that reduced arrhythmic episodes would also reduce the death rate. However, postmarketing trials showed that the active-treatment death rate with antiarrhythmic drugs could be twice higher than the placebo rate (DeGruttola and Tu, 1994). Another instance of a poorly validated surrogate came with the surge of the AIDS epidemic. The impressive early therapeutic results obtained with zidovudine, and the pressure for accelerated approval of new therapies, led to the use of CD4 blood count as a surrogate endpoint for time to clinical events and overall survival (OS) (Lagakos and Hoth, 1992), in spite of concerns about its limitations as a reliable predictor for clinically relevant endpoints (DeGruttola et al., 1997).

The main reason behind these historical failures was the incorrect assumption that surrogacy simply follows from the association between a potential surrogate endpoint and the corresponding clinical endpoint, the mere existence of which is insufficient for surrogacy (CAST, 1989). Even though the existence of an association between the potential surrogate and the clinical endpoint is a desirable property, what is required to replace the clinical endpoint by the surrogate is that the *effect* of the treatment on the surrogate endpoint reliably predicts the *effect* on the clinical endpoint. Owing to a lack of appropriate methodology, this condition was not checked for early putative surrogates, which in turn led to negative opinions about assessing the efficacy of new treatments on surrogates rather than on traditional clinical endpoints (CAST, 1989; Fleming, 1994; Ferentz, 2002).

Nowadays, the rapid advances in molecular biology, in particular the "-omics" revolution, are dramatically increasing the number of biomarkers available and hence potential surrogate endpoints. The advent of new drugs with well-defined mechanisms of action at the molecular level also allows drug developers to measure the effect of these drugs on relevant biomarkers (Lesko and Atkinson, 2001). If valid surrogate endpoints could be based on such biomarkers, the duration and size of clinical trials could be drastically reduced, subsets of responding patients could be more reliably identified, and the promise of personalized medicine could be closer to becoming a reality.

What do we mean by a *valid* surrogate? It is the question we will address in this chapter. We will use the terms *evaluation* and *validation* interchangeably. Evaluation or validation involves a host of considerations, ranging from statistical conditions to clinical and biological evidence (Schatzkin and Gail, 2002). Note that a surrogate endpoint can play different roles in different phases of drug development; hence, it could conceivably be considered valid for one goal but not for another. For instance, it may be more acceptable to use a surrogate in early phases of research, rather than as a substitute for the true endpoint in pivotal phase III trials, since the latter might imply replacing the true endpoint by a surrogate in all future studies, which is a far-reaching decision (as exemplified by the unfortunate example of antiarrhythmic drugs). For a biomarker to be used as a surrogate to establish the efficacy of new treatments, a number of conditions must be fulfilled. The ICH Guidelines on Statistical Principles for Clinical Trials state that

> In practice, the strength of the evidence for surrogacy depends upon (i) the biological plausibility of the relationship, (ii) the demonstration in epidemiological studies of the prognostic value of the surrogate for the clinical outcome, and (iii) evidence from clinical trials that treatment effects on the surrogate correspond to effects on the clinical outcome (ICH, 1998).

In the remainder of this chapter, we will focus on the latter two conditions, and we will propose statistical approaches that may be used to assess the extent to which these conditions are fulfilled.

We begin this chapter by general considerations on biomarkers, focusing on longitudinal biomarkers that can potentially be used to define surrogate endpoints (Section 18.2). We then discuss the evaluation of potential surrogates when data are available from a single trial (Section 18.3), or from multiple trials (Section 18.4). Implications for the prediction of the treatment effect in a new trial are sketched briefly (Section 18.5). The chapter closes with a few comments on two promising alternative validation paradigms, one based on information theory and the other on causal inference (Section 18.6). Many of the methods presented in this chapter are described in more detail in the book by Burzykowski et al. (2005).

18.2 Longitudinal Biomarkers

18.2.1 Definitions

The Biomarkers Definitions Working Group defines a biomarker as "a characteristic that is objectively measured and evaluated as an indicator of normal biological processes, pathogenic processes, or pharmacologic responses to a therapeutic intervention" (Table 18.1). Biomarkers can be contrasted with clinical endpoints, which capture information on how a patient feels, functions, or survives (Ellenberg and Hamilton, 1989; Biomarkers Definition Working Group, 2001).

Biomarkers can include physiological or electrophysiological measurements, biochemical or cellular markers, genetic markers (such as gene mutations, translocations, or amplifications), gene expression profiles, proteomic or metabolomics profiles, imaging markers, and so on and so forth. They can be measured once before a treatment is administered, or repeatedly before, during, and after the treatment is administered, in which case interest

TABLE 18.1
Definitions

Term	Definition
Biomarker	A characteristic that is objectively measured and evaluated as an indicator of normal biological processes, pathogenic processes, or pharmacologic responses to a therapeutic intervention
Prognostic biomarker	Biomarker that forecasts the likely course of disease irrespective of treatment
Predictive biomarker	Biomarker that forecasts the likely response to a specific treatment
Pharmacodynamic biomarker	Biomarker that reflects the effect of a treatment on a specific target
Clinical endpoint	Measurement that provides systematic information on how a patient feels, functions, or survives
Surrogate endpoint	Endpoint that provides early and accurate prediction of both a clinical endpoint, and the effects of treatment on this endpoint
Validation	Confirmation by robust statistical methods that a candidate biomarker fulfils a set of conditions that make it fit for its intended use in the clinic

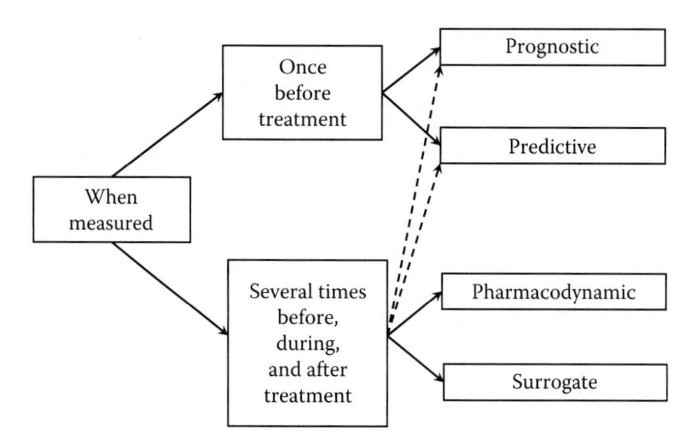

FIGURE 18.1
Biomarkers by type and time of measurement(s).

focuses on changes in the biomarker over time, possibly as a result of treatment. Figure 18.1 suggests a taxonomy of biomarkers.

Biomarkers that are measured once (typically *at baseline*, before treatment is administered) can have prognostic or predictive value. Prognostic biomarkers predict the likely course of disease irrespective of treatment, while predictive biomarkers forecast the likely response to a specific class of treatments. Examples of potent predictive biomarkers in oncology include gene mutations, rearrangements, and amplifications. For instance, some *KRAS* gene mutations are predictive of a poor response to the epidermal growth factor receptor (EGFR) inhibitors cetuximab and panitumumab in colorectal cancer, an *ALK* gene rearrangement is predictive of a good response to the tyrosine kinase inhibitor crizotinib in non–small-cell lung cancer, and the *HER2* gene amplification is predictive of good response to the monoclonal antibody trastuzumab or to the tyrosine kinase inhibitor lapatinib in advanced breast cancer.

Note that the term predictive can be misleading in so far as a prognostic factor is predictive of the outcome (but not of the effect of a specific treatment on this outcome). Some authors use *treatment effect modifiers, modulators,* or *theranostic biomarkers* to refer to predictive factors. However, in spite of the ambiguity, the term *predictive* has caught on and is now widely used in oncology. The identification, validation, and use of prognostic and predictive biomarkers are discussed in other chapters of this book; they are an integral component of personalized medicine.

In the present chapter, our interest will focus on biomarkers that are measured longitudinally. Examples of such biomarkers include prostate-specific antigen (PSA) in prostate cancer, carcinoembryonic antigen (CEA) in colorectal cancer, cancer antigen 125 (CA-125) in ovarian cancer, cancer antigen 19.9 (CA19.9) in pancreatic cancer, alpha-fetoprotein (AFP) in liver cancer, circulating tumor cells (CTCs) in several forms of advanced solid tumors, etc. Such biomarkers, specifically *changes* in these biomarkers, can have prognostic and predictive value. In this chapter, we will primarily discuss the potential use of these biomarkers to serve as early surrogate endpoints for clinical endpoints of interest that are measured much later in the course of the disease.

18.2.2 Example: Prostate-Specific Antigen (PSA)

Throughout this chapter, we will use PSA as an example of a longitudinal biomarker (Scher et al., 2004). PSA is one of the most extensively studied cancer biomarkers, in part because it is useful for the management of the disease. PSA is a glycoprotein produced by cells of the prostate gland, and shed in the bloodstream. PSA blood levels have been used to screen for prostate cancer, and to monitor disease progression in men with established prostate tumors. In patients with early disease, PSA serum concentrations at baseline have prognostic value, and decreases of PSA to normal levels indicate treatment benefit and are associated with good prognosis. Conversely, a rise in PSA predicts tumor recurrence and may call for intensified treatment regimens. In patients with androgen-sensitive metastatic prostate cancer, changes in PSA often antedate changes in bone scan, and they have long been used as an indicator of response to treatment (Section 18.2.3). Changes in PSA can also be used as a sensitive pharmacodynamic indicator of a treatment activity (Section 18.2.4). Many attempts have been made to validate PSA-based endpoints as surrogates for cancer-specific survival (in early disease) or OS (in metastatic disease), but so far, solid evidence for surrogacy is lacking. This chapter will discuss attempts to validate potential PSA-based surrogate endpoints when data are available from a single trial (Section 18.3.5) or from meta-analyses of several trials (Section 18.4.6).

18.2.3 PSA as a Prognostic Biomarker

We first show that changes in PSA can have prognostic value and, as such, are useful to guide treatment choice for individual patients. We use data from two trials in patients with androgen-sensitive metastatic prostate cancer who were randomized to receive an experimental or a control hormonal therapy (Renard et al., 2002b; Buyse et al., 2003).

Figure 18.2 shows the survival curves by randomized treatment and by PSA response, defined as a decrease of 50% or more in PSA compared with the baseline level, or a decrease in PSA to <4 ng/mL confirmed by a second PSA measurement at least 4 weeks later. Clearly, PSA response had a major prognostic impact on survival. In contrast, in these two trials, there was no significant effect of treatment on survival overall, neither among patients with PSA, nor among patients without such response. We will perform further analyses of these trials in Section 18.4.6. For now, our point is that PSA can be a very effective prognostic tool for deciding whether to continue, stop,

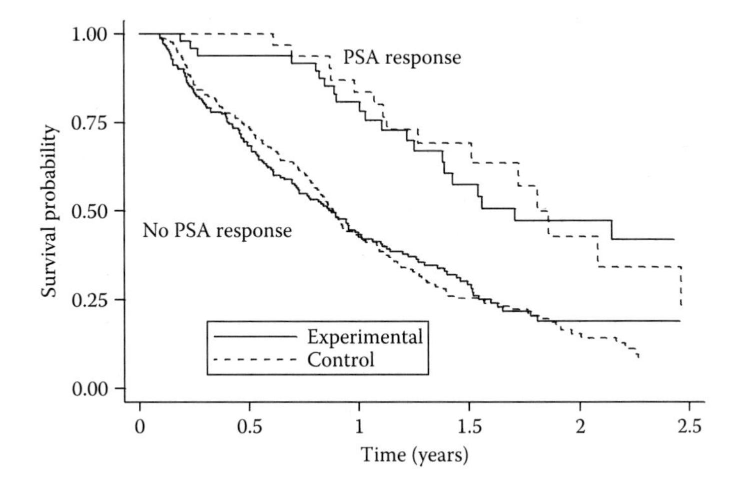

FIGURE 18.2
Survival by PSA response for patients with androgen-sensitive metastatic prostate cancer randomized to a control or an experimental hormonal therapy.

modify, or augment the treatment for individual patients, which is one of the central objectives of personalized medicine.

18.2.4 PSA as a Pharmacodynamic Biomarker

We now turn to the use of PSA as a pharmacodynamic biomarker of the effect of an investigational treatment. Here, we use data from a randomized phase II trial for patients who had undergone primary therapy with a curative intent (either surgery or radiation) and had progressive elevation of their PSA without documented evidence of metastatic disease (Dreicer et al., 2008). Outside of the trial, these patients would have been managed through observation until their clinical course dictated hormonal intervention. The trial was conducted to assess the clinical and biological effects of two different injection schedules of interleukin-2 plus a viral suspension of a recombinant vaccine containing the sequence coding for the human MUC1 antigen. Twenty-nine patients with histological documentation of MUC1 antigen expression were randomized to receive weekly ($N = 15$) or 3-weekly ($N = 14$) injections of the vaccine. In both arms, vaccination continued until progressive disease was documented or until toxicity required the cessation of treatment. The primary efficacy endpoint was PSA response, defined as a decrease of 50% or more in PSA compared with the baseline level, confirmed by a second PSA measurement 6 weeks later. Note that this definition of PSA response differs somewhat from the definition used in Section 18.2.3.

In a trial of this size (29 patients), PSA response or any other binary outcome only has power to detect a major, arguably unattainable, difference between the randomized groups. As it turns out, no patient achieved a PSA response in either treatment arm (Dreicer et al., 2008), so the trial could be considered negative. From a statistical point of view, however, a mixed-effects model on the longitudinal PSA measurements makes use of all the data available and is therefore quite sensitive to any treatment effect on the pharmacodynamic biomarker. For the ith patient ($i=1, \ldots, 29$), let T_i and W_i be indicators of whether the patient is in the 3-weekly or the weekly schedule, respectively; let P_i denote the period, taking the value −1 in case of prebaseline measurements, and 1 otherwise; and let PSA_{ij} be the PSA level measured at time point t_{ij} ($j=1, \ldots, n_i$). The mixed-effects model can be written as

$$\log\left(\text{PSA}_{ij}\right) = \beta_1 T_i + \beta_2 W_i + \beta_3 t_{ij} + \beta_4 P_i + \beta_5 P_i t_{ij} + \beta_6 T_i t_{ij} + \beta_7 T_i P_i + \beta_8 T_i P_i t_{ij} + b_{0i} + b_{1i} t_{ij} + \varepsilon_{ij}, \quad (18.1)$$

where

b_{0i} is a random intercept

b_{1i} a random slope

$\varepsilon_i \sim N\left(0, \sigma^2 I_{n_i}\right)$ is the vector of residual components

Figure 18.3 shows the model-fitted log(PSA) slopes, for the weekly and 3-weekly schedules. Visually, the log(PSA) slopes are (slightly) reduced when treatment is initiated. Indeed, there was a significant period effect (prebaseline versus postbaseline) for both schedules ($P<0.0001$), for the weekly schedule ($P<0.0001$) and for the 3-weekly schedule ($P=0.0003$). The effect of schedule (weekly versus 3-weekly) did not reach statistical significance ($P=0.20$). All in all, this example shows the exquisite sensitivity of longitudinal measurements of PSA as a pharmacodynamic biomarker, which resulted in a statistically convincing claim that the vaccination had a significant effect on PSA levels. The number of patients was however insufficient to reliably choose an optimal vaccination schedule. More importantly, a change in the PSA slope may or may not predict a clinical benefit in the long run, which is the central question in the remainder of this chapter. Specifically, does the effect of a treatment on PSA levels predict an effect of this treatment on long-term clinical endpoints such as survival?

18.3 Validation of a Surrogate Endpoint in a Single Trial

The most common situation for the evaluation of a potential surrogate endpoint is when data are available from a single randomized clinical trial. The notation and modeling concepts introduced here are useful to present and critically discuss the key ingredients of the Prentice–Freedman framework for surrogate evaluation, which is important conceptually and is still

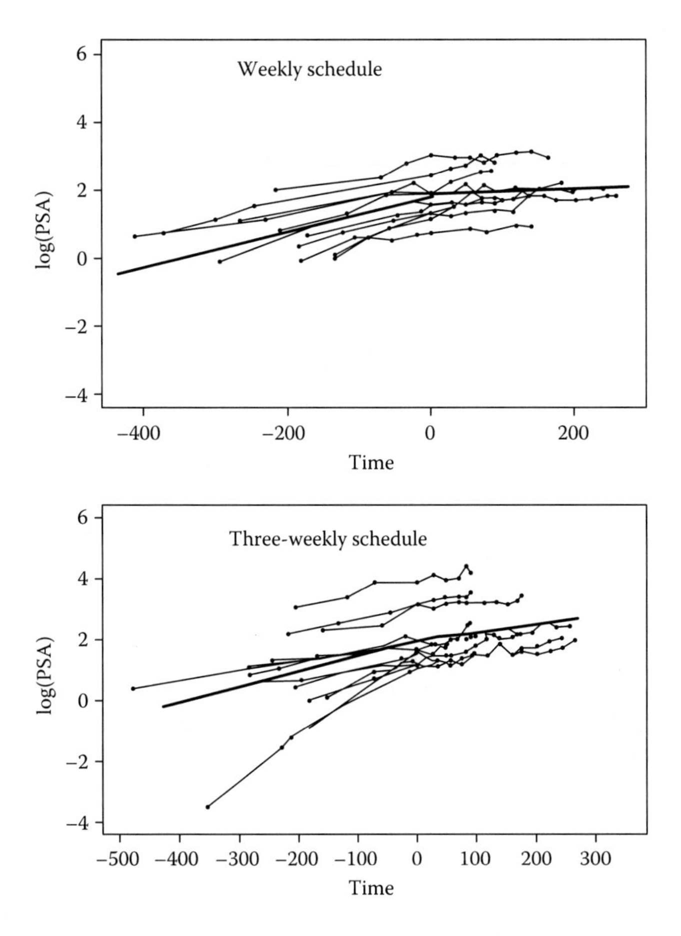

FIGURE 18.3
Individual log(PSA) observations over time and model-fitted log(PSA) slopes (thick lines) by vaccination schedule in a randomized phase II trial for patients with progressive elevation of their PSA without documented evidence of metastatic disease.

frequently used (Section 18.3.5), even though it will be shown to be insufficient to establish surrogacy (Section 18.3.4).

We adopt the following notation: T and S are random variables that denote the true and surrogate endpoints, respectively, and Z is an indicator variable for treatment. For now, and for ease of exposition, we assume that S and T are normally distributed. The effect of treatment on S and T can be modeled as follows:

$$S_j = \mu_s + \alpha Z_j + \varepsilon_{sj}, \tag{18.2}$$

$$T_j = \mu_T + \beta Z_j + \varepsilon_{Tj}, \tag{18.3}$$

where $j=1,\ldots,n$ indicates patients, and the error terms have a joint zero-mean normal distribution with variance-covariance matrix

$$\sum = \begin{pmatrix} \sigma_{SS} & \sigma_{ST} \\ & \sigma_{TT} \end{pmatrix}.$$

In addition, the relationship between S and T can be described by a regression of the form

$$T_j = \mu + \gamma S_j + \varepsilon_j. \tag{18.4}$$

18.3.1 Prentice's Definition and Criteria

Prentice (1989) proposed to define a surrogate endpoint as "a response variable for which a test of the null hypothesis of no relationship to the treatment groups under comparison is also a valid test of the corresponding null hypothesis based on the true endpoint" (Prentice, 1989, p. 432). In terms of our simple models (18.2) and (18.3), the definition states that for S to be a valid surrogate for T, α and β must simultaneously be equal to, or different from, zero. Note that this definition cannot be operationalized if data are available from a single trial only, since it would require multiple estimates of α and β to be available, preferably from a large number of experiments, some with treatment effects on both endpoints, and some without such effects. In the case of a single trial, Prentice suggested to use the following operational criteria:

1. Treatment has a significant impact on the surrogate endpoint (α differs significantly from zero in [18.2]).
2. Treatment has a significant impact on the true endpoint (β differs significantly from zero in [18.3]).
3. The surrogate endpoint has a significant impact on the true endpoint (γ differs significantly from zero in [18.4]).
4. The full effect of treatment upon the true endpoint is captured by the surrogate.

The last condition, often termed Prentice's fourth criterion, is verified through the conditional distribution of the true endpoint, given treatment *and* surrogate endpoint, derived from (18.2) to (18.3)

$$T_j = \tilde{\mu}_T + \beta_S Z_j + \gamma_Z S_j + \tilde{\varepsilon}_{Tj}, \tag{18.5}$$

where the treatment effect (corrected for the surrogate S), β_S, and the surrogate effect (corrected for treatment Z), γ_Z, are

$$\beta_S = \beta - \sigma_{TS}\sigma_{SS}^{-1}\alpha, \tag{18.6}$$

$$\gamma_Z = \sigma_{TS}\sigma_{SS}^{-1}, \tag{18.7}$$

and the variance of $\tilde{\varepsilon}_{Tj}$ is given by

$$\sigma_{TT} - \sigma_{TS}^{2}\sigma_{SS}^{-1}.$$

Prentice's fourth criterion requires that β_S be equal to zero, which implies that T does not depend on Z, given S. This criterion has been interpreted as implying that the effect of Z on T is completely captured by S. We shall however see in Section 18.3.4 that such an interpretation is problematic.

18.3.2 Freedman's Proportion Explained

Freedman et al. (1992) argued that Prentice's fourth criterion raises a conceptual difficulty, since it requires the statistical test for treatment effect on the true endpoint to be nonsignificant after adjustment for the surrogate. These authors argued that the nonsignificance of this test does not prove that the effect of treatment upon the true endpoint is *fully* captured by the surrogate, and therefore, they proposed to estimate the proportion of the treatment effect mediated by the surrogate

$$PE = \frac{\beta - \beta_S}{\beta},$$

with β_S and β obtained, respectively, from (18.5) to (18.3). In this paradigm, a valid surrogate would be one for which the proportion explained (PE) is equal to one. In practice, a surrogate would be deemed acceptable if the lower limit of the confidence interval of PE was *sufficiently* close to one.

Difficulties surrounding the PE have been discussed in the literature (Volberding et al., 1990; Choi et al., 1993; Lin et al., 1997; Buyse and Molenberghs, 1998; Flandre and Saidi, 1999; Molenberghs et al., 2002). The PE will tend to be unstable when β is close to zero, a situation that is likely to occur in actual situations. As Freedman et al. (1992) themselves acknowledged, the confidence limits of PE will tend to be rather wide (and sometimes even unbounded if Fieller confidence intervals are used), unless large sample sizes are available and/or a very strong treatment effect is observed on the true endpoint. Note that strong treatment effects are uncommon, but large sample sizes can be available in meta-analyses of randomized clinical trials, a situation we return to in Section 18.4. Several authors have noted that PE is not restricted to the unit interval (Lin et al., 1997; Buyse and Molenberghs, 1998; Molenberghs et al., 2002; Baker, 2006). Another serious issue arises when (18.5) is not the correct conditional model, and an interaction term between Z_j and S_j needs to be included. In that case, even the definition of *PE* becomes problematic.

18.3.3 Relative Effect and Adjusted Association

Buyse and Molenberghs (1998) proposed two other quantities for the evaluation of a surrogate endpoint: the relative effect (*RE*), which is the ratio of the effects of treatment upon the final and the surrogate endpoint,

$$RE = \frac{\beta}{\alpha},$$

and the treatment-adjusted association between the surrogate and the true endpoint, ρ_Z:

$$\rho_Z = \frac{\sigma_{ST}}{\sqrt{\sigma_{SS}\sigma_{TT}}}.$$

Molenberghs et al. (2002) showed that a simple relationship can be derived between *PE*, *RE*, and ρ_Z. Define $\lambda^2 = \sigma_{TT}\sigma_{SS}^{-1}$. It follows that $\lambda\rho_Z = \sigma_{ST}\sigma_{SS}^{-1}$ and, from (18.6), $\beta_S = \beta - \rho_Z\lambda\alpha$. As a result, we obtain

$$PE = \lambda\rho_Z \frac{\alpha}{\beta} = \lambda\rho_Z \frac{1}{RE}.$$

This relationship shows that *PE* has the undesirable property of depending on λ, which can take any arbitrary value by acting upon σ_{TT} or σ_{SS}. Begg and Leung (2000) used a similar argument to warn against the use of *PE*.

18.3.4 Limitations of Analyses Based on a Single Trial

The approaches described earlier all have serious limitations. Prentice's fourth criterion is very appealing, because it seems to provide a mathematical way of testing that there exists a biological mechanism through which the surrogate fully captures the effect of treatment on the true endpoint. In cancer trials, for example, if the surrogate (say, a change in PSA levels) was the unique mechanism in the causal chain leading from treatment exposure to the final endpoint (say, death), then any treatment effect on survival could be *causally* explained by the treatment effect on the surrogate. Unfortunately, fulfillment of Prentice's fourth criterion does not support a claim of causality. This is best illustrated through a simple example in which data are available on ten patients, five in a control group ($Z=0$) and five in a treatment group ($Z=1$). The surrogate endpoint S is a binary outcome (e.g., PSA response), with $S=0$ denoting failure and $S=1$ success. The true endpoint T is a continuous outcome (e.g., survival time, with complete observations for simplicity). Assume that treatment improves the surrogate, with three successes in the treatment arm *versus* two successes in the control arm. Assume that treatment also improves the true endpoint, with mean survival (denoted $\bar{T}$) equal to 16 in the treatment arm *versus* 14 in the control arm. Let δ be the treatment effect on survival, expressed as the difference between these means: overall, $\delta = \bar{T}(Z=1) - \bar{T}(Z=0) = 16 - 14 = 2$.

Two scenarios are presented in Table 18.2: in scenario A, the treatment effect on the true endpoint is completely captured by the treatment effect on the surrogate, while in scenario B, the treatment effect on the true endpoint is independent of the effect on the surrogate. Yet Prentice's fourth criterion is perfectly fulfilled in these two situations. Indeed, the mean survival difference, conditional on the surrogate value, is in both cases equal to zero: $\delta \mid \{S=0\} = \bar{T}(Z=1 \mid S=0) - \bar{T}(Z=0 \mid S=0) = 10 - 10 = 0$ and $\delta \mid \{S=1\} = \bar{T}(Z=1 \mid S=1) - \bar{T}(Z=0 \mid S=1) = 20 - 20 = 0$. This issue will arise when the probability that $S = 1$ depends on baseline prognostic factors. In this case, conditioning on S selects patients with different average prognosis in the two treatment groups, and the between-treatment comparison of T conditional on S is intrinsically biased. As a consequence, the fourth Prentice criterion may be misleading if prognostic factors are ignored.

In our simple example, imagine that the patients can be categorized as shown in the last column of Table 18.2: the patient in the first row of both treatment groups is of poor prognosis, the next three patients in both treatment groups are of intermediate prognosis, and the last patient in both treatment groups is of good prognosis. In scenario A, the effect of treatment is to improve the outcome of one patient for both S and T. In contrast, in scenario B, the treatment is deleterious or beneficial for T regardless of S.

TABLE 18.2

Two Scenarios in Which Prentice's Fourth Criterion Is Perfectly Fulfilled When the Patient Prognosis Is Ignored

$Z=0$		$Z=1$				
		Scenario A: Full Capture		**Scenario B: Independence**		
S	T	S	T	S	T	**Prognosis**
0	10	0	10	0	5	Poor
0	10	0	10	0	15	
0	10	1	20	1	5	Intermediate
1	20	1	20	1	15	
1	20	1	20	1	40	Good

Notes: The mean survival difference, conditional on the surrogate, is equal to zero. Scenario A, the treatment effect on T is fully captured by the treatment effect on S; scenario B, the treatment effect on T is independent of the treatment effect on S.

The survival comparison, conditional on *S*, includes patients of worse prognosis on average in the treatment group as compared with the control group, and is therefore biased toward the null in the presence of a beneficial treatment effect on *S* and *T*.

The bias can be removed by adjusting the analysis for the patient prognosis, for example, through stratification. Denote *P* the prognostic group used in the stratification, with strata p_1 denoting poor prognosis, p_2 intermediate prognosis, and p_3 good prognosis. In a stratified analysis, the mean survival difference, conditional on the surrogate value, is again equal to zero in scenario A: $\delta|\{S=0, P=p_i, i=1 \ldots 3\}=0$ and $\delta|\{S=1, P=p_i, i=1 \ldots 3\}=0$. In contrast, in a stratified analysis, the mean survival difference, conditional on the surrogate value, is *not* equal to zero in scenario B: $\delta|\{S=0, P=p_i, i=1 \ldots 3\}=0.5$ and $\delta|\{S=1, P=p_i, i=1 \ldots 3\}=1.0$. Hence a stratified analysis would suggest, correctly, that *S* is a good surrogate for *T* in scenario A, but not in scenario B. In general, the fourth Prentice criterion requires the strong and unverifiable assumption that there are no *unmeasured confounders* to provide evidence that a surrogate fully captures the effect of treatment on the true endpoint. When this criterion is used to assess surrogacy, the analysis should be adjusted for measured prognostic variables. Whether unmeasured prognostic variables would have an impact on the analysis can unfortunately not be tested; hence, the fourth Prentice criterion is never guaranteed to provide a valid test of surrogacy.

18.3.5 PSA as a Surrogate in a Single Trial

In locally advanced prostate cancer, various PSA-based endpoints have been proposed as potential surrogates for cancer-specific survival. The most popular is PSA doubling time, but others have been proposed: PSA nadir <0.5 ng/mL, PSA at the end of treatment <0.5 ng/mL, and time to biochemical failure, defined as the time from the end of treatment to an increase in PSA concentration ≥2 ng/mL above the posttreatment nadir value (Table 18.3). In androgen-independent metastatic disease, candidate surrogate endpoints for survival include the PSA rate of change or *velocity*, PSA declines, and PSA *normalization*, defined as a drop in PSA to ≤4 ng/mL (Table 18.4). PSA doubling times and velocities are usually estimated using least squares regressions of repeated measurements of log(PSA) over a relevant period of time. The PSA velocity is the slope of the regression line (expressed in ng/mL/month); the doubling time is equal to log(2) divided by the slope (expressed in months).

The PSA-based endpoints shown in Tables 18.3 and 18.4 have all been evaluated as surrogates for long-term clinical endpoints using data from single large randomized trials. These trials tested radiation and androgen deprivation therapy in locally advanced prostate cancer, and chemotherapy in androgen-independent prostate cancer. The long-term clinical endpoints of interest were cancer-specific survival in early disease and survival in

TABLE 18.3

Potential PSA-Based Surrogate Endpoints in Locally Advanced Prostate Cancer

Surrogate Endpoint	Surrogate Type	Validation Criteria	Reference
PSA DT	C	Prentice (adjusted)	Valicenti et al. (2006)
PSA DT TBF	C T	Prentice (adjusted) +PE	Denham et al. (2008)
PSA nadir PSA EOT	B B	Prentice +PE +PV	D'Amico et al. (2012)

Abbreviations: Surrogate endpoint: PSA DT, PSA doubling time; PSA EOT, PSA end of treatment; TBF, time to biochemical failure; surrogate type: B, binary; C, continuous; T, time to failure; validation criteria: PE, proportion of treatment effect explained; PV, proportion of variance explained.

TABLE 18.4

Potential PSA-Based Surrogate Endpoints in Androgen-Independent Metastatic Prostate Cancer

Surrogate Endpoint	Surrogate Type	Validation Criteria	Reference
PSA decline PSA velocity PSA normalization	C C B	PE	Petrylak et al. (2006)
PSA decline PSA velocity	C C	Prentice +PE +PV	Armstrong et al. (2007)

Abbreviations: Surrogate type: B, binary; C, continuous; validation criteria: PE, proportion of treatment effect explained; PV, proportion of variance explained.

advanced disease. The potential surrogate endpoints were of different types: binary (e.g., PSA nadir < 0.5 ng/mL), continuous (e.g., PSA declines), or failure time (e.g., time to biochemical failure). More complex types could have included longitudinal biomarkers (e.g., repeated measurements of PSA over time) or even multivariate longitudinal biomarkers (e.g., repeated joint measurements of PSA and CTCs over time). Complex types of biomarkers are rarely used in practice, probably because simple biomarker types are easier to use for clinical decision making. Even continuous biomarkers tend to be dichotomized; for instance, PSA declines were analyzed using a number of cutoffs ranging from 5% to 90% (Petrylak et al., 2006). It would be interesting to quantify the loss of information arising from using simple metrics instead of the full data available. We will return to this question in Section 18.4.6.

As shown in Tables 18.3 and 18.4, the PSA-based potential surrogate endpoints were evaluated using the Prentice criteria and/or the proportion of treatment explained. Some studies in locally advanced disease used models adjusted for baseline factors such as age, T stage, Gleason score, and initial PSA, which are known to be of major prognostic importance in this setting (Valicenti et al., 2006; Denham et al., 2008). Two studies also used proportions of variance explained as additional measures of surrogacy (Schemper, 1993). One of these studies (D'Amico et al., 2012) estimated the partial proportion of variance in T explained by model (18.5) when Z is added to model (18.4); for a good surrogate, this proportion is expected to be close to zero, in keeping with Prentice's fourth criterion. Another study (Armstrong et al., 2007) estimated the partial proportion of variance in T explained by model (18.5) when S is added to model (18.3); for a good surrogate, this proportion is expected to be *large* (keeping in mind that proportions of variance explained in survival models are typically quite low [Schemper, 1993]).

Four of the five studies referenced in Tables 18.3 and 18.4 claimed that PSA-based endpoints are acceptable surrogates. Only one study acknowledged that PSA doubling time did not meet all of Prentice's requirements for a surrogate of cancer-specific survival (Valicenti et al., 2006). In fact, all these analyses were based on a single trial, and as such they could only assess the association between the surrogate and the true endpoint (Collette et al., 2007). In order to fully validate a surrogate, it is also important to show that treatment effects on PSA are predictive of treatment effects on survival (ICH, 1998). This requires that data from multiple trials be analyzed, which is the topic of the next sections.

18.4 Validation of a Surrogate Endpoint in Multiple Trials

Several authors have proposed to use a meta-analysis of randomized trials to look for an association between the effects of treatment on a potential surrogate and on a clinical endpoint. An early paper used this approach to investigate whether tumor response can be used as a surrogate for survival in patients with advanced breast cancer (A'Hern et al., 1988). Another paper used a similar but more elaborate model to investigate whether tumor response can be used as a surrogate for survival in patients with advanced ovarian cancer, with due allowance for the fact that the treatment effects on both endpoints are estimated with error (Torri et al., 1992). Yet other authors used Bayesian methods to model the association between treatment effects on CD4 T-lymphocyte cell count and on the development of AIDS or death in patients with HIV infection (Daniels and Hughes, 1997). In the remainder of this section, we use a model that incorporates two levels of association, one between the surrogate and the true endpoint, and the other between the treatment effects on the surrogate and the true endpoint (Buyse et al., 2000; Gail et al., 2000; Korn et al., 2005). This meta-analytic approach was originally formulated for two continuous, normally distributed (Gaussian) outcomes, as outlined in Section 18.4.1. Even though the models in this case are relatively straightforward, they pose considerable computational challenges. Simplified modeling approaches are discussed in Section 18.4.2. In practice, the endpoints are often non-Gaussian variables. The meta-analytic model has been extended to a range of situations, in particular binary (Section 18.4.3), failure-time (Section 18.4.4), and longitudinally measured outcomes (Section 18.4.5). Applications of these models to PSA data are discussed in Section 18.4.6.

18.4.1 Meta-Analytic Model for Gaussian Endpoints

We use a hierarchical two-level model for the situation of a surrogate and a true endpoint that are jointly normally distributed. Let T_{ij} and S_{ij} be the random variables denoting the true and surrogate endpoints for the jth subject in the ith trial, respectively, and let Z_{ij} be the indicator variable for treatment. First, consider the following fixed-effects models:

$$S_{ij} = \mu_{Si} + \alpha_i Z_{ij} + \varepsilon_{Sij}, \tag{18.8}$$

$$T_{ij} = \mu_{Ti} + \beta_i Z_{ij} + \varepsilon_{Tij}, \tag{18.9}$$

where

μ_{Si} and μ_{Ti} are trial-specific intercepts

α_i and β_i are trial-specific effects of treatment Z_{ij} on the endpoints in trial i

ε_{Sij} and ε_{Tij} are correlated error terms, assumed to be zero-mean normally distributed with variance-covariance matrix

$$\Sigma = \begin{pmatrix} \sigma_{SS} & \sigma_{ST} \\ & \sigma_{TT} \end{pmatrix}. \tag{18.10}$$

In addition, we can decompose

$$\begin{pmatrix} \mu_{Si} \\ \mu_{Ti} \\ \alpha_i \\ \beta_i \end{pmatrix} = \begin{pmatrix} \mu_S \\ \mu_T \\ \alpha \\ \beta \end{pmatrix} + \begin{pmatrix} m_{Si} \\ m_{Ti} \\ a_i \\ b_i \end{pmatrix}, \tag{18.11}$$

where the second term on the right-hand side of (18.11) is assumed to follow a zero-mean normal distribution with variance-covariance matrix

$$D = \begin{pmatrix} d_{SS} & d_{ST} & d_{Sa} & d_{Sb} \\ & d_{TT} & d_{Ta} & d_{Tb} \\ & & d_{aa} & d_{ab} \\ & & & d_{bb} \end{pmatrix}. \tag{18.12}$$

A classical hierarchical, random-effects modeling strategy results from the combination of the aforementioned two steps into a single one:

$$S_{ij} = \mu_S + m_{Si} + \alpha Z_{ij} + a_i Z_{ij} + \varepsilon_{Sij}, \tag{18.13}$$

$$T_{ij} = \mu_T + m_{Ti} + \beta Z_{ij} + b_i Z_{ij} + \varepsilon_{Tij}, \tag{18.14}$$

where

- μ_S and μ_T are fixed intercepts
- α and β are fixed treatment effects
- μ_{Si} and μ_{Ti} are random intercepts
- a_i and b_i are random treatment effects in trial i for the surrogate and true endpoints, respectively

The vector of random effects (μ_{Si}, μ_{Ti}, a_i, b_i) is assumed to be mean-zero normally distributed with variance-covariance matrix (18.12).

The error terms ε_{Sij} and εT_{ij} follow the same assumptions as in the fixed effects models.

After fitting the aforementioned models, surrogacy is captured by means of two quantities: the *individual level* and *trial level* coefficients of determination, denoted respectively R^2_{indiv} and R^2_{trial}. R^2_{indiv} measures the association between S and T at the level of the individual patient, after adjustment for Z, while R^2_{trial} quantifies the association between the treatment effects on S and T at the trial level.

R^2_{indiv} is based on (18.10) and takes the following form:

$$R^2_{\text{indiv}} = R^2_{\varepsilon Tij|\varepsilon Sij} = \frac{\sigma^2_{ST}}{\sigma_{SS}\sigma_{TT}}.$$

R^2_{trial} is given by

$$R^2_{\text{trial}} = R^2_{b_i|m_{Si},a_i} = \frac{\begin{pmatrix} d_{Sb} \\ d_{ab} \end{pmatrix}^T \begin{pmatrix} d_{SS} & d_{Sa} \\ d_{Sa} & d_{aa} \end{pmatrix}^{-1} \begin{pmatrix} d_{Sb} \\ d_{ab} \end{pmatrix}}{d_{bb}}. \tag{18.15}$$

The aforementioned quantity is unitless and, if the corresponding variance-covariance matrix is positive definite, it lies within the unit interval.

A surrogate could be adopted when R^2_{indiv} and R^2_{trial} are both sufficiently close to one. Some authors (Lasserre et al., 2007) and health authorities (e.g., the German Institute for Quality and Efficiency in Health Care [IQWIG, 2011]) have proposed thresholds that need to be met by these measures of association before a surrogate is considered acceptable. While such thresholds provide useful guidance, there will always be clinical and other judgments involved in the decision process.

18.4.2 Simplified Modeling Strategies

R^2_{trial} is computed from the variance–covariance matrix (18.12). It is possible that this matrix be ill-conditioned and/or non–positive definite. In such cases, the resulting quantities computed based on this matrix may not be trustworthy. One way to assess the ill conditioning of a matrix is by reporting its condition number, that is, the ratio of the largest over the smallest eigenvalue. A large condition number is an indication of ill conditioning, which may be due to an insufficient number of trials, low sample sizes within trials, a narrow range in treatment effects, or a combination of all of these factors.

When such computational difficulties are encountered, the full models proposed earlier can be simplified. It is possible, for a start, to simplify models (18.8) and (18.9) by replacing the fixed trial-specific intercepts by a common one. Thus, the reduced mixed-effect models result from removing the random trial-specific intercepts m_{Si} and m_{Ti} from models (18.13) and (18.14). The R^2_{trial} for the reduced models then simplifies:

$$R^2_{\text{trial(r)}} = R^2_{b_i|a_i} = \frac{d^2_{ab}}{d_{aa}d_{bb}}.$$

Tibaldi et al. (2003) suggested other simplifications to overcome the computational challenges of hierarchical modeling. One can treat the trial-specific effects as fixed in the two-stage approach. The first-stage model takes the form (18.8) to (18.9) and at the second stage, the estimated treatment effect on the true endpoint is regressed on the treatment effect on the surrogate and the intercept associated with the surrogate endpoint:

$$\hat{\beta}_i = \hat{\lambda}_0 + \hat{\lambda}_1\hat{\mu}_{Si} + \hat{\lambda}_2\hat{\alpha}_i + \varepsilon_i.$$

The trial-level $R^2_{\text{trial(f)}}$ is obtained by regressing $\hat{\beta}_i$ on $\hat{\mu}_{Si}$ and $\hat{\alpha}_i$, whereas $R^2_{\text{trial(r)}}$ is obtained from regressing $\hat{\beta}_i$ on $\hat{\alpha}_i$ only.

Another major simplification consists of fitting separate models for the true and surrogate endpoints. If the trial-specific effects are considered fixed, models (18.8) to (18.9) are fitted separately, that is, the corresponding error terms in the two models are assumed independent. Similarly, if the trial-specific effects are considered random, models (18.13) and (18.14) are fitted separately. Such univariate models do not provide a direct estimate of R^2_{indiv}, but interest focuses here on R^2_{trial}. In addition, R^2_{indiv} can be estimated by making use of the correlation between the residuals from two separate univariate models.

When the univariate approach and/or the fixed-effects approach are chosen, there is a need to adjust for the heterogeneity in information content between trial-specific contributions. One common way of doing so is to use a weighted linear regression model in the second stage, with weights proportional to the trial sizes. However, measurement error models are required to account for the estimation error in the treatment effects on both S and T, and such models frequently do not converge.

Renfro et al. (2012) have taken a completely different route to address the computational challenges of the second stage of hierarchical modeling. They propose performing this second stage, trial-level evaluation within a Bayesian framework. They assume a vague multivariate normal prior for the mean treatment effects with a vague Wishart prior for the precision of these effects. They show, through simulations and real case studies, that the Bayesian approach yields estimates of R^2_{trial} when the likelihood-based approach does not (Renfro et al., 2012). Even though the choice of priors remains a key issue, it may be preferable to use a Bayesian approach to compute R^2_{trial} with due allowance for the variance–covariance of the estimated treatment effects, rather than to use an unadjusted R^2_{trial} that ignores the estimation error. Shkedy and Torres Barbosa (Chapter 15 in Burzykowski et al. [2005]) have also investigated the use of Bayesian methodology and conclude that even relatively noninformative prior have a strongly beneficial impact on the algorithms' performance.

18.4.3 Binary Endpoints

Renard et al. (2002a) have shown that extension to this situation is easily done using a latent variable formulation. That is, one posits the existence of a pair of continuously distributed latent variable responses $\left(\tilde{S}_{ij}, \tilde{T}_{ij}\right)$ that produce the actual values of (S_{ij}, T_{ij}). These unobserved variables are assumed to have a joint normal distribution and the realized values follow by double dichotomization. On the latent-variable scale, a model similar to (18.8) and (18.9) is obtained and in the matrix (18.10), the variances are set equal to unity in order to ensure identifiability. This leads to the following model:

$$\begin{cases} \Phi^{-1}\left(P\left[S_{ij}=1 \mid Z_{ij}, m_{S_i}, a_i, m_{T_i}, b_i\right]\right) = \mu_S + m_{S_i} + \left(\alpha + a_i\right) Z_{ij}, \\ \Phi^{-1}\left(P\left[T_{ij}=1 \mid Z_{ij}, m_{S_i}, a_i, m_{T_i}, b_i\right]\right) = \mu_T + m_{T_i} + \left(\beta + b_i\right) Z_{ij}, \end{cases}$$

where Φ denotes the standard normal cumulative distribution function. Renard et al. (2002a) used pseudolikelihood methods to estimate the model parameters. Similar ideas have been used in cases where one of the endpoints is continuous, with the other one is binary or categorical (Chapter 6 in Burzykowski et al. [2005]).

18.4.4 Failure-Time Endpoints

Assume now that S_{ij} and T_{ij} are failure-time endpoints. Models (18.8) and (18.9) are replaced by a model for two correlated failure-time random variables. Burzykowski et al. (2004) use copulas to this end and write the joint survivor function of (S_{ij}, T_{ij}) as

$$F(s,t) = P\left(S_{ij} \geq s, T_{ij} \geq t\right) = C_\delta\left\{F_{Sij}(s), F_{Tij}(t)\right\}, \quad s,t \geq 0,$$

where

(F_{Sij}, F_{Tij}) denote marginal survivor functions
C_δ is a copula, that is, a distribution function on $[0, 1]^2$ with $\delta \in R^1$

When the hazard functions are specified, estimates of the parameters for the joint model can be obtained using maximum likelihood. Shih and Louis (1995) discuss alternative estimation methods. Different copulas may be used, depending on assumptions made about the nature of the association between the surrogate and the true endpoint; such assumptions are generally unavailable, in which case, the best fitting copula may be chosen (Clayton, 1978; Dale, 1986; Hougaard, 1986). The association parameter is generally hard to interpret. However, it can be shown (Genest and McKay, 1986) that there is a link with Kendall's τ,

$$\tau = 4\int_0^1\int_0^1 C_\delta(u,v)C_\delta(du,dv) - 1,$$

providing an easy measure of surrogacy at the individual level. Spearman's rank correlation coefficient can also be used as a measure of association at the individual level for two time-related endpoints (Burzykowski et al., 2004).

At the second stage, R^2_{trial} can be computed based on the pairs of treatment effects estimated at the first stage. Similar ideas have been used in cases where one of the endpoints is categorical and the other is a survival endpoint (Burzykowski et al., 2004). In this case, one marginal distribution can be a proportional odds logistic regression, while the other is a proportional hazards model. If the Plackett copula (Dale, 1986) is chosen to capture the association between both endpoints, the global odds ratio is relatively easy to interpret the measure of association.

18.4.5 Longitudinal Endpoints

Frequently, a surrogate endpoint is based on longitudinal measurements of some outcome of interest, while the true endpoint is a failure-type endpoint. In most forms of advanced cancer, for instance, the size of the tumor is measured longitudinally, with tumor shrinkage indicating treatment benefit, and tumor growth lack of responsiveness to treatment. In this case, potential surrogates can be defined using simple metrics based on the longitudinal measures. The most common example is the so-called objective response in solid tumors (a reduction of at least 50% in the size of the surface area of the tumor measured by CT scan at any point in time, and maintained for at least one month). Such a simple binary endpoint is unlikely to be an acceptable surrogate in any form of advanced cancer; it has formally been shown not to be acceptable in advanced colorectal cancer (Buyse et al., 2008) and advanced breast cancer (Burzykowski et al., 2008). The question is whether use of the whole vector of tumor measurements over time might be a more promising alternative. In prostate cancer, which is the disease used to illustrate the various topics of this chapter, longitudinal measurements of PSA are typically used to define simple metrics (see Sections 18.3.5 and 18.4.6). Rather than using metrics that may waste valuable information, it seems desirable to be able to model the full vector of PSA measurements as a potential surrogate for long-term clinical endpoints.

Renard et al. (2002b) and Alonso et al. (2003) showed that going from a univariate setting to a multivariate setting is challenging. The R^2 measures proposed by Buyse et al. (2000) are no longer applicable. If treatment effect can be assumed constant over time, then (18.15) can still be useful to evaluate surrogacy at the trial level. However, the situation is different at the individual level, since R^2_{ind} is no longer uniquely defined. Renard et al. (2002b) propose to extend this measure through a function of time that captures the association between the longitudinal process underlying PSA and the hazard rate over time.

18.4.6 PSA as a Surrogate in Multiple Trials

Table 18.5 shows several PSA-based endpoints that have been evaluated as surrogates for survival in patients with androgen-sensitive metastatic prostate cancer. The analyses were based on two meta-analyses of patient-level data from five randomized trials testing experimental *versus* standard hormonal therapies (Renard et al., 2002b; Buyse et al., 2003; Collette et al., 2005). Since there were only two trials in one meta-analysis and three in the other, each trial was split by country into smaller *units* (i.e., groups of patients), to which the meta-analytic approach was applied. Note that the choice of appropriate units of analysis is a matter of debate. Technically, the optimal conditions are to have both a large number of units and a large

TABLE 18.5

Potential PSA-Based Surrogate Endpoints in Androgen-Sensitive Metastatic Prostate Cancer

Surrogate Endpoint	Surrogate Type	Individual-Level Surrogacy Measure	Reference
PSA response	B	Odds ratio	Buyse et al. (2003)
Time to PSA progression	T	Kendall's τ	
PSA repeated measures	L	$R^2_{\text{indiv}}(t)$	
PSA response	B	Odds ratio	Collette et al. (2005)
PSA normalization	B	Odds ratio	
Time to PSA progression	T	Kendall's τ	
PSA repeated measures	L	$R^2_{\text{indiv}}(t)$	

Abbreviations: Surrogate type: B, binary; L, longitudinal; T, time to failure.

number of patients per unit (Cortiñas Abrahantes et al., 2004). Splitting trials into smaller units may achieve the former condition at the expense of the latter. Some studies evaluating surrogates in a small number of trials have used clinical site as the unit of analysis (Burzykowski et al., 2001; Buyse et al., 2011; Laporte et al., 2013).

As indicated in Table 18.5, the PSA-based endpoints were of different types, calling for the use of methods specific to each variable type, as described in Sections 18.4.3 through 18.4.5. We discuss the results of one meta-analysis (Buyse et al., 2003), but the other meta-analysis showed very similar results (Collette et al., 2005). There was no significant difference in OS between the randomized treatment groups, so the Prentice criteria could not be used. In contrast, the meta-analytic approach could be used and was informative.

One of the potential surrogates was PSA response, defined in Section 18.2.3. At the individual level, there was a strong impact of PSA response on survival, as shown in Figure 18.2. Several measures can be used to quantify the individual level association. The survival odds ratio is one such measure: it is the ratio, assumed constant, of the odds of surviving beyond time t for PSA responders as compared with nonresponders. The survival odds ratio for PSA response was equal to 5.5 (95% CI 2.7 – 8.2). At the country level, there was no association between the treatment effects on PSA response and on survival ($R^2_{\text{country}} = 0.05$, Figure 18.4).

The treatment effects on other potential PSA-based surrogates such as PSA normalization or time to PSA progression did not reach much stronger associations with the treatment effects on survival at the country level. Even when the full vector of longitudinal PSA measurements was used for each patient as suggested in Section 18.4.5, the association between treatment effects remained quite weak (Figure 18.5), suggesting that PSA alone cannot be used to define a valid surrogate endpoint for survival in prostate cancer.

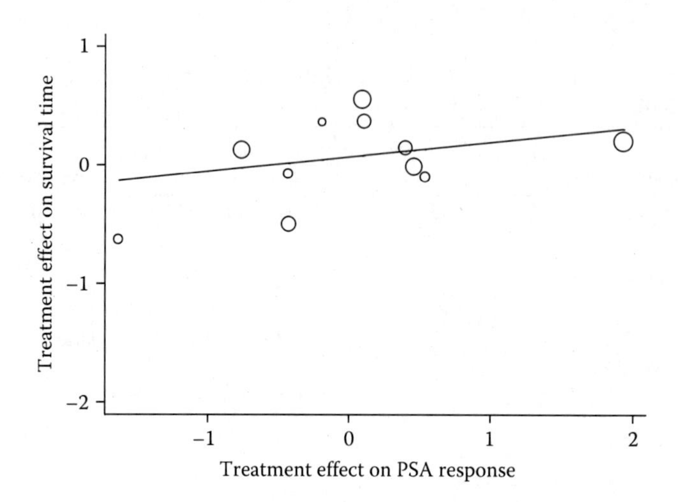

FIGURE 18.4
Association between treatment effects on PSA response and survival in patients with androgen-sensitive prostate cancer. Each bubble represents a country, with bubble size proportional to the sample size in the corresponding country.

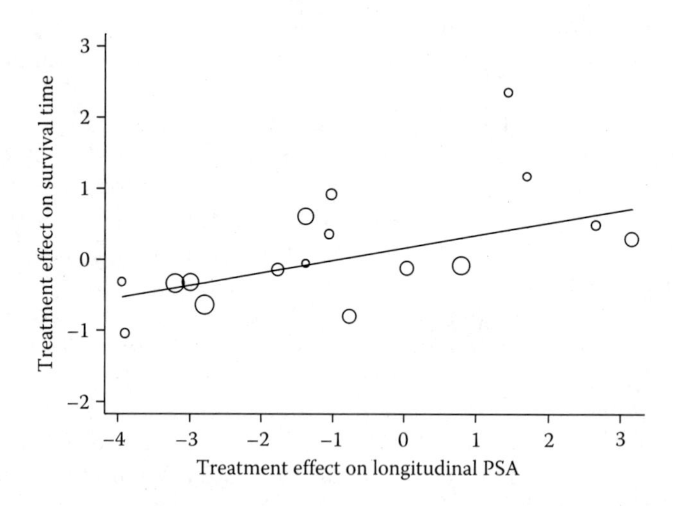

FIGURE 18.5
Association between treatment effects on longitudinal measurements of PSA and survival in patients with androgen-sensitive prostate cancer. Each bubble represents a country, with bubble size proportional to the sample size in the corresponding country.

18.5 Prediction of the Treatment Effect

The key motivation for validating a surrogate endpoint is the ability to predict the effect of treatment on the true endpoint based on the observed effect of treatment on the surrogate endpoint. Suppose that we have fitted the mixed-effects models (18.8) and (18.9) to data from a meta-analysis of N trials. Suppose further that a new trial is considered for which data are available on the surrogate endpoint but not on the true endpoint. It is essential to explore the quality of the prediction of the effect of Z on T in the new trial $i=0$, based on the information contained in the trials $i=1,\ldots, N$ used in the evaluation process, and the estimate of the effect of Z on S in the new trial. We can fit the following linear model to the surrogate outcomes S_{0j}:

$$S_{0j} = \mu_{S0} + \alpha_0 Z_{0j} + \varepsilon_{S0j}. \tag{18.16}$$

We are interested in an estimate of the effect $\beta + b_0$ of Z on T, given the effect of Z on S. To this end, one can observe that $(\beta + b_0 | m_{S0}, a_0)$, where m_{S0} and a_0 are, respectively, the surrogate-specific random intercept and treatment effect in the new trial, follows a normal distribution with mean linear in μ_{S0}, μ_S, α_0, and α, and variance

$$\mathrm{Var}\left(\beta + b_0 \middle| m_{S0}, a_0\right) = \left(1 - R^2_{\text{trial}}\right)\mathrm{Var}\left(b_0\right). \tag{18.17}$$

Here, $\mathrm{Var}(b_0)$ denotes the unconditional variance of the trial-specific random effect of Z on T. The smaller the conditional variance given by (18.17), the better is the precision of the prediction. Denote by ϑ the fixed-effects parameters and variance components related to the mixed-effects model (18.8) and (18.9), with $\hat{\vartheta}$ denoting the corresponding estimates. Fitting the linear model (18.16) to data on the surrogate endpoint from the new trial provides estimates for m_{S0} and a_0. The prediction variance can be written as

$$\begin{aligned}
&\mathrm{Var}\left(\beta + b_0 \middle| \mu_{S0}, \alpha_0, \vartheta\right) \\
&\quad \approx f\left\{\mathrm{Var}\left(\hat{\mu}_{S0}, \hat{\alpha}_0\right)\right\} + f\left\{\mathrm{Var}\left(\hat{\vartheta}\right)\right\} + \left(1 - R^2_{\text{trial}}\right)\mathrm{Var}\left(b_0\right),
\end{aligned} \tag{18.18}$$

where $f\left\{\mathrm{Var}\left(\hat{\mu}_{S0}, \hat{\alpha}_0\right)\right\}$ and $f\left\{\mathrm{Var}\left(\hat{\vartheta}\right)\right\}$ are functions of the asymptotic variance-covariance matrices of $\left(\hat{\mu}_{S0}, \hat{\alpha}_0\right)^T$ and $\hat{\vartheta}$, respectively. The third term on the right-hand side of (18.18), which is equivalent to (18.17), describes the prediction's variability if μ_{S0}, α_0, and ϑ were known. The first two terms describe the contributions to the variability due to the use of the estimates of these parameters, respectively, in the new trial (estimation of μ_{S0} and of α_0)

and in the meta-analysis (estimation of ϑ). Let us now consider some theoretical situations.

18.5.1 Some Theoretical Situations

In reality, the parameters of models (18.8) and (18.9) and (18.16) all have to be estimated, in which case, the prediction variance is given by the three terms on the right-hand side of (18.18). It is useful however to consider two theoretical situations:

1. *No estimation error*: If the parameters of the mixed-effects model (18.8) and (18.9) and the single-trial regression model (18.16) were known, the prediction variance for $\beta + b_0$ would only contain the last term on the right-hand side of (18.18). Thus, the variance would be reduced to (18.17) and the precision of the prediction would be driven entirely by the value R^2_{trial}. While this situation is of theoretical relevance only, as it would require an infinite number of trials and infinite sample sizes for the estimation in the meta-analysis and in the new trial, it provides important insights about the intrinsic quality of the surrogate, and shows that R^2_{trial} measures the *potential* validity of a surrogate endpoint at the trial level.
2. *Estimation error only in the meta-analysis*: This scenario is again possible only in theory, as it would require an infinite sample size in the new trial. But it can provide information of practical interest, since, with an infinite sample size, the parameters of the single-trial regression model (18.16) would be known and the first term on the right-hand side of (18.18), $f\left\{\text{Var}\left(\mu_{S0}, \alpha_0\right)\right\}$, would vanish. In this case, (18.18) would provide the minimum variance of the prediction of $\beta + b_0$ that is achievable when the size of the meta-analysis is finite. Gail et al. (2000) used this fact to point out that the use of a surrogate validated through a meta-analytic approach will always be less efficient than the direct use of the true endpoint. Even so, a surrogate can be of great use in terms of reduced sample size, shortened trial duration, or both.

In real-life situations, the question may be to design a new trial that uses the surrogate instead of the true endpoint. The sample size of this new trial may then be calculated using a measure of surrogacy that will be introduced in the next section.

18.5.2 Surrogate Threshold Effect

Burzykowski and Buyse (2006) have proposed the *surrogate threshold effect* (STE) as a useful measure of surrogacy when interest focuses on predicting the treatment effect on the true endpoint, having observed the treatment effect on the surrogate. Assume that the prediction of $\beta + b_0$ can be made independently of μ_{S0}. Under this assumption the conditional mean of $\beta + b_0$ is a linear function of α_0, the treatment effect on the surrogate. Assume further that α_0 is estimated without error. The conditional variance of $\beta + b_0$ can be written as

$$\text{Var}\left(\beta + b_0 \middle| \alpha_0, \vartheta\right) \approx f\left\{\text{Var}\left(\hat{\vartheta}\right)\right\} + \left(1 - R^2_{\text{trial(r)}}\right)\text{Var}\left(b_0\right). \tag{18.19}$$

Since in linear mixed models, the maximum likelihood estimates of the covariance parameters are asymptotically independent of the fixed effects parameters (Verbeke and Molenberghs, 2000), one can show that the prediction variance (18.19) can be expressed approximately as a quadratic function of α_0.

Consider a $(1 - \gamma)$ 100% prediction interval for $\beta + b_0$:

$$E\left(\beta + b_0 \middle| \alpha_0, \vartheta\right) \pm z_{1-\gamma/2}\sqrt{\text{Var}\left(\beta + b_0 \middle| \alpha_0, \vartheta\right)}, \tag{18.20}$$

where $z_{1-\gamma/2}$ is the $(1 - \gamma/2)$ quantile of the standard normal distribution. The limits of the interval (18.20) are functions of α_0. Define the lower and upper prediction limit functions of α_0 as

$$l\left(\alpha_0\right), u\left(\alpha_0\right) \equiv E\left(\beta + b_0 \middle| \alpha_0, \vartheta\right) \pm z_{1-\gamma/2}\sqrt{\text{Var}\left(\beta + b_0 \middle| \alpha_0, \vartheta\right)}.$$

One can then compute a value of α_0 such that $l(\alpha_0) = 0$. This value is called the STE. STE is the smallest treatment effect on the surrogate necessary to be observed to predict a significant treatment effect on the true endpoint. STE depends on the variance of the prediction. The larger is the variance, the larger the absolute value of STE. In practical terms, one would hope to get a value of STE that can realistically be achieved, given the range of treatment effects on surrogates observed in previous clinical trials. If STE was too large to be achievable, the surrogate would not be useful for the purposes of predicting a treatment effect on the true endpoint. In such a case, using the surrogate would not be reasonable, even if the surrogate were *potentially* valid, that is, with $R^2_{\text{trial(r)}} \simeq 1$. STE thus provides important information about the usefulness of a surrogate in practice.

18.5.3 Design of Trials Using Surrogate Endpoints

STE can be used to design clinical trials based on an accepted surrogate endpoint. Such trials should demonstrate a treatment effect on the surrogate that exceeds STE, which in turn would predict a significant treatment effect on the true endpoint. As mentioned earlier, STE cannot always be estimated. In the case of prostate cancer, the treatment effects on PSA-based endpoints are so poorly correlated with the treatment effects on OS that STE cannot be estimated for any of these endpoints. As a matter of fact, no biomarker-based surrogate endpoint has yet been identified in oncology; all the surrogate endpoints in current use are based on tumor recurrence or progression, and are therefore clinical endpoints in their own right. Consider gastric cancer as an example (Buyse et al., 2014). In patients with resectable tumors, disease-free survival (DFS) is an excellent surrogate for OS, with STE = 0.92 (Oba et al., 2013). Hence, a trial testing the effect of a new treatment on DFS should demonstrate a HR_{DFS} smaller than 0.92 in order to predict, with 95% confidence, a HR_{OS} smaller than 1 on survival. The size of this new trial can be calculated so that the 95% confidence interval of the estimated HR_{DFS} lies entirely under 0.92. In other words, the null and alternative hypotheses of interest for DFS are H_0: $HR_{DFS} \geq 0.92$ versus $H_A{:}HR_{DFS} < 0.92$. The test of hypothesis for DFS is more stringent than the test of hypothesis for OS, which is based on the conventional null and alternative hypotheses $H_0{:}HR_{OS} \geq 1.0$ versus $H_A{:}HR_{OS} < 1.0$. Even so, the test of hypothesis for DFS may require less patients and less follow-up time to reach the same statistical power than the test of hypothesis for OS, since the treatment effect may be larger on DFS than on OS, and the events are observed earlier.

In contrast to the situation of resectable tumors, progression-free survival (PFS) is not an acceptable surrogate for OS in patients with advanced gastric tumors, with STE = 0.56 (Paoletti et al., 2013). Hence, a trial testing the effect of a new treatment on PFS should demonstrate a HR_{PFS} smaller than 0.56 in order to predict, with 95% confidence, a HR_{OS} smaller than 1 on survival. Such a treatment effect is unlikely to be achieved, even with very effective treatments, and therefore, a trial using PFS as its endpoint does not seem a realistic option to pursue.

18.5.4 Constancy Assumption

The validation of surrogate endpoints is based on an implicit constancy assumption, whereby the relationship between the surrogate and the true endpoint, as well as between the treatment effects on the two endpoints, will be similar in the future as in historical trials used to evaluate the surrogate. This assumption constitutes a leap of faith at both levels, with limited guidance provided by statistical analysis. At the individual level, biology may be the best guide, absent further data, to predict whether the individual-level association between the surrogate and the true endpoint will continue to hold in the future. In prostate cancer, for instance, a better understanding of the disease process may suggest biomarkers such as CTCs that are strongly predictive of the clinical outcomes and may, as such, dominate PSA and render its use obsolete. At the trial level, it may be reasonable to assume that the surrogate can still be used if the new drug belongs to the same class of drugs as the ones in the evaluation datasets. Heterogeneity in the meta-analysis of historical trials is an asset in this respect: the more drugs were included in the meta-analysis, possibly with a wide range of treatment effects, the better. For new drugs having a substantially different mode of action, whether the surrogate would still be valid is an open question that may warrant another prospective evaluation. In advanced colorectal cancer, for instance, PFS was shown to be an acceptable surrogate for survival in the era of fluoropyrimidine-based therapies. However, some attenuation of the association between treatment effects on progression-free survival and survival was observed in trials using oxaliplatin (Buyse et al., 2007). A recent reevaluation of surrogacy using contemporary trials of chemotherapy and biological agents confirmed the weaker trial-level association (Shi et al., 2014). The association may have been weakened by the availability of active rescue treatments given to patients in progressive disease, but also by different mechanisms of action of the new drugs, which may fundamentally alter the way in which these drugs exert their effects on the true endpoint, directly or indirectly through the surrogate. One line of research based on causal inference purports to estimate direct and indirect effects and, as such, it holds great potential for the evaluation of surrogates in the future.

18.6 Other Approaches to Surrogacy

18.6.1 Variance Reduction and Information Theory

Alonso et al. (2003) used a two-stage approach to define further measures of surrogacy. They assumed that data are available from $i=1,\ldots, N$ trials, in the ith of which, $j=1,\ldots, n_i$ subjects are enrolled and observed at times t_{ijk}. If T_{ijk} and S_{ijk} represent the true and surrogate endpoints, respectively, and Z_{ij} is a binary indicator variable for treatment, then these authors followed Galecki (1994) and proposed the following joint model for both responses at the first stage:

$$T_{ijk} = \mu_{Ti} + \beta_i Z_{ij} + g_{Tij}\left(t_{ijk}\right) + \varepsilon_{Tijk},$$

$$S_{ijk} = \mu_{Si} + \alpha_i Z_{ij} + g_{Sij}\left(t_{ijk}\right) + \varepsilon_{Sijk},$$

where

μ_{Ti} and μ_{Si} are trial-specific intercepts
β_i and α_i are trial-specific effects of treatment Z_{ij} on the two endpoints
g_{Tij} and g_{Sij} are trial-subject-specific time functions that can include treatment-by-time interactions

They also assumed that the vectors collecting all information over time for patient j in trial i, $\tilde{\varepsilon}_{Tij}$ and $\tilde{\varepsilon}_{Sij}$, are correlated error terms, following a mean-zero multivariate normal distribution with variance–covariance matrix

$$\Sigma_i = \begin{pmatrix} \Sigma_{TTi} & \Sigma_{TSi} \\ \Sigma'_{TSi} & \Sigma_{SSi} \end{pmatrix} = \begin{pmatrix} \sigma_{TTi} & \sigma_{TSi} \\ \sigma_{TSi} & \sigma_{SSi} \end{pmatrix} \otimes R_i,$$

where R_i is a correlation matrix for the repeated measurements. It is important to realize that these longitudinal models were used as a convenient illustration only, and that they can be modified and extended according to the needs of a particular application.

Using ideas from multivariate analysis, Alonso et al. (2003) proposed the *variance reduction factor* (*VRF*) to capture individual-level surrogacy in this more elaborate setting. They quantify the relative reduction in the true endpoint variance after adjustment by the surrogate as

$$\text{VRF}_{\text{ind}} = \frac{\sum_i \left\{ \text{tr}(\Sigma_{TTi}) - \text{tr}\left(\Sigma_{(T|S)i}\right)\right\}}{\sum_i \text{tr}\left(\Sigma_{TTi}\right)},$$

where

$\Sigma_{(T|S)i}$ denotes the conditional variance–covariance matrix of $\tilde{\varepsilon}_{Tij}$ given $\tilde{\varepsilon}_{Sij} : \Sigma_{(T|S)i} = \Sigma_{TTi} - \Sigma_{TSi}\Sigma_{SSi}^{-1}\Sigma'_{TSi}$

Σ_{TTi} and Σ_{SSi} are the variance–covariance matrices associated with the true and surrogate endpoints respectively

Σ_{TSi} contains the covariances between the surrogate and the true endpoint

These authors showed that the VRF_{ind} ranges between zero and one, and that $\text{VRF}_{\text{ind}} = R^2_{\text{ind}}$ when the endpoints are measured only once (Alonso et al., 2003).

The VRF_{ind} can be estimated in the normal model, but extensions to non-normal settings are difficult. To overcome this limitation, Alonso et al. (2005) later introduced a new measure, R^2_Λ, to evaluate surrogacy at the individual level when both responses are measured over time or in general when multivariate or repeated measures are available

$$R^2_\Lambda = \frac{1}{N}\sum_i (1 - \Lambda_i),$$

where $\Lambda_i = |\Sigma_i| / \{|\Sigma_{TTi}| \quad |\Sigma_{SSi}|\}$. These authors proved that R^2_Λ ranges between zero and one, and that in the cross-sectional case $R^2_\Lambda = R^2_{\text{ind}}$ (Alonso et al., 2005).

Alonso and Molenberghs (2007) have pushed the search for universal measures of surrogacy a step further, and propose a unifying approach to surrogate evaluation based on information theory. Their proposal avoids the need for a joint, hierarchical model, which as discussed earlier can be computationally demanding. Moreover, surrogate measures based on the concept of entropy allow for unification across different types of endpoints. The theory behind entropy is beyond the scope of this chapter; details are available in Alonso and Molenberghs (2007).

18.6.2 Principal Stratification and Causal Inference

Frangakis and Rubin (2004) proposed a completely different approach to surrogate evaluation based on principal stratification. Drawing from the causality literature, Robins and Greenland (1992), Pearl (2001), and Taylor et al. (2005) suggested use of the concepts of direct/indirect effect for surrogacy evaluation. Joffe and Greene (2008) proposed a useful overview of similarities and differences between the various paradigms. They identified two important dimensions. First, some methods are based on a single trial, while others use several trials. Second, some approaches study association, while others, briefly mentioned at the end of Section 18.5.4, study causation. In the meta-analytic framework presented in Section 18.4, the surrogate is evaluated using association measures estimated from multiple trials. Joffe and Green (2008) point out that the meta-analytic approach is essentially causal in so far as the treatment effects observed in all trials are average causal effects. If a meta-analysis of several trials is not possible, there are serious limitations in using an association approach using a single trial, as discussed in Section 18.3.4. In this case, a more promising approach may be to estimate causal effects for individual patients, which requires strong and unverifiable assumptions to be made. Some authors have used a Bayesian approach to estimate individual causal effects (Li et al., 2010, 2011), but further research is warranted to develop less arduous estimation methods.

The relationship between individual causal effects (which are of interest in the causal framework) and expected causal effects (which are of interest in the meta-analytic framework) has recently been investigated by Alonso et al. (2013). These authors consider the quadruple $Y_{ij} = [T_{ij}(Z_{ij}=0), T_{ij}(Z_{ij}=1), S_{ij}(Z_{ij}=0), S_{ij}(Z_{ij}=1)]'$, which is observable only if patient j in trial i can be assessed under both control and experimental treatment (e.g., in a cross-over trial). Clearly, this is generally not possible and hence, half of the outcomes in the quadruple are generally *counterfactual*. Alonso et al. (2013) assume a multivariate normal for Y_{ij} to derive insightful expressions. They show that, under broad circumstances, when a surrogate is considered acceptable from a meta-analytic perspective at both the individual and trial levels, it can be expected to be acceptable from the causal inference perspective as well. However, a surrogate that is valid from a single-trial framework perspective, using individual causal effects, may not pass the test from a meta-analytic point of view. More work is needed, especially for endpoints of different types, but it seems comforting that, when based on multiple trials, the two frameworks appear to show a good level of agreement.

18.7 Concluding Remarks

Over the years, various strategies have been proposed for the evaluation of surrogate endpoints. Attempts to validate a surrogate endpoint using data from a single trial have been shown insufficient in so far as they focus solely on the individual-level association. Indeed none of these attempts have, to the best of our knowledge, successfully identified an acceptable surrogate endpoint for use in the clinic. In the case of the biomarker considered throughout this chapter, some endpoints based on longitudinal PSA measurements such as the PSA doubling time (in locally advanced prostate cancer) or PSA declines (in metastatic prostate cancer) have been shown to fulfill the Prentice criteria, but none of these endpoints are currently considered a valid surrogate for cancer-specific survival or OS. Combinations of several longitudinal biomarkers and laboratory values may hold more potential to define useful surrogate endpoints, for instance, a combination of PSA, CTCs, hemoglobin, alkaline phosphatase, and lactate dehydrogenase in prostate cancer (Scher et al., 2011). An evaluation of these potential surrogates will clearly need to go beyond the Prentice criteria to be convincing.

Today, much of the attention has shifted to the meta-analytic setting in which data are available from several trials; hence, investigation of the trial-level association is possible as well as the individual-level association (or the Prentice criteria). A number of surrogacy measures have been proposed, depending on the types of endpoints considered (i.e., continuous, binary, time-to-event, or longitudinal). When one or more longitudinal biomarkers are available, potential surrogate endpoints can be defined as summary measures of the longitudinal data, although it seems generally preferable, from a statistical point of view, to use the full vector of measurements as the surrogate. Fitting fully specified hierarchical models is challenging, but simplified modeling strategies can be used. The information-theoretic approach, which is both general and simple to implement, provides a unified theory that can be broadly applied. Approaches based on causal inference offer promising alternatives or complementary routes to evaluate potential surrogates, but use of these newer approaches has been limited in oncology so far.

While quantifying surrogacy is important, so is prediction of the treatment effect in a new trial based on the surrogate. The STE addresses this issue and has been shown informative in validating surrogate endpoints in ovarian (Burzykowski et al., 2001), colorectal (Buyse et al., 2007), lung (Laporte et al., 2013), and gastric cancers (Oba et al., 2013; Paoletti et al., 2013). Finally, the validity of a surrogate rests in large part on the constancy assumption, which may or may not be valid when new treatments are developed that have a substantially different mechanism of action than the treatments used in historical trials. The search for valid surrogates is, therefore, an open-ended quest that will continue to require constant reevaluation.

Acknowledgments

The authors gratefully acknowledge support from IAP research Network P7/06 of the Belgian Government (Belgian Science Policy). They thank the Janssen Research Foundation for permission to use data from two clinical trials in patients with advanced prostate cancer. Software implementations for the methods described in this chapter are available at www.ibiostat.be/software.

References

A'Hern, R., Ebbs, S.R., and Baum, M. 1988. Does chemotherapy improve survival in advanced breast cancer? A statistical overview. *British Journal of Cancer*, 57:615–618.

Alonso, A., Geys, H., Molenberghs, G., and Vangeneugden, T. 2003. Validation of surrogate markers in multiple randomized clinical trials with repeated measurements. *Biometrical Journal*, 45:931–945.

Alonso, A. and Molenberghs, G. 2007. Surrogate marker evaluation from an information theoretic perspective. *Biometrics*, 63:180–186.

Alonso, A., Molenberghs, G., Geys, H., and Buyse, M. 2005. A unifying approach for surrogate marker validation based on Prentice's criteria. *Statistics in Medicine*, 25:205–211.

Alonso, A., Van der Elst, W., Molenberghs, G., Buyse, M., and Burzykowski, T. 2013. On the relationship between the causal-inference and meta-analytic paradigms for the validation of surrogate endpoints. Biometrics, 63:180–186.

Armstrong, A.J., Garrett–Mayer, E., Yang, Y.C.O. et al. 2007. Prostate-specific antigen and pain surrogacy analysis in metastatic hormone-refractory prostate cancer. *Journal of the Clinical Oncology*, 25:3965–3970.

Baker, S.G. 2006. Surrogate endpoints: Wishful thinking or reality? *Journal of the National Cancer Institute*, 98:502–503.

Begg, C. and Leung, D. 2000. On the use of surrogate endpoints in randomized trials. *Journal of the Royal Statistical Society, Series A*, 163:26–27.

Biomarkers Definition Working Group. 2001. Biomarkers and surrogate end-points: Preferred definitions and conceptual framework. *Clinical Pharmacological Therapy*, 69:89–95.

Burzykowski, T. and Buyse, M. 2006. Surrogate threshold effect: An alternative measure for meta-analytic surrogate endpoint validation. *Pharmaceutical Statistics*, 5:173–186.

Burzykowski, T., Buyse, M., Piccart-Gebhart, M.J. et al. 2008. Evaluation of tumor response, disease control, progression-free survival, and time to progression as potential surrogate endpoints in metastatic breast cancer. *Journal of Clinical Oncology*, 26:1987–1992.

Burzykowski, T., Molenberghs, G., and Buyse, M. 2004. The validation of surrogate endpoints using data from randomized clinical trials: A case-study in advanced colorectal cancer. *Journal of the Royal Statistical Society, Series A*, 167:103–124.

Burzykowski, T., Molenberghs, G., and Buyse, M. 2005. *The Evaluation of Surrogate Endpoints*. Springer, New York.

Burzykowski, T., Molenberghs, G., Buyse, M., Geys, H., and Renard, D. 2001. Validation of surrogate endpoints in multiple randomized clinical trials with failure-time endpoints. *Journal of the Royal Statistical Society, Series C*, 50:405–422.

Buyse, M., Burzykowski, T., Carroll, K. et al. 2007. Progression-free survival is a surrogate for survival in advanced colorectal cancer. *Journal of Clinical Oncology*, 25:5218–5224.

Buyse, M., Michiels, S., Squifflet, P. et al. 2011. Leukemia-free survival as a surrogate endpoint for overall survival in the evaluation of maintenance therapy for patients with acute myeloid leukemia in complete remission. *Haematologica*, 96:1106–1112.

Buyse, M. and Molenberghs, G. 1998. Criteria for the validation of surrogate endpoints in randomized experiments. *Biometrics*, 54:1014–1029.

Buyse, M., Molenberghs, G., Burzykowski, T., Renard, D., and Geys, H. 2000. The validation of surrogate endpoints in meta-analyses of randomized experiments. *Biostatistics*, 1:49–68.

Buyse, M., Molenberghs, G., Paoletti, X., Oba, K., Alonso, A., Van der Elst, W., and Burzykowski, T. 2014. Validation of surrogate endpoints with examples from cancer clinical trials. *Biometrical Journal*, in press.

Buyse, M., Thirion, P., Carlson, R.W. et al. 2008. Relation between tumour response to first-line chemotherapy and survival in advanced colorectal cancer: A meta-analysis. *Lancet*, 356:373–378.

Buyse, M., Vangeneugden, T., Bijnens, L. et al. 2003. Validation of Biomarkers as Surrogates for Clinical Endpoints. In: *Biomarkers in Clinical Drug Development* (Bloom JC and Dean RA, eds.), pp. 149–168. Marcel Dekker, New York.

Cardiac Arrhythmia Suppression Trial (CAST) Investigators. 1989. Preliminary Report: Effect of encainide and flecainide on mortality in a randomized trial of arrhythmia suppression after myocardial infarction. *New England Journal of Medicine*, 321:406–412.

Choi, S., Lagakos, S., Schooley, R.T., and Volberding, P.A. 1993. CD4+ lymphocytes are an incomplete surrogate marker for clinical progression in persons with asymptomatic HIV infection taking zidovudine. *Annals of Internal Medicine*, 118:674–680.

Clayton, D.G. 1978. A model for association in bivariate life tables and its application in epidemiological studies of familial tendency in chronic disease incidence. *Biometrika*, 65:141–151.

Collette, L., Burzykowski, T., and Buyse, M. 2007. Are prostate-specific antigen changes valid surrogates for survival in hormone-refractory cancer? A meta-analysis is needed! [Letter to the Editor]. *Journal of Clinical Oncology*, 25:5673–5674.

Collette, L., Burzykowski, T., Carroll, K. et al. 2005. Is prostate-specific antigen a valid surrogate end point for survival in hormonally treated patients with metastatic prostate cancer? *Journal of Clinical Oncology*, 23:6139–6148.

Cortiñas Abrahantes, J., Molenberghs, G., Burzykowski, T., Shkedy, Z., and Renard, D. 2004. Choice of units of analysis and modeling strategies in multilevel hierarchical models. *Computational Statistics and Data Analysis*, 47:537–563.

Dale, J.R. 1986. Global cross ratio models for bivariate, discrete, ordered responses. *Biometrics*, 42:909–917.

D'Amico, A.V., Chen, M.H., de Castro, M. et al. 2012. Surrogate endpoints for prostate cancer-specific mortality after radiotherapy and androgen suppression therapy in men with localized or locally advanced prostate cancer: An analysis of 2 randomized trials. *Lancet Oncology*, 13:189–195.

Daniels, M.J. and Hughes, M.D. 1997. Meta-analysis for the evaluation of potential surrogate markers. *Statistics in Medicine*, 16:1515–1527.

DeGruttola, V., Fleming, T.R., Lin, D.Y., and Coombs, R. 1997. Validating surrogate markers—Are we being naive? *Journal of Infectious Diseases*, 175:237–246.

DeGruttola, V. and Tu, X.M. 1994. Modelling progression of CD-4 lymphocyte count and its relationship to survival time. *Biometrics*, 50:1003–1014.

Denham, J.W., Steigler, A., Wilcox, C. et al. 2008. Time to biochemical failure and prostate-specific antigen doubling time as surrogates for prostate cancer-specific mortality: Evidence from the TROG 96.01 randomised controlled trial. *Lancet Oncology*, 9:1058–1068.

Dreicer, R., Stadler, W.M., Ahmann, F.R. et al. 2008. MVA-MUC 1-IL2 vaccine immunotherapy (TG4010) improves PSA doubling time in patients with prostate cancer with biochemical failure. *Invest New Drugs*, 27:379–86.

Ellenberg, S.S. and Hamilton, J.M. 1989. Surrogate endpoints in clinical trials: Cancer. *Statistics in Medicine*, 8:405–413.

Ferentz, A.E. 2002. Integrating pharmacogenomics into drug development. *Pharmacogenomics*, 3:453–467.

Flandre, P. and Saidi, Y. 1999. Letter to the editor: Estimating the proportion of treatment effect explained by a surrogate marker. *Statistics in Medicine*, 18:107–115.

Fleming, T.R. 1994. Surrogate markers in AIDS and cancer trials. *Statistics in Medicine*, 13:1423–1435.

Fleming, T.R. and DeMets, D.L. 1996. Surrogate end points in clinical trials: Are we being misled? *Annals of Internal Medicine*, 125:605–613.

Frangakis, C.E. and Rubin, D.B. 2004. Principal stratification in causal inference. *Biometrics*, 58:21–29.

Freedman, L.S., Graubard, B.I., and Schatzkin, A. 1992. Statistical validation of intermediate endpoints for chronic diseases. *Statistics in Medicine*, 11:167–178.

Gail, M.H., Pfeiffer, R., van Houwelingen, H.C., and Carroll, R.J. 2000. On meta-analytic assessment of surrogate outcomes. *Biostatistics*, 1:231–246.

Galecki, A. 1994. General class of covariance structures for two or more repeated factors in longitudinal data analysis. *Communications in Statistics: Theory and Methods*, 23:3105–3119.

Genest, C. and McKay, J. 1986. The joy of copulas: Bivariate distributions with uniform marginals. *American Statistician*, 40:280–283.

Hougaard, P. 1986. Survival models for heterogeneous populations derived from stable distributions. *Biometrika*, 73:387–396.

Institut fűr Qualitat und Wirtschaftlichkeit im Gesundheitswesen. 2011. Validity of surrogate endpoints in oncology. (https://www.iqwig.de/download/A10-05_Rapid_Report_Version_1-1_Surrogatendpunkte_in_der_Onkologie.pdf), IQWiG Reports—Commission, No. A10-05 (accessed November 18, 2014).

International Conference on Harmonisation of technical requirements for registration of pharmaceuticals for human use. 1998. ICH Harmonised Tripartite Guideline. Statistical principles for clinical trials. (http://www.ich.org/fileadmin/Public_Web_Site/ICH_Products/Guidelines/Efficacy/E9/Step4/E9_Guideline.pdf), Federal Register 63, No. 179, 49583 (accessed November 18, 2014).

Joffe, M.M. and Greene, T. 2008. Related causal frameworks for surrogate outcomes. *Biometrics*, 64:1–10.

Korn, E.L., Albert, P.S., and McShane, L.M. 2005. Assessing surrogates as trial endpoints using mixed models. *Statistics in Medicine*, 24:163–182.

Lagakos, S.W. and Hoth, D.F. 1992. Surrogate markers in AIDS: Where are we? Where are we going? *Annals of Internal Medicine*, 116:599–601.

Laporte, S., Squifflet, P., Baroux, N. et al. 2013. Prediction of survival benefits from progression-free survival benefits in advanced non small cell lung cancer: evidence from a pooled analysis of 2334 patients randomized in 5 trials. *BMJ Open*, 3:3.03.

Lassere, M., Johnson, K., Boers, M. et al. 2007. Definitions and validation criteria for biomarkers and surrogate endpoints: Development and testing of a quantitative hierarchical levels of evidence schema. *Journal of Rheumatology*, 34:607–615.

Lesko, L.J. and Atkinson, A.J. 2001. Use of biomarkers and surrogate end-points in drug development and regulatory decision making: Criteria, validation, strategies. *Annual Review of Pharmacological Toxicology*, 41:347–366.

Li, Y., Taylor, J.M.G., and Elliott, M.R. 2010. A Bayesian approach to surrogacy assessment using principal stratification in clinical trials. *Biometrics*, 58:21–9.

Li, Y., Taylor, J.M.G., Elliott, M.R., and Sargent, D.R. 2011. Causal assessment of surrogacy in a meta-analysis of colorectal clinical trials. *Biostatistics*, 12:478–492.

Lin, D.Y., Fleming, T.R., and DeGruttola, V. 1997. Estimating the proportion of treatment effect explained by a surrogate marker. *Statistics in Medicine*, 16:1515–1527.

Molenberghs, G., Buyse, M., Geys, H., Renard, D., and Burzykowski, T. 2002. Statistical challenges in the evaluation of surrogate endpoints in randomized trials. *Controlled Clinical Trials*, 23:607–25.

Oba, K., Paoletti, X., Alberts, S. et al. On behalf of the GASTRIC group. 2013. Disease-free survival as a surrogate for overall survival in adjuvant trials of gastric cancer: A meta-analysis. *Journal of the National Cancer Institute*, 5:1600–1607.

Paoletti, X., Oba, K., Bang, Y.J. et al. On behalf of the GASTRIC group. 2013. Progression-free survival as a surrogate for overall survival in patients with advanced/recurrent gastric cancer: A meta-analysis. *Journal of the National Cancer Institute*, 5:1608–1612.

Pearl, J. 2001. *Causality: Models, Reasoning, and Inference.* Cambridge University Press, Cambridge, U.K.

Petrylak, D.P., Ankerst, D.P., Jiang, C.S. et al. 2006. Evaluation of prostate-specific antigen declines for surrogacy in patients treated on SWOG 99–16. *Journal of the National Cancer Institute*, 98:516–521.

Prentice, R.L. 1989. Surrogate endpoints in clinical trials: Definitions and operational criteria. *Statistics in Medicine*, 8:431–440.

Renard, D., Geys, H., Molenberghs, G., Burzykowski, T., and Buyse, M. 2002. Validation of surrogate endpoints in multiple randomized clinical trials with discrete outcomes. *Biometrical Journal*, 44:1–15.

Renard, D., Geys, H., Molenberghs, G. et al. 2002. Validation of a longitudinally measured surrogate marker for a time-to-event endpoint. *Journal of Applied Statistics*, 30:235–247.

Renfro, L.A., Shi, Q., Sargent, D.J., and Carlin, B.P. 2012. Bayesian adjusted R^2 for the meta-analytic evaluation of surrogate time-to-event endpoints in clinical trials. *Statistics of Medicine*, 31:743–761.

Robins, J.M. and Greenland, S. 1992. Identifiability and exchangeability for direct and indirect effects. *Epidemiology*, 3:143–155.

Schatzkin, A. and Gail, M. 2002. The promise and peril of surrogate end points in cancer research. *Nature Reviews Cancer*, 2:19–27.

Schemper, M. 1993. The relative importance of prognostic factors in studies of survival. *Statistics in Medicine*, 12:2377–2382.

Scher, H.I., Eisenberger, M., D'Amico, A.V. et al. 2004. Eligibility and outcomes reporting guidelines for clinical trials for patients in the state of a rising prostate-specific antigen: Recommendations from the Prostate-Specific Antigen Working Group. *Journal of Clinical Oncology*, 22:537–556.

Scher, H.I., Heller, G., Molina, A. et al. 2011. Evaluation of Circulating Tumor Cells (CTCs) as an efficacy response biomarker of overall survival (OS) in metastatic castration-resistant prostate cancer (mCRPC): Planned final analysis (FA) of COU-AA-301, a randomized, double-blind, placebo-controlled, phase III study of Abiraterone Acetate (AA) plus low-dose Prednisone (P) post docetaxel. *ASCO Meeting Abstract*, 29, LBA4517.

Shi, Q. de Gramont, A., Grothey, A. et al. 2014. Individual patient data analysis of progression-free versus overall survival as a first-line endpoint for metastatic colorectal cancer in modern randomized trials: Findings from 16,700 patients from the ARCAD database. *Journal of Clinical Oncology*, DOI: 10.1200/JCO.2014.56.5887.

Shih, J.H. and Louis, T.A. 1995. Inferences on association parameter in copula models for bivariate survival data. *Biometrics*, 51:1384–1399.

Taylor, J.M.G., Wang, Y., and Thiébaut, R. 2005. Counterfactual links to the proportion of treatment effect explained by a surrogate marker. *Biometrics*, 61:1102–1111.

Tibaldi, F.S., Cortiñas Abrahantes, J., and Molenberghs, G. et al. 2003. Simplified hierarchical linear models for the evaluation of surrogate endpoints. *Journal of Statistical Computation and Simulation*, 73:643–658.

Torri, V., Simon, R., Russek-Cohen, E. et al. 1992. Statistical model to determine the relationship of response and survival in patients with advanced ovarian cancer treated with chemotherapy. *Journal of the National Cancer Institute*, 84:407–414.

Valicenti R.K., DeSilvio M., Hanks G.E. et al. 2006. Posttreatment prostatic-specific antigen doubling time as a surrogate endpoint for prostate cancer-specific survival: An analysis of Radiation Therapy Oncology Group Protocol 92–02. *International Journal Radiation Oncology Biology Physics*, 66:1064–1071.

Verbeke, G. and Molenberghs, G. 2000. *Linear Mixed Models for Longitudinal Data*. Springer, New York.

Volberding, P.A., Lagakos, S.W., Koch, M.A. et al. 1990. Zidovudine in asymptomtic human immunodeficiency virus infection: A controlled trial in persons with fewer than 500 CD4-positive cells per cubic millimeter. *New England Journal of Medicine*, 322:941–949.

Index

H

I

K

L

M

N

O

P

R

S

T